Second Edition

practice management and EHR

A TOTAL PATIENT ENCOUNTER

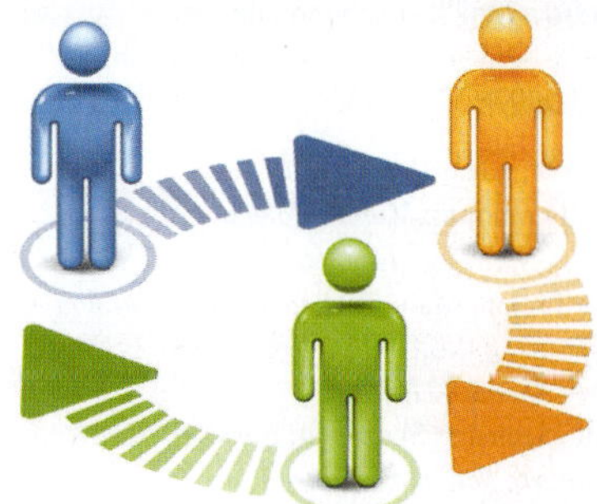

Amy L. Ensign, MBA, BHSA, CMA (AAMA), RMA (AMT)

Tammy M. Berger, BHSA, CPC, CMA (AAMA), RMA (AMT)

Mc Graw Hill

PRACTICE MANAGEMENT AND EHR: A TOTAL PATIENT ENCOUNTER. SECOND EDITION

Published by McGraw Hill LLC, 1325 Avenue of the Americas, New York, NY 10019.

This book is printed on acid-free paper.

1 2 3 4 5 6 7 8 9 LMN 28 27 26 25 24 23

ISBN 978-0-07-786207-7 (bound edition)
MHID 0-07-786207-4 (bound edition)
ISBN 978-1-260-46522-8 (loose-leaf edition)
MHID 1-260-46522-5 (loose-leaf edition)

Portfolio Manager: *Marah Bellegarde*
Product Developer: *Monica Toledo*
Marketing Manager: *Tami Hodge*
Content Project Managers: *Jane Mohr and Ron Nelms*
Manufacturing Project Manager: *Sandy Ludovissy*
Designer: *David W. Hash*
Content Licensing Specialist: *Lorraine Buczek*
Cover Image: *PopTika/Shutterstock*
Compositor: *Straive*

All credits appearing on page or at the end of the book are considered to be an extension of the copyright page.

Library of Congress Cataloging-in-Publication Data

Cataloging-in Publication Data has been requested from the Library of Congress.

LCCN: 2022051172

about the authors

Amy L. Ensign, MBA, BHSA, CMA (AAMA), RMA (AMT), has worked in health care for over 25 years, working clinically, administratively, and in higher education. Beginning her career as a medical assistant with Michigan's Henry Ford Health System, she moved into a leadership role working with senior management and supervising medical assistants, eventually becoming a medical assistant adjunct faculty member for Baker College. She has been in academics for 16 years and is currently the Director of Online Academics for Ross College, working with online and hybrid medical assistant, billing and coding, dental assistant, pharmacy technician, and health care administration programs. She previously held positions as program director for medical assistant, medical administrative assistant, and health service administration diploma, associate, and bachelor degree programs at Baker College.

She is an active member of the AAMA. On the chapter level, Amy has served as treasurer and secretary of Michigan's AAMA Macomb Chapter.

Amy lives in Sterling Heights, Michigan, with her husband and two sassy huskies; they have two adult sons and two beautiful granddaughters.

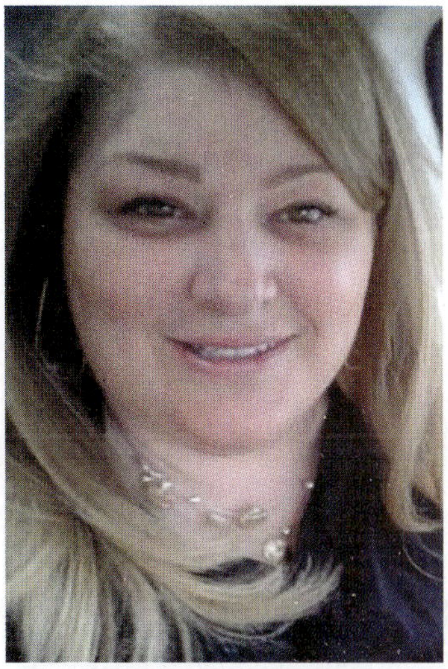

Amy Ensign, MBA, BHSA, CMA (AAMA), RMA (AMT)
Courtesy of Amy Ensign

Tammy M. Berger, BHSA, CPC, CMA (AAMA), RMA (AMT), worked in health care for over 25 years. She began her career as a medical assistant with Michigan's Henry Ford Health System. In 2004, she transitioned to administration roles in billing and coding. She held positions as a biller, back-end coder, documentation educator, emergency department (ED) coding coordinator and educator, and the ED coding manager. In 2006, she became a medical assistant adjunct faculty instructor at Baker College, and later joined Ross College-Online, teaching a variety of classes in the medical assisting and medical billing and coding programs.

Tammy was an active member of the AAPC and served as president, education officer, and member development officer for the Macomb Township, Michigan, chapter. She was also selected to be on the board of directors for the AAPC Chapter Association for the 2021–2023 term. She spoke at national conferences on a variety of topics.

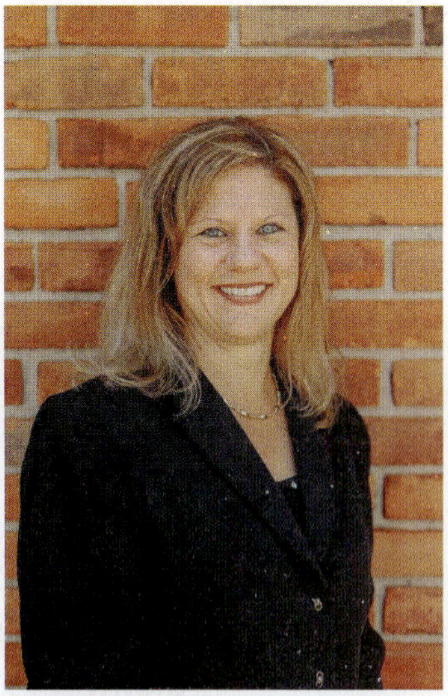

Tammy Berger, BHSA, CPC, CMA (AAMA), RMA (AMT)
Courtesy of Tammy Berger

brief contents

> ***This book is dedicated to the memory of Tammy (Vannatter) Berger, who will forever be in our hearts. Tammy, you accomplished so much in such a short time and will be missed more than you know. This project wouldn't have been possible without you!***
>
> **–Amy**

contents

part 1 Managing the Revenue Cycle 1

part 2 Documenting Patient Encounters 91

part 3 Charge Capture and Billing Patient Encounters 235

part 4 Producing Reports and Following Up 351

part 5 PM and EHR Practical Applications 433

preface

Practice Management and Electronic Health Records (EHR) Without the Hassles of Software Installation!

Welcome to *Practice Management and EHR: A Total Patient Encounter*! This is an exciting time to be participating in the health professions. Employment opportunities in health care are plentiful, and taking steps toward diplomas, degrees, and certifications in this field is commendable.

PMEHR provides the experience students need to understand the medical billing cycle and become familiar with the seamless integration of patient clinical records in that cycle. By completing the activities in *Connect*, students will learn transferable skills that will prepare them for success in the medical office, regardless of what program their practice uses.

With widespread implementation of EHRs, there continues to be a growing need for qualified health information technology workers. Every health care professional who comes into contact with patient records–from medical coders to billers, from medical assistants to doctors–must have an understanding of EHR. With a highly skilled workforce, EHR helps to improve the quality of health care for everyone.

PMEHR provides a comprehensive introduction to integrated practice management and EHR, providing hands-on experience to clinical health care workers as well as to their administrative and financial colleagues. Congratulations on embarking on this exciting new adventure!

Here's What Instructors and Students Can Expect from *PMEHR*

- One completely integrated solution with instruction on how practice management software works with EHR software, illustrating the complete patient encounter
- The opportunity to learn not only how to use a combined practice management and EHR solution, but also the why behind learning those skills
- The opportunity to learn a transferable skill
- No need for software installation–all EHRclinic applications will be completed within *Connect*
- The opportunity to complete EHRclinic exercises in *Connect* via Demo, Practice, and Assessment simulations
- Use of supporting source documents to add real-world experience to EHRclinic simulations

Organization of *PMEHR*

PMEHR is divided into six parts:

Part	Coverage
1. Managing the Revenue Cycle	Part 1 sets the stage for understanding the uses of an integrated practice management and electronic health record program in the medical practice. An overview of patient care and reimbursement is provided, as well as the basics about electronic health records and about maintaining the privacy and security of these records. maintaining the privacy and security of these records. EHRclinic software is introduced.
2. Documenting Patient Encounters	Part 2 presents the use of the PM/EHR during the patient encounter, covering scheduling, check-in, intake, exam documentation, electronic orders, and coding.
3. Charge Capture and Billing Patient Encounters	Part 3 presents the use of the PM/EHR to capture the charges resulting from the patient encounter and then collecting time-of-service (TOS) payments, creating and following up on claims, posting payments from payers and patients, and creating statements.
4. Producing Reports and Following Up	Part 4 covers the final steps in the PM/EHR cycle, focusing on financial and clinical reports as well as patient collections. Administrative and health information management tasks are also covered, including management of databases, data backup and recovery, messaging, coding compliance, and data analysis.
5. PM and EHR Practical Applications	Part 5 allows students to demonstrate mastery of the practical applications covered throughout the book. Students will complete exercises related to a scenario throughout an entire patient encounter.
6. Source Documents	Part 6 provides the source documents—patient information forms, electronic encounter forms, and remittance advice forms—needed to complete the exercises in Part 5 (Chapter 19).

Content Highlights of *PMEHR* by Chapter

(Information about the book's pedagogical elements appears in the Walkthrough starting on page xvi.)

- **Chapter 1** compares practice management (PM) programs and electronic health records (EHR). This chapter covers the steps in the medical documentation and billing cycle and the uses of clinical information gathered during patient encounters. The chapter also explains the roles of professional health care and administrative staff in implementing HIT in physician practices.
- **Chapter 2** explains the purpose of medical records and discusses the implementation and use of EHRs and practice management programs in healthcare, including both inpatient and outpatient settings. This chapter also covers how EHR data is captured and recorded while introducing EHRclinic, a program that combines practice management with electronic health record functions.
- **Chapter 3** defines the legal medical record and provides an overview of key health care regulation, including HIPAA and HITECH. It explores

Medical Documentation and Billing Cycle

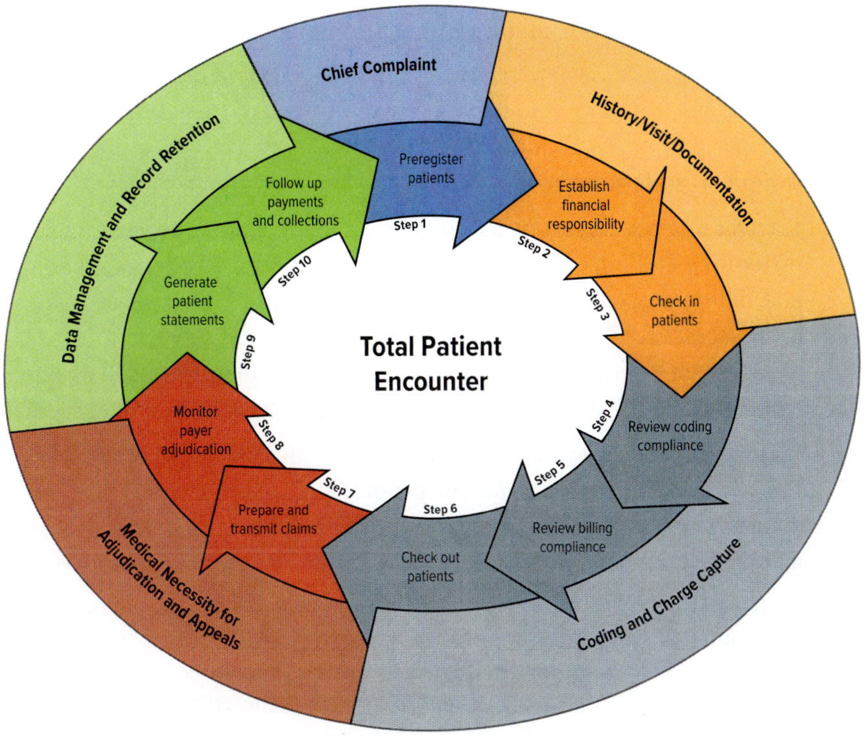

privacy and security concerns associated with electronic health information. The chapter also covers fraud and abuse to help office staff complete tasks in a PM/EHR in compliance with regulatory obligations.

- **Chapter 4** marks the beginning of the patient experience in an office visit encounter. The chapter presents the knowledge and skills needed to use a PM/EHR to create appointments for new and established patients and to reschedule appointments, as well as to add provider breaks, create recall lists, and verify insurance eligibility.
- **Chapter 5** explains the patient registration process and describes how patient data elements are organized in EHRclinic. The chapter also covers the skills needed to use a PM/EHR to check balances, collect patients, and electronically track patients during a visit.
- **Chapter 6** introduces the stages of the patient flow and describes the main sections of the patient chart in EHRclinic. The student learns how to use an EHR to record a patient's history, allergies, medications, vital signs, and chief complaint.
- **Chapter 7** describes methods used to enter documentation in an EHR, including the use of dictation and transcripts, voice recognition software, and templates. Students practice entering progress notes with and without the use of a template. The chapter covers the SOAP format and describes the elements of SOAP as they relate to office visit documentation.
- **Chapter 8** explains the benefits of E-Prescribing, including the use of medication reconciliation, drug interaction checkers, safety checks, and formularies. The chapter also covers electronic order entry in an EHR and discusses how orders are monitored and followed up.
- **Chapter 9** introduces students to the charge capture process in an office using integrated PM/EHR. This is followed by a discussion of the role

of EHR in reimbursement and the relationship between documentation and coding. The chapter covers HIPAA required code sets; the use of diagnostic, procedure, and E&M coding; and medical necessity.

- **Chapter 10** describes order processing in the flow of clinical check-out procedures. Encounter follow-up is also discussed, including patient referrals and patient education. The purpose and use of a clinical visit summary is identified.
- **Chapter 11** provides an overview of the charge capture process, including coding and billing compliance. Strategies to avoid common coding and billing problems and errors to the coding and billing process are also discussed. The chapter covers the various types of patient payments, such as copayments and coinsurance payments, as well as different types of charges and real-time adjudication.
- **Chapter 12** compares the major features of health plans and discusses third-party payment methods. The chapter describes the organization and regulation of employer-sponsored group health plans, self-insured health plans, and government-sponsored and disability insurance programs.
- **Chapter 13** explains the content and format of electronic and paper claims, and then illustrates the flow of claims from the PM/EHR to a clearinghouse and on to the payer. Students gain the skills required to create, submit, and monitor insurance claims through the claim adjudication process.
- **Chapter 14** describes how to interpret a remittance advice (RA) from a health plan and to enter and apply insurance payments in a PM/EHR. The process of appealing claims and postpayment audits are discussed. Students also learn how to create patient statements and process patient payments.
- **Chapter 15** provides an overview of the accounts receivable follow-up process, including the process for handling nonsufficient funds. The correct procedures for collections, including payment plans and the write-offs of uncollectable balances, are described.
- **Chapter 16** explains the contents of standard reports and how they are used to help generate and monitor practice revenue as well as to improve the delivery of health care, including the use of reports in PM/EHR to demonstrate quality standards. The chapter also discusses the use of aging reports to aid in patient and insurance collections.
- **Chapter 17** describes how emails and telephone encounters are used in the EHR. The various types of written communication are covered, and the student will learn strategies for effective message documentation and professional letter-writing. The chapter also covers task management in an EHR and use of the patient recall list.
- **Chapter 18** provides an overview of health information management (HIM) tasks, including the use of practice databases for maintaining billing information, updating referral facilities, adding new employees, and developing patient education libraries. The chapter discusses the purpose for backing up and restoring PM/EHR data and identifies the use of the EHR for auditing patients' health records. The use of data for practice analysis and the importance of monitoring coding compliance is also discussed.
- **Chapter 19** provides students with the opportunity to demonstrate mastery of their skills in a PM/EHR. Throughout 24 unique EHRclinic

exercises, students will apply their knowledge by completing a scenario that takes them through the entire medical documentation and billing process. By using source documents and references to earlier chapters, students will use their critical-thinking skills to complete the simulated exercises related to the scenario.

McGraw Hill connect Connect for *PMEHR*

McGraw Hill Connect for *PMEHR* includes:

- All end-of-chapter questions.
- Testbank questions.
- EHRclinic blends the best of both worlds with simulated Demo and Practice mode exercises and a sandbox approach to the Assessment mode exercises–all of which are auto-graded and accessible through *Connect.*
- Application-Based Activities in *Connect* are highly interactive, assignable exercises that provide students a safe space to apply the concepts they have learned to real-world, course-specific problems. Each Application-Based Activity involves the application of multiple concepts, allowing students to synthesize information and use critical thinking skills to solve realistic scenarios.

Instructors' Resources

You can rely on the following materials to help you and your students work through the exercises in the book. The following supplements can be found with the Instructor Resources, located through the Library tab on Connect:

- Instructor's Manual that contains everything to organize your course, complete with lesson plans and answer keys for end-of-chapter questions.
- A PowerPoint slide presentation for each chapter, containing teaching notes keyed to Learning Outcomes. Each presentation seeks to reinforce key concepts and provide a visual for students. The slides are excellent for in-class lectures.
- A Competency Correlation grid mapping chapters and Learning Outcomes to competencies for ABHES, CAAHEP, and CAHIIM.
- Sample syllabi according to course length to help plan your course.
- A comprehensive Asset Map breaks down all of the resources available through the book and Connect by chapter and by Learning Outcome to help you identify *what* you want to include in your course and *where* to find it.
- Instructor and student guides for EHRclinic containing directions on assigning EHRclinic, best practices, and user tutorials.

Need Help? Contact the McGraw-Hill Education Customer Experience Group (CXG)

Visit the CXG website at www.mhhe.com/support. Browse our frequently asked questions (FAQs) and product documentation and/or contact a CXG representative.

walkthrough

Many pedagogical tools have been incorporated throughout the book to help students learn.

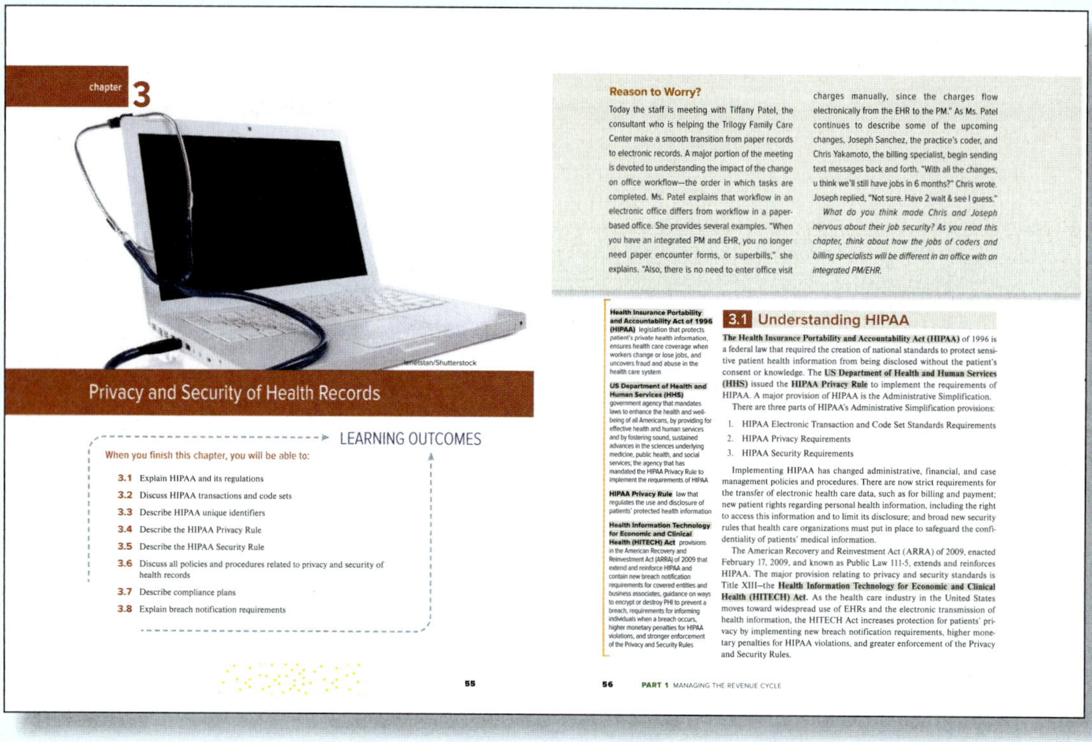

chapter 3

Shutterstock

Privacy and Security of Health Records

LEARNING OUTCOMES

When you finish this chapter, you will be able to:

3.1 Explain HIPAA and its regulations
3.2 Discuss HIPAA transactions and code sets
3.3 Describe HIPAA unique identifiers
3.4 Describe the HIPAA Privacy Rule
3.5 Describe the HIPAA Security Rule
3.6 Discuss all policies and procedures related to privacy and security of health records
3.7 Describe compliance plans
3.8 Explain breach notification requirements

55

Reason to Worry?

Today the staff is meeting with Tiffany Patel, the consultant who is helping the Trilogy Family Care Center make a smooth transition from paper records to electronic records. A major portion of the meeting is devoted to understanding the impact of the change on office workflow—the order in which tasks are completed. Ms. Patel explains that workflow in an electronic office differs from workflow in a paper-based office. She provides several examples. "When you have an integrated PM and EHR, you no longer need paper encounter forms, or superbills," she explains. "Also, there is no need to enter office visit charges manually, since the charges flow electronically from the EHR to the PM." As Ms. Patel continues to describe some of the upcoming changes, Joseph Sanchez, the practice's coder, and Chris Yakamoto, the billing specialist, begin sending text messages back and forth. "With all the changes, u think we'll still have jobs in 6 months?" Chris wrote. Joseph replied, "Not sure. Have 2 wait & see I guess."

What do you think made Chris and Joseph nervous about their job security? As you read this chapter, think about how the jobs of coders and billing specialists will be different in an office with an integrated PM/EHR.

Health Insurance Portability and Accountability Act of 1996 (HIPAA) legislation that protects patient's private health information, ensures health care coverage when workers change or lose jobs, and uncovers fraud and abuse in the health care system

US Department of Health and Human Services (HHS) government agency that mandates laws to enhance the health and well-being of all Americans, by providing for effective health and human services and by fostering sound, sustained advances in the sciences underlying medicine, public health, and social services; the agency that has mandated the HIPAA Privacy Rule to implement the requirements of HIPAA

HIPAA Privacy Rule law that regulates the use and disclosure of patients' protected health information

Health Information Technology for Economic and Clinical Health (HITECH) Act provisions in the American Recovery and Reinvestment Act (ARRA) of 2009 that extend and reinforce HIPAA and contain new breach notification requirements for covered entities and business associates, guidance on ways to encrypt or destroy PHI to prevent a breach, requirements for informing individuals when a breach occurs, higher monetary penalties for HIPAA violations, and stronger enforcement of the Privacy and Security Rules

3.1 Understanding HIPAA

The Health Insurance Portability and Accountability Act (HIPAA) of 1996 is a federal law that required the creation of national standards to protect sensitive patient health information from being disclosed without the patient's consent or knowledge. The **US Department of Health and Human Services (HHS)** issued the **HIPAA Privacy Rule** to implement the requirements of HIPAA. A major provision of HIPAA is the Administrative Simplification.

There are three parts of HIPAA's Administrative Simplification provisions:

1. HIPAA Electronic Transaction and Code Set Standards Requirements
2. HIPAA Privacy Requirements
3. HIPAA Security Requirements

Implementing HIPAA has changed administrative, financial, and case management policies and procedures. There are now strict requirements for the transfer of electronic health care data, such as for billing and payment; new patient rights regarding personal health information, including the right to access this information and to limit its disclosure; and broad new security rules that health care organizations must put in place to safeguard the confidentiality of patients' medical information.

The American Recovery and Reinvestment Act (ARRA) of 2009, enacted February 17, 2009, and known as Public Law 111-5, extends and reinforces HIPAA. The major provision relating to privacy and security standards is Title XIII–the **Health Information Technology for Economic and Clinical Health (HITECH) Act**. As the health care industry in the United States moves toward widespread use of EHRs and the electronic transmission of health information, the HITECH Act increases protection for patients' privacy by implementing new breach notification requirements, higher monetary penalties for HIPAA violations, and greater enforcement of the Privacy and Security Rules.

56 PART 1 MANAGING THE REVENUE CYCLE

Chapter Opener

The **chapter opener** sets the stage for what will be learned in the chapter.

Learning Outcomes

Learning Outcomes are written to reflect Bloom's Taxonomy and to establish the key points the student should focus on in the chapter. In addition, major chapter headings are structured to reflect the Learning Outcomes and are numbered accordingly.

Case Opener

A brief case study is presented so students can better understand how the content will apply to their future experiences in the health care profession.

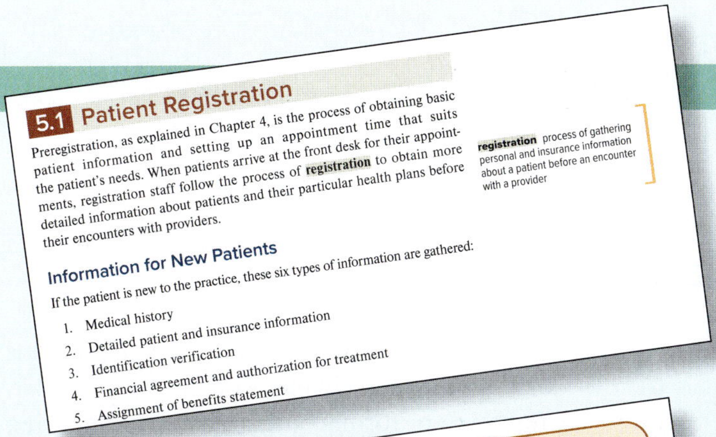

5.1 Patient Registration

Preregistration, as explained in Chapter 4, is the process of obtaining basic patient information and setting up an appointment time that suits the patient's needs. When patients arrive at the front desk for their appointments, registration staff follow the process of **registration** to obtain more detailed information about patients and their particular health plans before their encounters with providers.

registration process of gathering personal and insurance information about a patient before an encounter with a provider

Information for New Patients

If the patient is new to the practice, these six types of information are gathered:

1. Medical history
2. Detailed patient and insurance information
3. Identification verification
4. Financial agreement and authorization for treatment
5. Assignment of benefits statement

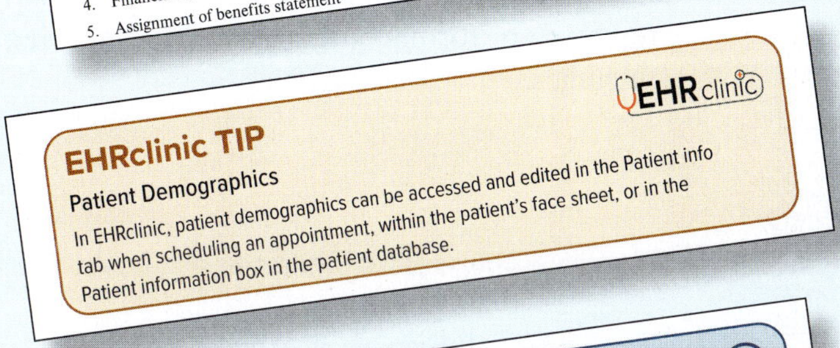

EHRclinic TIP

Patient Demographics

In EHRclinic, patient demographics can be accessed and edited in the Patient info tab when scheduling an appointment, within the patient's face sheet, or in the Patient information box in the patient database.

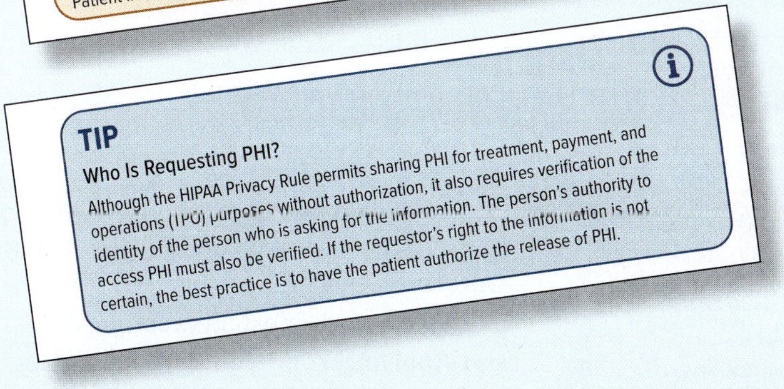

TIP

Who Is Requesting PHI?

Although the HIPAA Privacy Rule permits sharing PHI for treatment, payment, and operations (TPO) purposes without authorization, it also requires verification of the identity of the person who is asking for the information. The person's authority to access PHI must also be verified. If the requestor's right to the information is not certain, the best practice is to have the patient authorize the release of PHI.

Learning Aids

Key Terms

Key terms are called out at the beginning of each chapter and are set in bold throughout the text to further promote the mastery of Learning Outcomes.

Glossary

The **Glossary** at the back of the book also makes it easy to find a term's definition.

Tips

Tips (billing, coding, practice management tips) located throughout the chapters highlight important information for students. **EHRclinic Tips** suggest ways to be a more efficient user of the software.

Exercises

Thinking It Through

Thinking It Through exercises at major points in the chapter challenge students to stop and think through the information that has been presented.

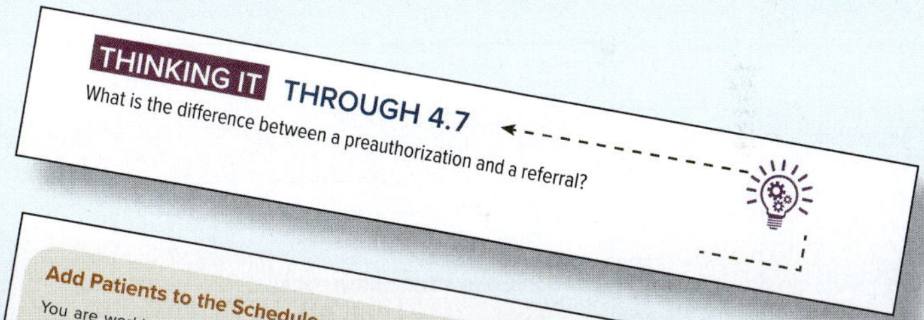

THINKING IT THROUGH 4.7

What is the difference between a preauthorization and a referral?

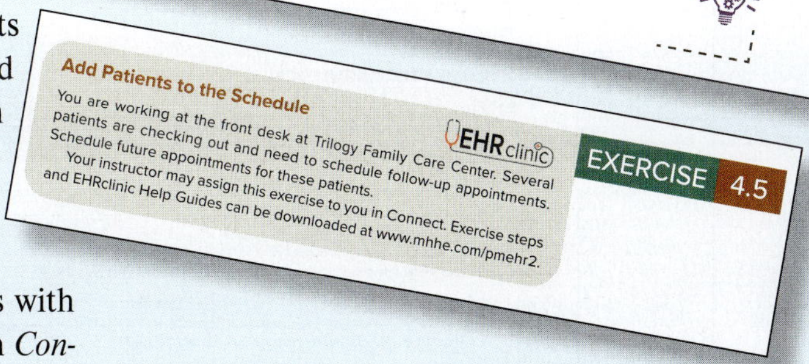

EXERCISE 4.5

Add Patients to the Schedule

You are working at the front desk at Trilogy Family Care Center. Several patients are checking out and need to schedule follow-up appointments. Schedule future appointments for these patients.

Your instructor may assign this exercise to you in Connect. Exercise steps and EHRclinic Help Guides can be downloaded at www.mhhe.com/pmehr2.

Chapter Exercises

Exercises within the chapter provide students with hands-on practice using EHRclinic through *Connect* Demo, Practice, and Assessment modes.

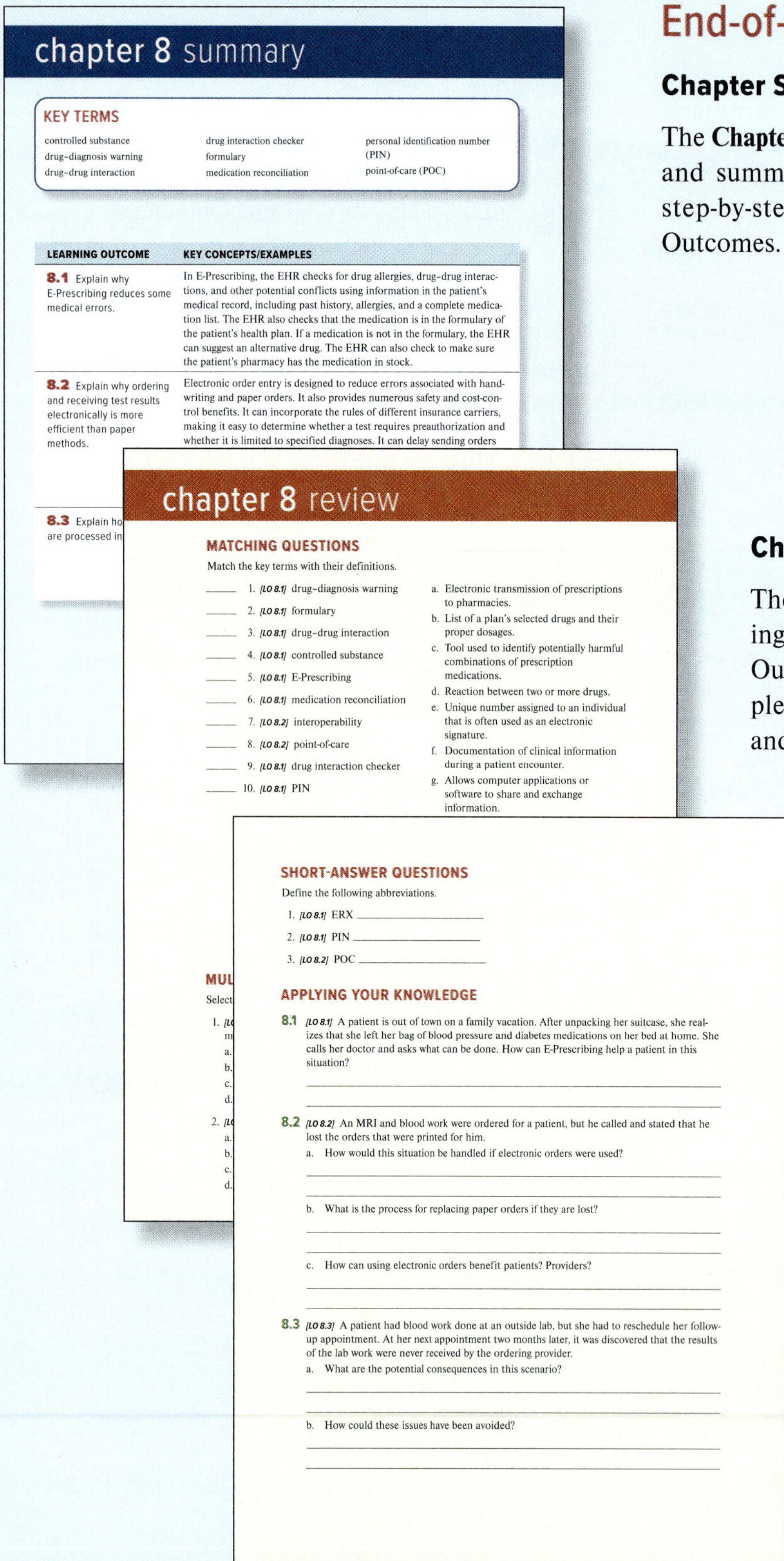

chapter 8 summary

KEY TERMS

controlled substance
drug-diagnosis warning
drug-drug interaction
drug interaction checker
formulary
medication reconciliation
personal identification number (PIN)
point-of-care (POC)

LEARNING OUTCOME	KEY CONCEPTS/EXAMPLES
8.1 Explain why E-Prescribing reduces some medical errors.	In E-Prescribing, the EHR checks for drug allergies, drug-drug interactions, and other potential conflicts using information in the patient's medical record, including past history, allergies, and a complete medication list. The EHR also checks that the medication is in the formulary of the patient's health plan. If a medication is not in the formulary, the EHR can suggest an alternative drug. The EHR can also check to make sure the patient's pharmacy has the medication in stock.
8.2 Explain why ordering and receiving test results electronically is more efficient than paper methods.	Electronic order entry is designed to reduce errors associated with handwriting and paper orders. It also provides numerous safety and cost-control benefits. It can incorporate the rules of different insurance carriers, making it easy to determine whether a test requires preauthorization and whether it is limited to specified diagnoses. It can delay sending orders

chapter 8 review

MATCHING QUESTIONS

Match the key terms with their definitions.

_____ 1. [LO 8.1] drug-diagnosis warning
_____ 2. [LO 8.1] formulary
_____ 3. [LO 8.1] drug-drug interaction
_____ 4. [LO 8.1] controlled substance
_____ 5. [LO 8.1] E-Prescribing
_____ 6. [LO 8.1] medication reconciliation
_____ 7. [LO 8.2] interoperability
_____ 8. [LO 8.2] point-of-care
_____ 9. [LO 8.1] drug interaction checker
_____ 10. [LO 8.1] PIN

a. Electronic transmission of prescriptions to pharmacies.
b. List of a plan's selected drugs and their proper dosages.
c. Tool used to identify potentially harmful combinations of prescription medications.
d. Reaction between two or more drugs.
e. Unique number assigned to an individual that is often used as an electronic signature.
f. Documentation of clinical information during a patient encounter.
g. Allows computer applications or software to share and exchange information.

SHORT-ANSWER QUESTIONS

Define the following abbreviations.

1. [LO 8.1] ERX ____________
2. [LO 8.1] PIN ____________
3. [LO 8.2] POC ____________

APPLYING YOUR KNOWLEDGE

8.1 [LO 8.1] A patient is out of town on a family vacation. After unpacking her suitcase, she realizes that she left her bag of blood pressure and diabetes medications on her bed at home. She calls her doctor and asks what can be done. How can E-Prescribing help a patient in this situation?

8.2 [LO 8.2] An MRI and blood work were ordered for a patient, but he called and stated that he lost the orders that were printed for him.

a. How would this situation be handled if electronic orders were used?

b. What is the process for replacing paper orders if they are lost?

c. How can using electronic orders benefit patients? Providers?

8.3 [LO 8.3] A patient had blood work done at an outside lab, but she had to reschedule her follow-up appointment. At her next appointment two months later, it was discovered that the results of the lab work were never received by the ordering provider.

a. What are the potential consequences in this scenario?

b. How could these issues have been avoided?

End-of-Chapter Resources

Chapter Summary

The **Chapter Summary** includes a list of key terms and summarizes chapter content in a tabular, step-by-step format organized by Learning Outcomes.

Chapter Review

The **Chapter Review** contains the following exercises, all tagged with Learning Outcomes: terminology exercises, multiple-choice and short-answer questions, and Applying Your Knowledge exercises.

digital tools for your success

Proctorio

Remote Proctoring & Browser-Locking Capabilities

Remote proctoring and browser-locking capabilities, hosted by Proctorio within Connect, provide control of the assessment environment by enabling security options and verifying the identity of the student.

Seamlessly integrated within Connect, these services allow instructors to control the assessment experience by verifying identification, restricting browser activity, and monitoring student actions.

Instant and detailed reporting gives instructors an at-a-glance view of potential academic integrity concerns, thereby avoiding personal bias and supporting evidence-based claims.

ReadAnywhere®

Read or study when it's convenient for you with McGraw Hill's free ReadAnywhere® app. Available for iOS or Android smartphones or tablets, ReadAnywhere gives users access to McGraw Hill tools, including the eBook and SmartBook® 2.0 or Adaptive Learning Assignments in Connect. Take notes, highlight, and complete assignments offline–all of your work will sync when you open the app with Wi-Fi access. Log in with your McGraw Hill Connect username and password to start learning–anytime, anywhere!

OLC-Aligned Courses

Implementing High-Quality Instruction and Assessment through Preconfigured Courseware

In consultation with the Online Learning Consortium (OLC) and our certified Faculty Consultants, McGraw Hill has created preconfigured courseware using OLC's quality scorecard to align with best practices in online course delivery. This turnkey courseware contains a combination of formative assessments, summative assessments, homework, and application activities, and can easily be customized to meet an individual instructor's needs and desired course outcomes. For more information, visit https://www.mheducation.com/highered/olc.

Tegrity: Lectures 24/7

Tegrity in Connect is a tool that makes class time available 24/7 by automatically capturing every lecture. With a simple one-click start-and-stop process, you capture all computer screens and corresponding audio in a format that is easy to search, frame by frame. Students can replay any part of any class with easy-to-use, browser-based viewing on a PC, Mac, or mobile device.

Educators know that the more students can see, hear, and experience class resources, the better they learn. In fact, studies prove it. Tegrity's unique search feature helps students efficiently find what they need, when they need it, across an entire semester of class recordings. Help turn your students' study time into learning moments immediately supported by your lecture. With Tegrity, you also increase intent listening and class participation by easing students' concerns about note-taking. Using Tegrity in Connect will make it more likely you will see students' faces, not the tops of their heads.

Test Builder in Connect

Available within Connect, Test Builder is a cloud-based tool that enables instructors to format tests that can be printed, administered within a Learning Management System, or exported as a Word document. Test Builder offers a modern, streamlined interface for easy content configuration that matches course needs, without requiring a download.

Test Builder allows you to:

- access all test bank content from a particular title.
- easily pinpoint the most relevant content through robust filtering options.
- manipulate the order of questions or scramble questions and/or answers.
- pin questions to a specific location within a test.
- determine your preferred treatment of algorithmic questions.
- choose the layout and spacing.
- add instructions and configure default settings.

Test Builder provides a secure interface for better protection of content and allows for just-in-time updates to flow directly into assessments.

Writing Assignment

Available within Connect and Connect Master, the Writing Assignment tool delivers a learning experience to help students improve their written communication skills and conceptual understanding. As an instructor, you can assign, monitor, grade, and provide feedback on writing more efficiently and effectively.

Create

Your Book, Your Way

McGraw Hill's Content Collections Powered by Create® is a self-service website that enables instructors to create custom course materials–print and eBooks–by drawing upon McGraw Hill's comprehensive, cross-disciplinary content. Choose what you want from our high-quality textbooks, articles, and cases. Combine it with your own content quickly and easily, and tap into other rights-secured, third-party content such as readings, cases, and articles.

Content can be arranged in a way that makes the most sense for your course, and you can include the course name and information as well. Choose the best format for your course: color print, black-and-white print, or eBook. The eBook can be included in your Connect course and is available on the free ReadAnywhere® app for smartphone or tablet access as well. When you are finished customizing, you will receive a free digital copy to review in just minutes! Visit McGraw Hill Create®—www.mcgrawhillcreate.com—today and begin building!

acknowledgments

The efforts of many people are needed to develop and improve a product. Among these people are the reviewers and consultants who point out areas of concern, cite areas of strength, and make recommendations for change. Suggestions have been received from faculty and students throughout the country. We would like to thank these reviewers and contributors for their assistance in developing content, offering suggestions, and shaping this revision. Many of the additions, improvements, and changes are due directly to their feedback. We appreciate their insight and commitment to helping us provide information that is relevant and valuable to students.

Acknowledgments from the Authors

To the students and instructors who will use this book, your feedback and suggestions will be greatly appreciated.

We want to thank our talented McGraw Hill team–Marah Bellegarde, Executive Portfolio Manager; Krystal Faust, Lead Product Developer; Monica Toledo, Product Developer; Jane Mohr, Lead Core Content Project Manager; Lorraine Buczek, Content Licensing Specialist; and David Hash, Lead Designer–for their belief in our vision for *PMEHR 2e* and for their tireless support throughout.

This text is dedicated to our families who have continually supported us in so many indescribable ways, Their flexibility, encouragement, and patience truly spurred us on through the authoring process.

part one

Managing the Revenue Cycle

chapter 1

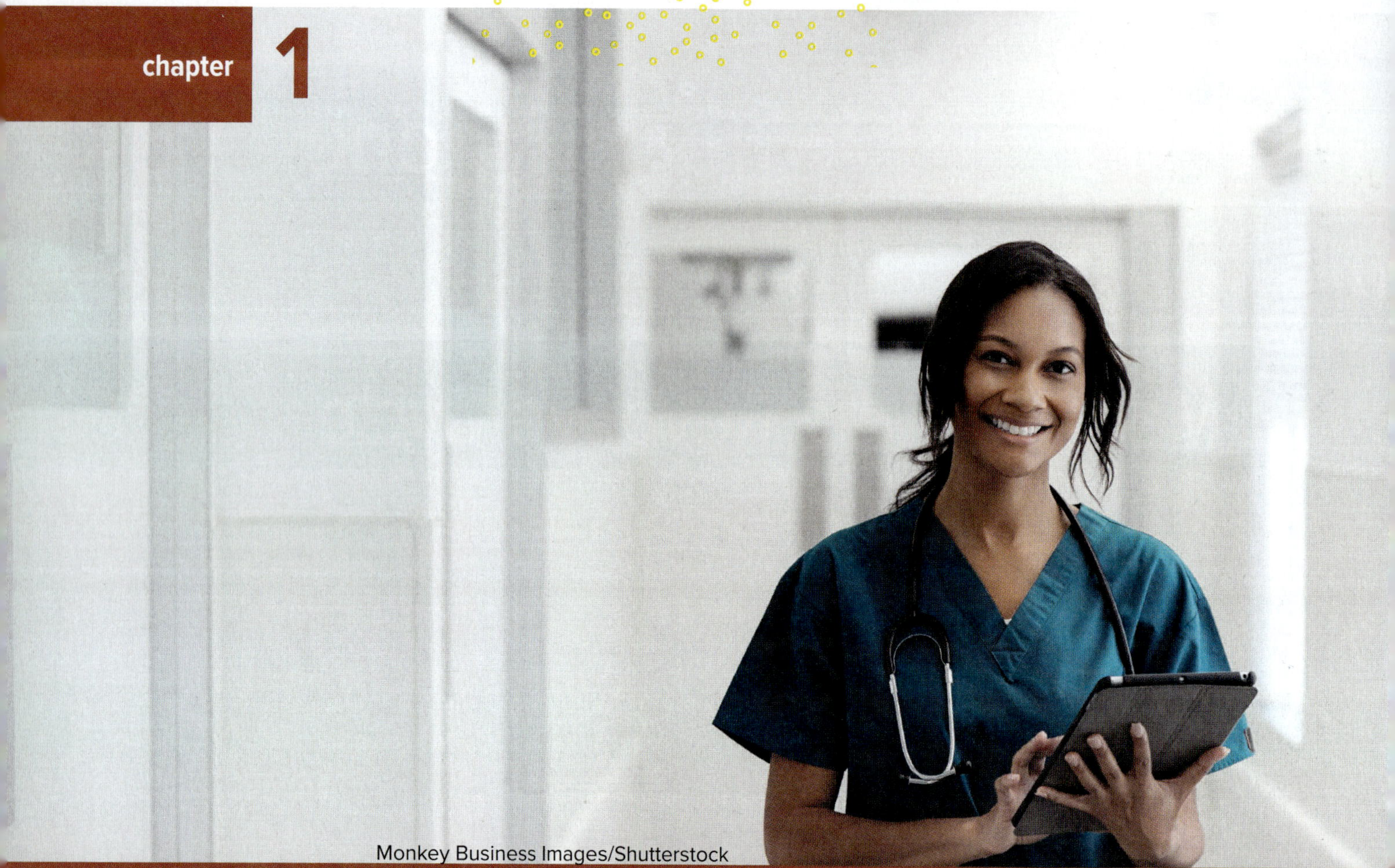

Monkey Business Images/Shutterstock

Patient Care and Reimbursement in the Medical Office

LEARNING OUTCOMES

When you finish this chapter, you will be able to:

1.1 Compare practice management (PM) programs and electronic health records (EHRs).

1.2 List the steps in the medical documentation and billing cycle.

1.3 List the eight facts that are documented in the medical record for an ambulatory patient encounter.

1.4 Identify the additional uses of clinical information gathered in patient encounters.

1.5 Compare the roles and responsibilities of clinical and administrative personnel on the physician practice health care team.

1.6 Explain how professional certification and lifelong learning contribute to career advancement in medical administration.

The New Program . . .

On his way out of the office Friday afternoon, Dr. Rudner stuck his head into Dr. McGrath's office. "Are you ready? Monday is the big day." "Yes, I'm actually looking forward to Tiffany's visit," Dr. McGrath replied. Tiffany Patel is a certified RHIA and an EHR implementation specialist with Trilogy Family Care Center. She will be spending several days in the office to set up the practice's new EHR and to train staff members.

"I think once the staff is trained and gets some hands-on experience, we'll be good to go," said Dr. McGrath.

Dr. Rudner responded, "I'm wondering how it's going to impact our cash flow and patient flow . . . and workflow. But since our staff had a part in selecting EHRclinic, we have everyone on board. And you know our staff is top notch. Breanna is a terrific medical assistant, Chris knows billing inside and out, and Joseph is a coding pro."

"I'm sure it will be challenging, but in the end, we'll be able to provide better care to our patients," Dr. McGrath replied.

"That's the bottom line. See you Monday," Dr. Rudner said as he left Dr. McGrath's office and headed down the hall.

1.1 Health Information Technology: Tools for a Total Patient Encounter

Do you remember what it was like to make a call from a pay phone or to wait for the bank to open to withdraw cash or make a deposit? If you needed cash when the bank was closed, you were out of luck. This is almost unimaginable today; we are used to having access to our money twenty-four hours a day, seven days a week. Perhaps you are too young to remember life before cell phones, ATMs, and the Internet. Look at Table 1.1. How many of the

TABLE 1.1 Activities Then and Now

What Do You Want to Do?	Then	Now
Get your mail	Wait for the post office to deliver it	Check your email online
Pay some bills	Write a check and mail it or go to a utility company to pay	Pay over the Internet
Make a phone call away from home	Look for a pay phone booth	Use a cell phone
See a movie	Go to a theater	Download and stream through your computer, mobile device, or TV
Buy some music	Go to a store that sells CDs	Download or stream music
Find out how to get to a restaurant	Call the restaurant and ask for directions, making sure to write them down	Enter the restaurant's address in your GPS
Get in touch with a friend	Make a phone call from home or a pay phone	Send a text message or use social media
Take some photographs	Buy film, load your camera, take pictures, unload film, bring film to a store to have it developed	Use a cell phone or digital camera

activities listed in the "Then" column do you remember doing, or perhaps someone has told you about?

We have become accustomed to using technology in our daily lives, and most of us would not want to go back to the old way of doing things. Technology saves time, gives us more choices, and generally makes life easier.

Technology has also become a part of daily life in the medical office. Innovations are changing the way medicine is practiced. Diabetes patients measure their blood glucose levels at home and wirelessly transmit readings to their physician. X-rays no longer require film, and they are available for almost instant reading with digital imaging. A paramedic performs an ECG on an incoming patient in the back of an ambulance and wirelessly transmits the images to the emergency room before the patient arrives. When a boy on vacation in Florida experiences unusual shortness of breath, the doctor at the walk-in clinic in Florida is able to view his medical record on the computer, even though the boy's pediatrician is in a different state. These are just a few examples of the ways in which technology is changing the delivery of health care.

Practice Management Programs and Electronic Health Records

health information technology (HIT) the use of computers and electronic communications to manage medical information and its secure exchange

The use of computers and electronic communications to manage medical information and its secure exchange is known as **health information technology (HIT)**. Physicians and facilities use HIT to help them accomplish many of the tasks they do each day. To receive payment for their services, physicians use software known as practice management (PM) programs, which will be discussed further in Chapter 2. These programs perform administrative and financial functions, such as scheduling patients' appointments, billing patients and health plans, receiving and recording payments, and managing collections. Since the software transmits data electronically, physicians receive payment in less time than when they send in paper claims and wait for checks to arrive in the mail. As they recognized some of the benefits that PMs could provide, they made the transition from paper to computer. Today, most practices no longer write patients' names in an appointment book and fill in paper claim forms. Figure 1.1 displays a sample appointment entry screen from a practice management program.

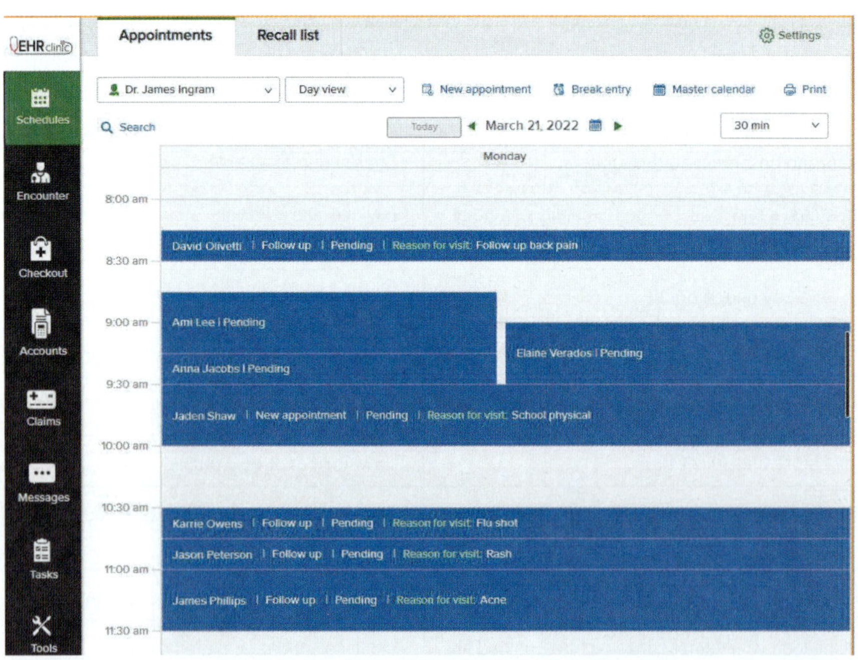

Figure 1.1 Sample Appointment Entry Screen from Practice Management Program

So while patients' financial records have been electronic for over a decade, clinical records—the information about a patient's health entered by doctors, nurses, and other health care professionals–are still primarily stored in paper charts. In the last several years, however, more and more physicians are converting paper charts to computerized records. An **electronic health record (EHR)** is a computerized lifelong health care record for an individual that incorporates data from all sources that provide treatment for the individual.

While EHRs are intended to replace paper records, their capabilities go beyond that of their paper equivalent. Since EHRs include information entered by all health care professionals who treat the patient, the programs make it easier to access and share patient information. Doctors, nurses, therapists, and other health care professionals can access the patient record via computer, regardless of whether they are in the same office, several miles away, or across the country. Figure 1.2 is a sample screen from a patient's facesheet in an electronic health record. In this example, you'll see that the categories are collapsed. When they are expanded, health care professionals can access the information in the patient's chart.

electronic health record (EHR) a computerized lifelong health care record for an individual that incorporates data from all sources that provide treatment for the individual

health informatics knowledge required to optimize the acquisition, storage, retrieval, and use of information in health and biomedicine

Health Informatics

Although access to information is a major advantage, EHRs provide even more benefits. With the push of a button, a physician can access the most recent treatment guidelines or check whether a new prescription might interact with existing medications before electronically sending it to the patient's pharmacy. Many people in government positions, as well as leaders in health care, believe that EHRs have the potential to improve the quality of health care, prevent many medical errors, and reduce health care costs.

It is for this reason that the field of **health informatics** (also known as *medical informatics*) grew by 20 percent through 2018. The U.S. Bureau of Labor Statistics predicts this field will maintain its current workforce and continue to grow 9 percent from 2020 to 2030. A vast array of health organizations–from physician practices, clinics, hospitals, and other institutions to insurance companies and public health education groups–require knowledgeable employees who can use technology efficiently, safely, and

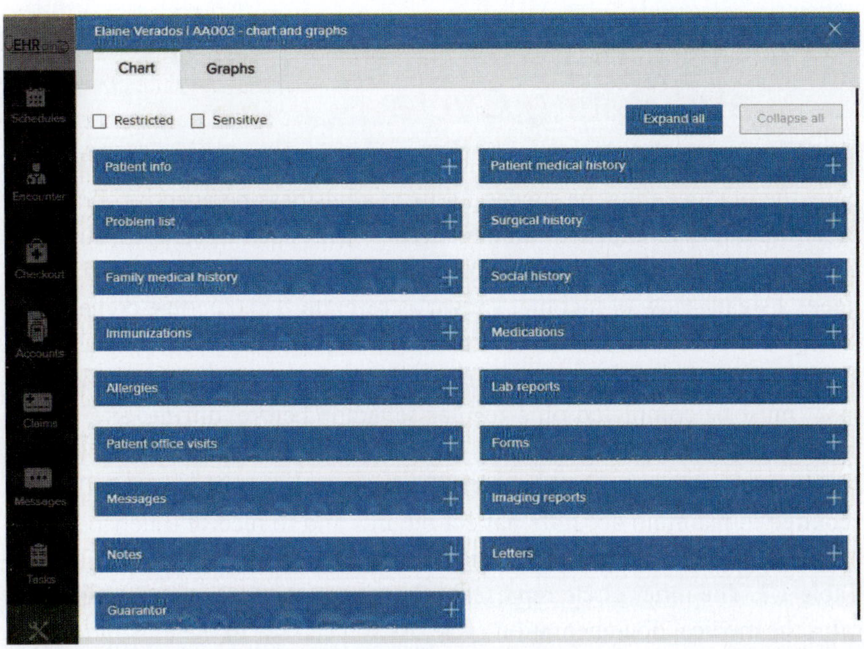

Figure 1.2 Sample Patient Facesheet in an EHR

THINKING IT THROUGH 1.1

A seventy-six-year-old man with a history of heart disease experiences chest pain while on vacation. He calls 911 and is transported to the nearest hospital. When he arrives in the emergency room, he is conscious and able to communicate with doctors. He tells the staff that he had prior heart attacks and that he had his six-month checkup with his cardiologist just before he left for vacation.

- How would an EHR enable doctors to determine a course of action in less time than was possible in a paper record-keeping environment?
- What information might the emergency room doctors be able to access from the cardiologist's EHR?

Figure 1.3 Health Informatics Skills

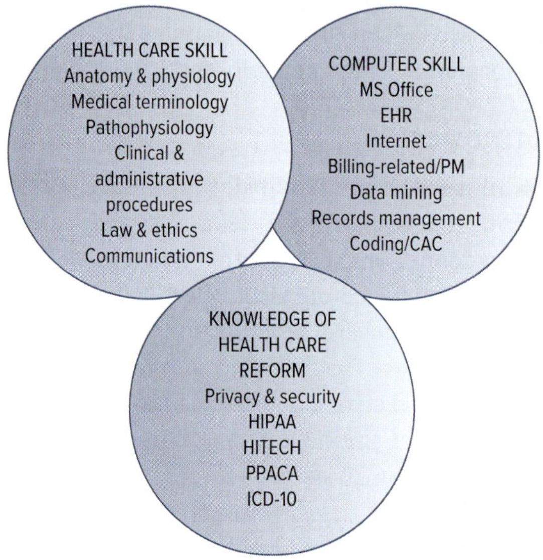

effectively. As shown in Figure 1.3, these new employees need health care skill, computer skill, and knowledge of health care reform in order to have the greatest opportunities for advancement in their careers.

1.2 The Medical Documentation and Billing Cycle

A physician practice's main focus is to care for patients, but to provide this care, the practice must be successful from a business perspective. Practices incur a number of expenses on a recurring basis, such as salaries, supplies, utilities, insurance, and equipment leasing. To meet its expenses, a practice needs a steady flow of income, known as revenue. This income comes from billing and collecting for services provided to patients. To maintain a regular **cash flow**—the movement of monies into or out of a business—specific tasks must be completed on a regular schedule before, during, and after a patient visit.

cash flow the movement of monies into and out of a business

medical documentation and billing cycle a ten-step process that results in timely payment for medical services

The **medical documentation and billing cycle** consists of ten steps that are required to maintain accurate patient records and to receive timely payment for services. This cycle is illustrated in Figure 1.4 with the steps listed in Table 1.2. The inner circle represents the billing cycle; the outer circle contains the medical documentation cycle. As you can see in the illustration, the

Medical Documentation and Billing Cycle

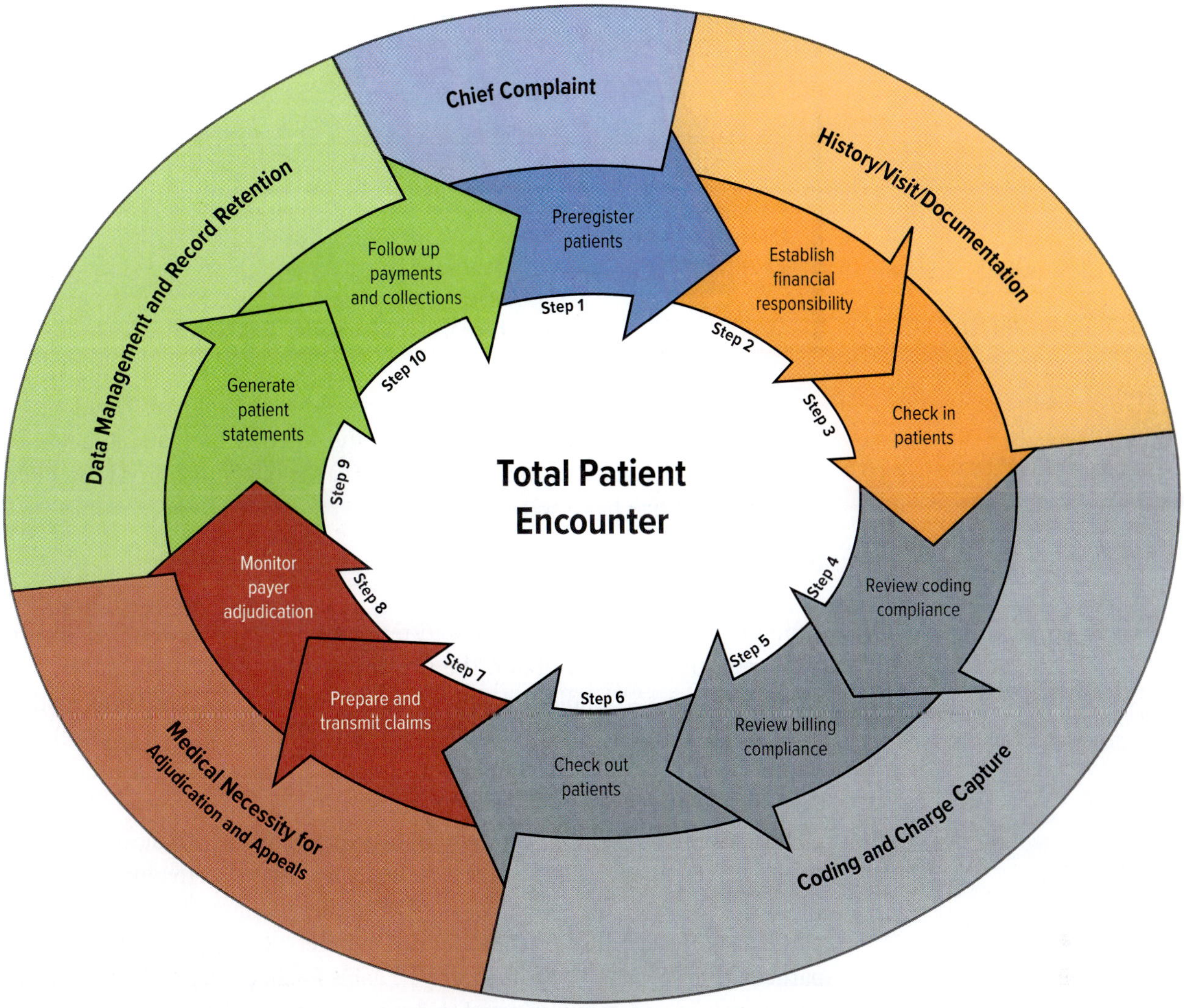

Figure 1.4 The Medical Documentation and Billing Cycle

two cycles are interrelated. For example, during Step 1, Preregistration, a new patient phones for an appointment. Both billing and clinical information must be collected during the phone call. From a billing perspective, the office wants to know whether the patient has insurance that will cover some or all of the cost of the visit, or whether the patient will pay for the visit. From a health or medical perspective, the staff wants to know the reason the person needs to see the doctor, known as the chief complaint. As the medical documentation and billing cycle continues, so does the interaction between the two types of information.

Steps in the Medical Documentation and Billing Cycle

Step 1: Preregister Patients

The first step in the cycle is to gather information so patients can be preregistered before their office visit. This information includes the patient's name,

TABLE 1.2	Steps in the Medical Documentation and Billing Cycle
Before the encounter	Step 1: Preregister patients
During the encounter	Step 2: Establish financial responsibility Step 3: Check in patients Step 4: Review coding compliance Step 5: Review billing compliance Step 6: Check out patients
After the encounter	Step 7: Prepare and transmit claims Step 8: Monitor payer adjudication Step 9: Generate patient statements Step 10: Follow up payments and collections

contact information, the chief complaint, and whether the patient is new to the practice. The information is obtained over the telephone or via the Internet, if the practice has a website.

Step 2: Establish Financial Responsibility for Visit

Most patients are covered by some type of health plan. While scheduling the appointment, it is important to determine whether the patient has health insurance and, if so, to obtain the identification number, plan name, and name of the person who is the policyholder. Once the insurance information is obtained, the patient's current eligibility and benefits are verified with the payer. Verification may be done by telephone, but most often it is done via the Internet and takes a matter of seconds.

It is also important to make sure that the health plan's conditions for payment, such as advance approval requirements for particular treatments or procedures, are met before treatment is provided. In addition, physicians usually participate in some health plans and not in others. If the physician does not participate in the plan, the patient may be liable for all charges. All of this must be determined and communicated to the patient before the appointment.

Step 3: Check In Patients

When patients arrive in the office, they are asked to complete or update patient information forms that have the personal, employment, and medical insurance data needed to collect payment for services. Most offices ask all patients to update this information periodically to ensure that it is current and accurate. As practices move from paper to electronic documents, a patient information form may be electronic. The advantage to using electronic forms is that they can be completed online before an office visit. Some offices provide a computer in a private area near the waiting room where patients can complete the electronic form if they do not have access to a computer at home. During check-in, it is also common practice to photocopy or scan the patient's insurance identification card and photo ID.

Patient coinsurance or copayments, as required under the policy of the patient's health plan, may be paid during check-in or check-out, depending on the medical practice's procedures. In addition, if a patient owes a balance from a previous visit, this amount may also be collected. A coinsurance is a partial payment of the office visit charges as determined by the health plan; the amount of the partial payment is the estimated patient responsibility for the procedure or service provided. For example, a patient may have an 80–20 coinsurance, meaning that the health plan covers 80% of the charges and the patient is responsible for 20% of the charges. Copayments are fixed fees, also under the policy of the patient's health plan, and are typically collected at the time of service (check-in or check-out). For example, a patient may have a $25 copayment, and this is the amount collected at the time of service regardless of the cost of service charges.

New patients receive information about the practice's financial policy at the time of their first visit, so they understand that they are responsible for payment of charges that are not paid by their health plans. Most practices accept checks, cash, and debit and credit cards for payment. Some practices also offer payment plans to patients.

During the office visit, a physician evaluates, treats, and documents a patient's condition. The visit documentation varies depending on a number of factors, including whether the patient is new or established. A provider who sees a patient for the first time obtains the patient's medical history. Once the patient is established, the visit documentation focuses more on the current medical needs of the patient.

Step 4: Review Coding Compliance

The physician records the procedures performed and/or treatments provided, as well as the determination of the patient's diagnoses. Then the physician (or medical assistant/coder) converts these written diagnoses and procedures to medical codes for reporting to health plans for payment.

The patient's primary complaint (the illness or condition that is the reason for the visit) is assigned a **diagnosis code** from the *International Classification of Diseases,* Tenth Revision, *Clinical Modification* (ICD-10-CM) (this process is explained in Chapter 9).

diagnosis code a code that represents the physician's determination of a patient's primary illness

procedure code a code that represents the particular service, treatment, or test provided by a physician

EXAMPLES

The ICD-10-CM code for Alzheimer's disease, unspecified is G30.9.

The ICD-10-CM code for influenza with other respiratory manifestations is J10.1.

Similarly, each procedure the physician performs is assigned a **procedure code** that stands for the particular service, treatment, or test. This code is selected from the *Current Procedural Terminology* (CPT) (see Chapter 9). A large group of codes covers the physician's evaluation and management of a patient's condition during office visits or visits at other locations, such as nursing homes. Other codes cover groups of specific procedures, such as surgery, pathology, and radiology. Yet another group of codes covers supplies and other services.

EXAMPLES

99460 is the CPT code for the physician's examination of a normal newborn infant in a hospital or birthing center.

27130 is the CPT code for a total hip replacement operation.

These codes are stored and before the practice submits them to an insurance plan for payment, they must be reviewed for compliance. In the area of coding, compliance requires checking that the codes are up to date and follow the official guidelines of the American Hospital Association and the American Medical Association (AMA). Also, the diagnosis and the medical services that are documented in the patient's medical record should be logically connected, so that the **medical necessity** of the charges is clear to the health plan. In billing, making this connection is known as *code linkage.* The AMA has defined medical necessity as "services or products that a prudent physician would provide to a patient for the purpose of preventing, diagnosing, or treating an illness, injury, or its symptoms in a manner that is:

medical necessity treatment that is in accordance with generally accepted medical practice

1. In accordance with generally accepted standards of medical practice
2. Clinically appropriate in terms of type, frequency, extent, site, and duration
3. Not primarily for the convenience of the patient, physician, or other health care provider."

If medical necessity is not met, the physician will not receive payment from the health plan.

Step 5: Review Billing Compliance

Medical practices bill numerous health plans and government payers. The provider's fees for services are listed on the medical practice's fee schedule. Most medical practices have standard fee schedules listing their usual fees. Each charge, or fee, is related to a specific procedure code.

However, the fees listed on the practice's master fee schedule are not necessarily the amount the provider will be paid. Instead, each of the health plans and government payers reimburses the practice according to its own negotiated or government-mandated fee schedule. Many providers enter into contracts with health plans that require a discount from standard fees. In addition, although there is a separate fee associated with each code, each code is not necessarily billable. Whether it can be billed depends on the payer's particular rules. Following these rules when preparing claims results in billing compliance, which will be discussed further in Chapter 11.

Step 6: Check Out Patients

Check-out is the last step that occurs when the patient is still in the office. The medical codes have been assigned and checked, and the amounts to be billed have also been verified according to payers' rules.

The PM/EHR then is used to calculate the charges for the visit and to ask for payment for the types of charges usually collected at time of service:

- Previous balances
- Copayments or coinsurance
- Noncovered or overlimit fees
- Charges of nonparticipating providers
- Charges for self-pay patients
- Deductibles

(Each of these charges is explained in Chapter 11.) A receipt is prepared for the payments made by the patients, and follow-up work is scheduled as ordered by the physician.

Step 7: Prepare and Transmit Claims

To receive payment, medical practices must produce documents for health plans and patients. One kind of document is an insurance claim. For a health plan to pay a claim, certain information about the patient must be shared. For example, a health plan needs to know the procedures the provider performed while the patient was in the office, the patient's diagnosis, and the date and location of the encounter.

Health plans also require basic information about the provider who is treating the patient, including the provider's name and identification number. Beyond the basic information requirements that are common to all payers, there are differences in what information is required on an insurance claim. A payer lists the required information in a provider's manual that is available to the medical office. In general, the information needed to create a claim is found on two documents–the patient information form and the encounter form. These documents are increasingly electronic rather than paper-based. The majority of health care claims are transmitted electronically.

Step 8: Monitor Payer Adjudication

When the payer receives the claim, it goes through a series of steps designed to determine whether the claim should be paid, a process called *adjudication.* Claims may be paid in full, partially paid, or denied. The results of the claim review, including an explanation of why charges were not paid in full or were denied entirely, are sent to the provider along with the payment. This information is reviewed for accuracy by a member of the billing staff, such as a medical insurance specialist, who compares each payment and explanation with the claim to check that:

- All procedures that were listed on the claim also appear on the payment transaction
- Any unpaid charges are explained
- The codes on the payment transactions match those on the claim
- The payment listed for each procedure is as expected

If any discrepancies are found, a request for a review of the claim is filed with the payer. If no issues are discovered, the amount of the payment is recorded. The payment may be in the form of a paper check, or it may be sent electronically to the practice's bank. Depending on the rules of the health plan, the patient may be billed for an outstanding balance. In other circumstances, an adjustment is made and the patient is not billed for a remainder balance. Occasionally, an overpayment may be received, and a refund check is issued by the medical practice.

Step 9: Generate Patient Statements

If charges are billed to the patient, a statement is created and sent to the patient. The statement lists all services performed, along with the charges for each. The statement lists the amount paid by the health plan and the remaining balance that is the responsibility of the patient. Some practices send statements electronically, but the majority still create and mail paper documents.

Most medical practices have a regular schedule, referred to as a billing cycle, for sending statements to patients. For example, some practices bill half the patients on the fifteenth of the month and the other half on the thirtieth.

accounts receivable (A/R) monies that are coming into a practice

accounts payable (A/P) monies going out of a business or medical practice, such as to pay staff, lease/rent, utilities, supplies, and equipment

revenue cycle management (RCM) management of the activities associated with a patient encounter to ensure that the provider receives full payment for services

Step 10: Follow Up Payments and Collections

A practice must track **accounts receivable (A/R)**—monies that are coming into the practice—and produce financial reports that provide information about its financial health. Some reports are produced on a daily basis, while others are created on a monthly or an annual basis. This financial information also helps a practice with **accounts payable (A/P)**, such as deciding whether to buy or lease new equipment, adopting new technology, expanding to a larger office, adding staff members, and so on. Financial reports can tell a practice which payers are denying more claims than others or are paying less than the expected amount. This information can be used in deciding whether to renew a contract with a payer, renegotiate the contract, or adjust fees.

Increasing Patient Financial Responsibility

In the past, physicians received the majority of their revenue from health plans, so collecting payments from patients was not a high priority. If the patient owed a balance after the insurance paid, the amount was likely to be small. For a number of reasons, this has begun to change. The ever-rising cost of health insurance has forced many employers to change the plans they offer to their employees. The new plans require employees to carry a greater share of the cost burden than in the past.

Out-of-pocket expenses, those that the patient pays before the health plan contributes, for average families are expected to rise due to the rising costs of health care. When health plans pay less, patients pay more. Accordingly, the amount of revenue that physicians receive from health plans is shrinking, and the amount that they receive from patients is growing. For this reason, physicians are seeking new ways to ensure that they receive payments from their patients.

It is much more difficult (and expensive) to try to obtain payment after a patient has left the office than to do so while the patient is in the office, so some practices estimate a patient's portion of visit charges during check-in and collect payment at that time. Managing the activities associated with a patient encounter to ensure that the provider receives full payment for services is known as **revenue cycle management (RCM)**. RCM is not just concerned with collecting payment from patients; it also focuses on improving cash flow from health plans.

Activities associated with managing the revenue cycle to improve cash flow include:

- Gathering complete and accurate information at registration
- Verifying insurance eligibility before the patient sees the provider
- Educating patients about the practice's financial policy and their own insurance benefits
- Increasing the number of payments collected at check-in
- Ensuring that all services performed by the provider are included on a claim
- Improving the accuracy of procedural and diagnostic coding
- Minimizing the time between submission of claims and receipt of payment
- Reducing the number of claims that are not paid or are not paid in full
- Reducing the number of overdue patient accounts

THINKING IT THROUGH 1.2

Alan West is checking in at the front desk for his appointment. The medical practice recently instituted a new financial policy that requires patients to make an estimated payment upon check-in. The receptionist checks his eligibility and benefits and sees that he is responsible for 20 percent of covered charges under his Blue Cross and Blue Shield plan. After checking the appointment schedule and determining that the estimated charge for today's visit is $160, she asks Mr. West for a payment of $32. Mr. West replies that he did not know he was expected to pay up-front, and asks the receptionist to mail him a bill.

- What should have been done before implementing the new financial policy?
- How should the receptionist handle Mr. West's request to mail the bill?

Data Management and Records Retention

The information collected throughout the medical documentation and billing cycle must be managed and retained. The data stored by a medical practice come from a variety of different databases, including practice management programs, electronic health record programs, and financial systems that process payroll and manage accounts receivable and payable. Information from all the databases is loaded into a **data warehouse**, a collection of data that includes all areas of an organization's operations. It does not replace the individual databases, which are still used for the day-to-day operations of the practice. Rather, it facilitates the storage, maintenance, and analysis of large amounts of data by creating a single source of stored data.

Data mining is the process of analyzing large amounts of data to discover patterns or knowledge. The results are used in many areas of the health care organization, from choosing the best course of treatment for a patient to identifying insurance plans that reimburse at below-average rates. Health information management professionals perform data warehousing and data mining activities. You will read about careers in health information management later in this chapter.

A physician practice must also establish a records retention schedule to ensure that patients' medical information is available for medical, legal, research, and other uses. A **records retention schedule** is a plan for the management of records, listing types of records and how long they should be kept. Retention schedules must comply with state and federal laws. While many states require physicians to maintain medical records for seven years, some states, including Hawaii, require records to be retained for twenty-five years after the last entry. The federal government specifies retention limits for some types of information. For example, laboratory pathology tests must be maintained for ten years, and other lab records for just two years. Because these laws vary by state, it is important to research the record retention requirements when establishing a practice's records retention schedule.

data warehouse a collection of data that includes all areas of an organization's operations

data mining the process of analyzing large amounts of data to discover patterns or knowledge

records retention schedule a plan for the management of records that lists types of records and indicates how long they should be kept

encounter the meeting of a patient with a physician or other medical professional for the purpose of providing health care (also known as a visit)

patient examination an examination of a person's body in order to determine his or her state of health

1.3 Documenting the Patient Encounter

An **encounter**, also known as a visit, is the meeting of a patient with a physician or other medical professional for the purpose of providing health care. At the heart of the encounter is the **patient examination**. After the patient is escorted to the exam room, the medical assistant gathers information such as the patient's current medications and allergies and the reason for the visit. The patient's vital signs–blood pressure, body temperature, oxygen level, heart rate (pulse), and respirations–are measured and recorded, as are other data such as height and weight. The medical assistant then notifies the provider that the patient is ready to be seen. After reviewing the patient's record, the provider enters the room, discusses the patient's reason for the visit and medical history, and completes a physical examination.

If the visit is for routine preventive services such as an annual physical examination, the provider makes an assessment of the patient's condition. If symptoms are present that must be managed, the provider develops a differential diagnosis–a mental list of all the possible causes of the patient's condition or symptoms. The provider may write orders for lab work, diagnostic tests, medications, or further visits with specialists to confirm or rule out particular diagnoses. Based on the suspected or confirmed diagnosis, a treatment plan is determined by the provider.

Types of Clinical Encounters

Health care providers supply preventive and acute care to patients, as well as ongoing treatment for chronic illnesses. Care to keep diseases from occurring or to enable early detection and treatment is known as *preventive care;* it includes routine annual physical examinations, immunizations, screening tests, and behavioral counseling. *Acute care* is provided for illnesses with a sudden onset that are time limited–not expected to continue more than a few days or weeks, such as a recovery from a broken bone. *Chronic* illnesses, on the other hand, must be treated over the long term. A patient with a chronic illness requires some level of ongoing medical treatment for a lengthy period of time, in some cases for a lifetime. Chronic diseases, such as heart disease, diabetes, asthma, and AIDS, are the leading causes of death and disability in the United States. Consider these facts:

- Seventy-five percent of the $2.3 trillion–over $7,000 per person–that the United States spends on health care goes toward treating chronic conditions like diabetes, heart disease, and cancer.
- Two-thirds of elderly patients have five or more chronic conditions, so the number of patients with chronic conditions will increase dramatically in proportion to the aging population of the United States.
- In particular, diabetes is gaining; it is estimated that by 2034, nearly twice as many Americans as today will suffer from diabetes, and spending on the disease will triple.

Figure 1.5 illustrates the past, present, and projected future incidence of chronic disease.

The Medical Record

Patient encounters, whether for acute, chronic, or preventive health care, generate clinical information about the patients' conditions and courses of treatment. Clinical information is used by health care professionals and patients to make judgments and decisions about patients' health care. For this reason, every time a health care provider treats a patient, a record, known

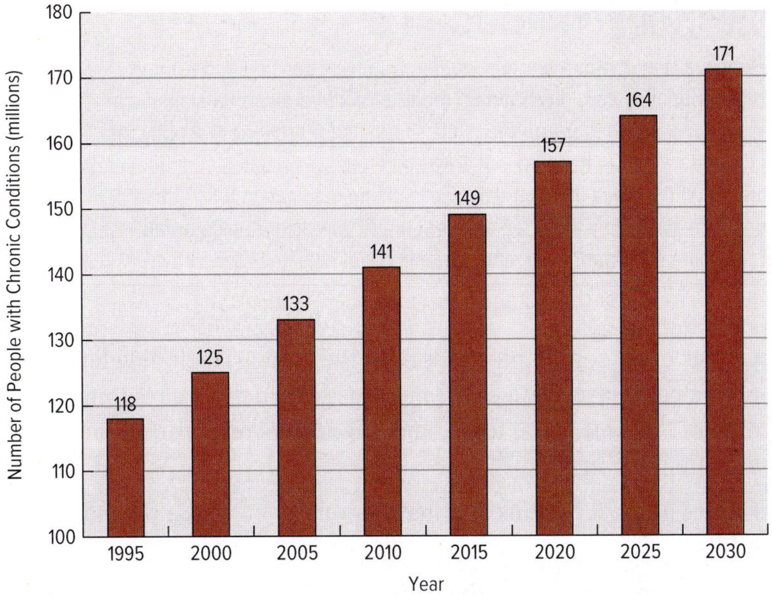

Figure 1.5 Rising Number of Americans with Chronic Conditions

as **documentation**, is made of the encounter. This chronological **medical record**, or chart, includes information that the patient provides, such as medical history, as well as the physician's assessment, diagnosis, and treatment plan. Records also contain laboratory test results, X-rays and other diagnostic images, lists of medications prescribed, and reports that indicate the results of operations and other medical procedures.

documentation the record created when a physician provides treatment to a patient

medical record a chronological health care record that includes information that the patient provides, such as medical history, as well as the physician's assessment, diagnosis, and treatment plan

The contents of medical records vary depending on the setting in which they are created and used, such as whether they are for acute care or ambulatory care. Acute care is most often provided in a hospital, which treats patients with urgent problems that cannot be handled in another setting. A patient in this setting is expected to require an overnight stay, and so is called an inpatient. *Ambulatory care* refers to treatment that is provided without admission to a hospital in settings such as physician practices, hospital emergency rooms, and clinics for outpatients.

Physicians' office charts tend to track the ongoing health and wellness needs of the individual. Eight data points are included in an ambulatory care medical record:

1. Patient's name
2. Encounter date and reason
3. Appropriate history and physical examination
4. Review of all tests that were ordered
5. Diagnosis
6. Plan of care, or notes on procedures or treatments that were given
7. Instructions or recommendations that were given to the patient
8. Signature of the provider who saw the patient

In addition, a patient's medical record contains:

- Biographical and personal information (also known as *demographics*), including the patient's full name, Social Security number, date of birth, full address, marital status, home and work telephone numbers, and employer information as applicable

THINKING IT THROUGH 1.3

Jane Mendoza is a fifty-four-year-old woman with hypertension and asthma. She visits her primary care physician for monitoring of her hypertension and a pulmonary specialist for her asthma. While shopping for groceries recently, she fell on the ice and broke her ankle. She was taken to the hospital, admitted, and had surgery on the ankle the next day. She is taking medication for all three conditions, prescribed by the three different physicians. Is her ankle break a chronic or acute condition? How many chronic conditions does Jane have?

- Copies of all communications with the patient, including letters, telephone calls, faxes, and email messages; the patient's responses; and a note of the time, date, topic, and physician's response to each communication
- Copies of prescriptions and instructions given to the patient, including refills
- Original documents that the patient has signed, such as an authorization to release information and an advance directive about end-of-life care
- Medical allergies and reactions, or their absence
- Up-to-date immunization record and history if appropriate, such as for a child
- Previous and current diagnoses, test results, health risks, and progress
- Copies of referral or consultation letters
- Hospital admissions and release documents
- Records of any missed or canceled appointments
- Requests for information about the patient (from a health plan or an attorney, for example), and a detailed log listing to whom information was released

continuity of care coordination of care received by a patient over time and across multiple health care providers

Whether created in a physician practice or in a hospital, the medical record allows health care professionals involved in the patient's care to provide continuity of care to individual patients. **Continuity of care** refers to coordination of care received by a patient over time and across multiple health care providers.

1.4 Other Uses of Clinical Information

Although the primary use of clinical information is to provide effective health care to the patient, clinical information also has several important secondary uses. These uses involve legal issues, quality review, research, education, public health and homeland security, and billing and reimbursement.

Legal Issues

Clinical information may be used as evidence in a legal matter involving a patient or a provider. For example, an individual may bring a lawsuit against another driver's automobile insurance plan as a result of back injuries sustained in an accident. The automobile insurance plan would require access to the clinical information to determine whether the individual was being treated for back problems before the accident.

Clinical information is also important in protecting the physician from accusations of **medical malpractice**, the provision of medical services at a less than acceptable level of professional skill that results in injury or harm to a patient. A patient who feels that a physician has made an error in diagnosis or treatment may bring a lawsuit known as a malpractice claim. Such claims include alleging that the wrong medication was prescribed and accusing physicians of failing to follow up on ordered tests. Accurate and complete documentation is an important part of a defense against the accusation that a patient was not treated appropriately, as it shows that the physician followed the medical standards of care that apply in the state. The standard of care is the actions or measures that a reasonable health care professional in the same location would take in similar circumstances. Health care providers are liable (that is, legally responsible) for providing this level of care to their patients.

medical malpractice the provision of medical services at a less than acceptable level of professional skill that results in injury or harm to a patient

Merit-Based Incentive Payment System (MIPS) program that determines Medicare payment adjustments through the Quality Payment Program

Quality Payment Program (QPP) the Medicare value-based reimbursement system

Quality Review

Individuals and institutions in the health care field must regularly evaluate the adequacy and appropriateness of the care they deliver. Clinical data are analyzed to obtain a measure of the quality of the services provided to the patient. Increasingly, data on quality are being linked to physician reimbursement. An example is the **Merit-Based Incentive Payment System (MIPS)** track of the **Quality Payment Program (QPP)**. MIPS provides financial incentives to eligible clinicians who provide evidence-based treatments to their patients and report health care quality data to the Centers for Medicare and Medicaid Services (CMS). Evidence-based medicine is medical care that uses the latest and most accurate clinical research in making decisions about the care of patients. For example, a hospital that is in the top 10 percent of statistics on the fewest post-surgery infections could receive additional compensation from a payer. In the physician office, a provider might be financially rewarded for significantly increasing the number of women over the age of sixty-five who are screened for osteoporosis.

Research

Clinical information collected during a patient visit is used by medical researchers to develop new methods of treatment and to compare the effectiveness of existing treatments. For example, researchers who are conducting clinical trials of a new medication need access to clinical information to validate that patients meet the criteria for the study.

Education

Case studies that are used to train a wide range of health professionals are developed with information from patient encounters. For example, medical students are presented with cases during their training. In these cases, the patient's identity is removed from the record, so patient confidentiality is not at risk.

Public Health and Homeland Security

The records of physicians and hospitals are also important in determining the incidence of disease and in developing methods to improve the health of the population. The incidence and spread of disease can be followed closely using health records. For example, in the event of an influenza pandemic, data from physician visits would be critical in detecting the outbreak early and in containing its effects.

THINKING IT THROUGH 1.4

The Quality Payment Program (QPP) rewards physicians who follow the latest medical evidence when providing care to patients. This evidence often is in the form of generally agreed upon guidelines written by experts in the field. For example, physicians may be rewarded if a certain percentage of their patients have LDL cholesterol readings below 100. Scientific evidence indicates that individuals with LDL levels below 100 are less likely to develop coronary artery disease.

- Can you think of any reasons why physicians may not be in favor of incentive programs?
- How might incentive programs affect the physician–patient relationship?

Billing and Reimbursement

It is important to understand that physician practices are businesses as well as centers for patient care. In addition to the uses already described, the medical record is also the main source of information for physician reimbursement. Most patients have some form of medical insurance to help them pay for medical services. In order for the insurer to make payment, the physician's documentation in the medical record must show that the service provided was warranted given the patient's condition. Reimbursement may be denied if this clinical information is incomplete or inaccurate.

1.5 The Physician Practice Health Care Team: Roles and Responsibilities

It takes a talented, dedicated group of health care professionals to care for patients and to run a successful health care business. Staff members who provide treatment to patients are known as clinicians, while those who manage the business aspects of health care are called administrative staff. Administrative staff, including medical billers and coders, receptionists, practice managers, compliance officers, and anyone else who works behind the scenes in a medical office, do not provide medical treatment or testing. Some administrative workers, such as schedulers, do interact with patients, but they do not provide medical care.

In large practices, administrative roles are likely to be specialized. For example, one person schedules appointments, another processes Medicare claims, and another follows up on patient accounts. Small offices usually combine several of these tasks into one staff role. The person who processes claims may also be required to collect on patient accounts. The best preparation for medical office work is to gain a broad understanding of the different clinical and administrative staff roles.

Physicians

Physicians (MDs and DOs) are the primary clinicians in the practice. They diagnose illness and injury, prescribe and administer treatment, and advise patients about how to prevent and manage disease.

Advanced Practice Providers

Advanced practice providers (APPs), such as physician assistants (PAs) and nurse practitioners (NPs) are formally trained to provide diagnostic, therapeutic, and preventive health care services under the supervision of a physician. They take medical histories, examine and treat patients, order and interpret laboratory tests and X-rays, make diagnoses, and prescribe medications. They also treat minor injuries by suturing, splinting, and casting. In most states, PAs may prescribe medications.

Nurses

Nurses perform a wide range of clinical and nonclinical duties. When caring for patients, nurses develop care plans or contribute to existing plans. Plans may include numerous activities, such as administering medication; starting, maintaining, and discontinuing intravenous (IV) lines for fluid, medication, blood, and blood products; administering therapies and treatments; observing patients and recording their observations; and consulting with physicians and other health care clinicians.

Medical Assistants

medical assistant (MA) health care professional who performs both administrative and certain clinical tasks in physician offices

Medical assistants (MAs) are trained to perform both administrative and certain clinical tasks in physician offices. MAs assist physicians by taking patient medical histories and vital signs, providing patient education, collecting specimens and performing basic medical laboratory tests, and administering medications. They prepare for and assist with examinations and procedures.

The range and scope of their tasks depends on the amount and type of training as well as the location, size, and specialty of the practice. In small practices, medical assistants perform many different clinical and administrative tasks. In large practices, they tend to specialize in particular areas. Some MAs may focus on the clinical areas, while others pursue certification as medical coders or billers, as explained below.

The scope of clinical practice also depends upon state laws that regulate the duties of medical assistants. For example, tasks such as drawing blood, giving injections, and starting or disconnecting IVs are permissible in some states and not in others.

According to the U.S. Department of Labor, the clinical tasks that medical assistants may perform include:

- Taking medical histories and recording vital signs
- Preparing patients for examinations
- Assisting physicians during examinations
- Collecting and preparing laboratory specimens
- Performing basic laboratory tests
- Explaining treatment procedures to patients
- Instructing patients about medications and special diets
- Preparing and administering medications as directed
- Correctly disposing of contaminated supplies
- Sterilizing medical instruments

The administrative duties of medical assistants include:

- Scheduling and managing appointments
- Scheduling inpatient and outpatient admissions and procedures
- Performing bookkeeping duties such as preparing bank deposits and posting payments and adjustments
- Processing insurance claims

Medical Billers and Coders

medical biller health care professional who performs administrative tasks throughout the medical billing cycle

medical coder medical office staff member with specialized training who handles the diagnostic and procedural coding of medical records

The term **medical biller** describes all the tasks that are completed by administrative staff members during the medical billing cycle. Typically, front office staff members handle duties such as reception (registration) and scheduling. Back office staff duties are related to billing, insurance, and collections. Job titles in common use are billing clerk, insurance specialist, reimbursement specialist, and claims specialist.

Common tasks are:

- Verifying patient insurance information and eligibility before medical services are provided
- Collecting payments that are due, such as copayments, at the time of service
- Maintaining up-to-date information about health plans' billing guidelines
- Following federal, state, and local regulations on maintaining the confidentiality of information about patients
- Abstracting information from patients' records for accurate billing
- Billing health plans and patients, maintaining effective communication to avoid problems or delayed payments
- Assisting patients with insurance information and required documents
- Processing payments and requests for further information about claims and bills
- Maintaining financial records
- Updating the forms and computer systems the practice uses for patient information and health care claims processing

TIP

Medical billing tasks may be handled by a medical billing specialist, a medical insurance specialist, a medical coder, or an administrative medical assistant. This text uses the term *medical biller* to include any administrative tasks.

Medical coders are trained in the correct use of standard medical code sets (covered in Chapter 9). In larger practices, a medical coder or a coding team handles coding, while the medical biller or billing group handles billing and claims processing.

Practice or Office Manager

Practice managers or office managers are responsible for directing the successful business operation of physician practices. A large practice may employ a practice manager who has graduate education in business and sometimes a clinical background as well. Smaller offices are commonly managed by an office manager well versed in running a practice with fewer clinicians.

The practice manager's duties include budgeting office revenues and expenses; monitoring performance against budgets; performing payroll and accounting tasks; planning usage space; determining office and clinical policies, procedures, and guidelines; and hiring and managing office employees. Individuals wishing to pursue a career in health care management must be knowledgeable about all aspects of practice operations. Although many practice managers have backgrounds in a clinical specialty or training in health care administration, some enter these jobs with a general business education.

Compliance Officer

Federal regulations also require the designation of a team member to serve as the practice compliance officer. This person is often either a physician or the practice manager. The compliance officer in a physician practice investigates and resolves all compliance issues relating to coding, billing, documentation, and reimbursement. Compliance officers' duties are based on HIPAA/ARRA rules, as covered in Chapter 3.

Working as a Team

Collecting payment for services is not the sole responsibility of the administrative staff. All personnel—both administrative and clinical—play key roles in the process, and each must communicate critical information to other staff members for reimbursement to occur. Without complete information, health claims created after the office visit will not be paid by health plans.

Staff members who schedule patient appointments start the reimbursement process by collecting necessary information from patients, such as current phone numbers and insurance identification numbers. Before the appointment, a staff member checks the patient's eligibility and benefits.

Data collected during the scheduling phone call is confirmed once the patient arrives in the office. The front desk collects payment from the patient based on the information obtained in the eligibility and benefits check.

The physician, physician assistant, nurse, and medical assistant also have responsibilities for ensuring that the practice receives reimbursement for services. Documenting the patient encounter is primary among these responsibilities. The documentation must be complete and must demonstrate medical necessity to the health plan. The appropriate procedure and diagnosis codes must be assigned and recorded on an encounter form, which may be paper or electronic.

Referring to the information on the encounter form, staff working the check-out desk determine whether the patient owes any additional payment, even if payment was collected during check-in. The patient is responsible for charges if the services are not covered by his or her health plan. If the encounter form does not contain the appropriate diagnosis and procedure codes, payment cannot be collected at check-out.

The billing and coding staff are responsible for generating and transmitting insurance claims, but first they must review the information on the

THINKING IT THROUGH 1.5

John Guastella is a medical biller responsible for analyzing why claims are not paid as expected. He spends his days researching each claim and determining the cause of the partial payment. A few weeks ago, the practice manager asked him to begin creating weekly reports that list each claim, the dollar amount not collected, and the source of the problem. He emails the report to the practice manager, who reviews the contents and follows up with office staff. Last week, John noticed that some staff members avoided him in the lunchroom. He feels uncomfortable preparing a report that pinpoints which staff members have made mistakes—even if their errors resulted in the practice not receiving payment.

- Why is John being avoided?
- What could be done to change the way unpaid claims are handled in the office?

encounter form. In addition, they must use their knowledge of each health plan's rules and regulations to determine whether all necessary information has been captured on the claim. Once the claim has been submitted, they are responsible for following up to ensure the claim is paid. If a claim is rejected, they review the reason for the rejection and follow up with the relevant staff member.

When payments arrive, a medical biller reviews the amounts to make sure they are as expected, and then posts the payments in the practice management program. Next, patient statements must be created and mailed. Finally, staff must follow up on unpaid accounts and initiate collections activities when appropriate.

Everyone working in the medical office plays a key role in the billing cycle. Successful reimbursement requires a team effort. If one team member does not do a good job, there is a chance that the practice will not be paid as expected. In addition, team members need to share information. The front office, back office, and clinical staff all need to communicate if the practice is to receive timely payment for services in situations such as the following:

- A claim is rejected because the patient's identification number is incorrect; the biller must talk to the scheduler or front desk person who collected that information.
- An encounter form is missing a diagnosis code; the biller needs to speak with the physician.
- The billing staff notices that information a payer requires is missing from a claim; the biller needs to obtain the missing information from the appropriate staff member.
- An eligibility check reveals that the patient is not covered by the health plan; the scheduler needs to contact the patient to review the information on file.
- A claim is not paid because the patient's plan does not cover the treatment provided; the biller needs to check with the staff member who performed the eligibility and verification check to determine what went wrong.

1.6 Administrative Careers Working with Integrated PM/EHR Programs

Health care is information-intensive. Every encounter someone has with the health care system–from seeing a physician, to having blood drawn at a lab, to picking up a prescription at a pharmacy–is documented and stored. The accuracy and availability of this information plays a major role in determining the outcome of a patient's health care experience.

On its own, health information technology does little to ensure a positive outcome for the patient. The usefulness and value of the information depend on a workforce of skilled professionals capable of creating, managing, and analyzing the data. To manage the information effectively, health care workers, regardless of their specific job roles, need information technology skills. The knowledge required extends beyond basic computer literacy to:

- Using word processing and presentation software
- Searching, retrieving, and managing data from internal sources, external databases, and the Internet
- Communicating using email, instant messaging, listservs, and file transfers
- Understanding and following security measures such as access control and data security

An office that has made the transition to an integrated practice management program and electronic health record program also requires a staff that is familiar with health information technology. Two major curricula, Registered Health Information Technician and Registered Health Information Manager, are available under the guidance of the American Health Information Management Association (AHIMA) to provide a strong foundation in health information management (HIM).

The technician level is an associate degree program intended to prepare students to examine medical records for accuracy, report patient data for reimbursement, and help provide information for medical research and statistical data. The manager level is a baccalaureate degree program that produces graduates skilled in the collection, interpretation, and analysis of patient data who can interact with all levels of an organization–clinical, financial, and administrative–that employ patient data in decision making. The graduate is trained to assume managerial positions related to these functions.

Whether or not students choose to specialize in HIT, every graduate of an allied health program will be required to use health information technology on the job. As the United States has implemented the use of electronic health records as an industry standard, the demand for allied health graduates with skills in information technology and familiarity with computers exceeds the supply.

Gaining Certification in Your Field

As in other medical fields, individuals with certification generally have an easier time finding employment and advancing on the job than do those without certification. **Certification** acknowledges that an individual has mastered

certification a nationally recognized designation that acknowledges that an individual has mastered a standard body of knowledge and meets certain competencies

a standard body of knowledge and meets certain competencies. Employers look for certification when filling open positions, and certified individuals usually earn higher salaries than those who are not certified. Certification is offered in most allied health specialties. The field of health information technology offers a number of certifications, including the following:

- Registered Health Information Technician (RHIT) certification is offered by the American Health Information Management Association (AHIMA; www.ahima.org).
- Registered Health Information Administrator (RHIA) certification is also offered by AHIMA.
- The American Association of Medical Assistants (AAMA) offers a Certified Medical Assistant (CMA) designation to individuals who pass an examination after earning a diploma in medical assisting from an accredited school (AAMA; www.aama-natl.org).
- Medical assistants may, alternatively, acquire the Registered Medical Assistant (RMA) designation from the American Medical Technologists (AMT; www.americanmedtech.org).
- The Certified Professional in Healthcare Information and Management Systems (CPHIMS) designation is offered by the Healthcare Information and Management Systems Society (HIMSS; www.himss.org). It is intended for health care information and management systems professionals who possess a combination of educational and work experience.
- Certification in Healthcare Privacy and Security (CHPS) is offered by AHIMA and signifies competence in designing, implementing, and administering privacy and security measures. A minimum of a baccalaureate degree is required to be considered for the certification.
- Health IT Certification (www.healthitcertification.com) offers a Certified Professional in Electronic Health Records (CPEHR) credential. Individuals who pass the certification examination demonstrate competency in the planning, implementation, and operation of electronic health record systems.
- A Certified Professional in Health Information Technology (CPHIT) credential offered by Health IT Certification indicates mastery in planning, selecting, implementing, using, and managing health information technology (HIT) and electronic health record (EHR) applications.
- The Certified Professional in Health Information Exchange (CPHIE) credential, also offered by Health IT Certification, is awarded to individuals who have mastered a body of knowledge about exchanges of electronic information among organizations.
- A number of certifications in medical coding are available from AHIMA and from the American Academy of Professional Coders (AAPC; www.aapc.com). A coder who completes an education program may become an apprentice coder, but full certification is reserved for individuals with additional education and on-the-job experience.
- The American Association of Professional Coders (AAPC) in conjunction with the National Alliance of Medical Auditing Specialists (NAMAS) offers a Certified Professional Medical Auditor (CPMA) credential

THINKING IT THROUGH 1.6

Read the following help wanted advertisement:

We are a large, multispecialty physician practice seeking an enthusiastic, self-motivated college graduate looking for an administrative position. We prefer a candidate who was involved in extracurricular school activities or held a leadership role in a club or an organization. The individual selected for this position will work with the physicians, medical assistants, the accounts receivable department, and scheduling staff. The position requires computer proficiency, outstanding communication skills (both verbal and written), health care experience, and a professional image. Flexibility and the ability to multitask are essential components for success in this role.

- Why is the practice interested in whether the person participated in extracurricular activities?
- Do you think participation in extracurricular activities is relevant to the position?

related to EHRs. This certification focuses on federal regulations as they pertain to physician practices (www.healthitcertification.com).

- The Certified Tumor Registrar (CTR) certification in tumor registry is available from the National Cancer Registrars Association (NCRA; www.ncra-usa.org).

A Commitment to Lifelong Learning

The field of health care is always changing. This makes it an exciting area for employment, but it also presents challenges. To keep pace with rapid change, professionals must keep their knowledge and skills current. Education does not end with the awarding of a certificate or a degree; in the health care field, it is a lifelong commitment. Most professional organizations require certified members to keep up to date by taking annual training courses to refresh or extend their knowledge. Continuing education sessions are assigned course credits by the credentialing organizations, and satisfactory completion of a test on the material is often required. Employers often approve attendance at seminars that apply to the practice's goals and ask the person who attends to update other staff members.

Technology makes it easy to access information from many different sources. A wide range of information is available on the Internet, including up-to-date professional information. Sources of information include:

- **Websites** Locations on the Internet that contain a collection of linked documents, images, and files.
- **Blogs** Websites with regular entries of commentary, descriptions of events, or other materials such as videos.
- **Newsfeeds** Listings of news headlines and excerpts that are sent automatically to subscribers.
- **Webinars and podcasts** Educational sessions delivered via the Internet. A podcast is an audio recording in digital format that can be played back on a computer or a mobile device.
- **e-Books** Digital versions of books that can be viewed using a computer, an e-book reader, or a mobile device.

- **Videos** A wide range of videos can be viewed online or downloaded and viewed, many with educational content.
- **Listservs** Electronic mailing lists for groups interested in a common topic. Emails sent to the list are automatically delivered to individuals who sign up to receive them.
- **Social networking sites** Online communities of people who share common interests and/or activities. In health care and other businesses, these networks can be used to share knowledge, exchange ideas, and find job opportunities, among other things.

chapter 1 summary

KEY TERMS

accounts receivable (A/R)
accounts payable (A/P)
cash flow
certification
continuity of care
data mining
data warehouse
diagnosis code
documentation
electronic health record (EHR)
encounter
health informatics
health information technology (HIT)
medical assistant (MA)
medical biller
medical coder
medical documentation and billing cycle
medical malpractice
medical necessity
medical record
Merit-based Incentive Payment System (MIPS)
patient examination
procedure code
Quality Payment Program (QPP)
records retention schedule
revenue cycle management (RCM)

LEARNING OUTCOME	KEY CONCEPTS/EXAMPLES
1.1 Compare practice management (PM) programs and electronic health records (EHRs).	• A practice management program performs administrative and financial functions, such as scheduling patients' appointments, billing patients and health plans, receiving and recording payments, and managing collections. • An electronic health record is a computerized lifelong health care record for an individual that incorporates data from all sources that provide treatment for the individual.
1.2 List the steps in the medical documentation and billing cycle.	• The steps in the medical documentation and billing cycle are: 1. Preregistering patients 2. Establishing financial responsibility 3. Checking in patients 4. Reviewing coding compliance 5. Reviewing billing compliance 6. Checking out patients 7. Preparing and transmitting claims 8. Monitoring payer adjudication 9. Generating patient statements 10. Following up on patient payments and collections

LEARNING OUTCOME	KEY CONCEPTS/EXAMPLES
1.3 List the eight facts that are documented in the medical record for an ambulatory patient encounter.	• The eight facts documented in medical records are: 1. Patient's name 2. Encounter date and reason 3. Appropriate history and physical examination 4. Review of all tests that were ordered 5. Diagnosis 6. Plan of care, or notes on procedures or treatments that were given 7. Instructions or recommendations that were given to the patient 8. Signature of the provider who saw the patient
1.4 Identify the additional uses of clinical information gathered in patient encounters.	• Additional uses of clinical information include legal issues, quality review, research, education, public health and homeland security, and billing and reimbursement.
1.5 Compare the roles and responsibilities of clinical and administrative personnel on the physician practice health care team.	• Clinical personnel provide treatment to patients, while administrative personnel manage the business aspects of health care. Administrative staff work behind the scenes in a medical office and do not provide medical treatment or testing. Some administrative workers, such as schedulers, do interact with patients.
1.6 Explain how professional certification and lifelong learning contribute to career advancement in medical administration.	• Individuals with certification generally have an easier time finding employment and advancing on the job than do those without certification. Certification acknowledges that an individual has mastered a standard body of knowledge and meets certain competencies. Employers look for certification when filling open positions, and certified individuals usually earn higher salaries than those who are not certified. • Most professional organizations require certified members to keep up to date by taking annual training courses to refresh or extend their knowledge. Continuing education sessions are assigned course credits by the credentialing organizations, and satisfactory completion of a test on the material is often required.

chapter 1 review

MATCHING QUESTIONS

Match the key terms with their definitions.

_____ 1. *[LO 1.2]* medical necessity

_____ 2. *[LO 1.2]* cash flow

_____ 3. *[LO 1.1]* health information technology

_____ 4. *[LO 1.2]* revenue cycle management

_____ 5. *[LO 1.6]* certification

_____ 6. *[LO 1.3]* patient examination

_____ 7. *[LO 1.4]* Quality Payment Program

_____ 8. *[LO 1.3]* encounter

_____ 9. *[LO 1.1]* health informatics

_____ 10. *[LO 1.1]* electronic health record

a. Oversight of the activities associated with a patient encounter to ensure that the provider receives full payment for services.

b. An examination of a person's body in order to determine his or her state of health.

c. Meeting of a patient with a medical professional for the purpose of providing health care.

d. Treatment that is in accordance with generally accepted medical practice.

e. Provision of financial incentives to physicians who provide evidence-based treatments to their patients.

f. Using computers and electronic communications to manage medical information.

g. Computerized lifelong health care record with data from all sources.

h. Movement of monies into and out of a business.

i. Knowledge required to optimize the acquisition, storage, retrieval, and use of information in health and biomedicine.

j. Nationally recognized designation that acknowledges that an individual has mastered a standard body of knowledge and meets certain competencies.

MULTIPLE-CHOICE QUESTIONS

Select the letter that best completes the statement or answers the question.

1. *[LO 1.1]* Specialized programs that help process patients' appointments, billing, payments, and collections are called_________.
   a. electronic health records
   b. clinical encounters
   c. practice management programs
   d. pay-for-performance programs

2. *[LO 1.2]* The federal law that protects patients' private health information, ensures coverage during job changes, and uncovers fraud and abuse is the ________.
   a. Health Insurance Portability and Accountability Act of 1996
   b. Medicare Prescription Drug, Improvement, and Modernization Act of 2003
   c. Physician Quality Reporting Initiative
   d. American Recovery and Reinvestment Act of 2009

3. *[LO 1.3]* Which of the following must be included in medical office records for patients?
   a. parent's name
   b. country of birth
   c. diagnosis
   d. educational history

4. *[LO 1.5]* Which of the following is *not* a concern when a physician practice is implementing an EHR?
   a. changes to the practice workflow
   b. the inability to share information due to a lack of clinical standards
   c. cost
   d. revenue management

5. *[LO 1.4]* Medical care that uses the latest and most accurate clinical research in making decisions about the care of patients is known as ________.
   a. medical malpractice
   b. evidence-based medicine
   c. quality care initiative(s)
   d. clinical quality reporting

6. *[LO 1.2]* The purpose of managing the revenue cycle is to generate ________.
   a. cash flow
   b. patient encounters
   c. coding
   d. medical records

7. *[LO 1.1]* Practice management programs are used to ________.
   a. create electronic prescriptions
   b. provide continuity of care
   c. manage payments from payers electronically
   d. exchange health information

8. *[LO 1.1]* Electronic health records contain information that ________.
   a. is maintained by the patient
   b. may be entered by a number of physicians and other providers
   c. is entered only by the patient's primary care physician
   d. records patient billing and payments

9. *[LO 1.6]* Administrative personnel on the health care team ________.
   a. are considered clinical staff
   b. may include physician assistants and nurses
   c. may include medical clinical assistants
   d. may include medical administration assistants and billers

10. *[LO 1.6]* Professional certification is maintained over time by requirements for ________.
   a. graduate-level education
   b. ongoing continuing education
   c. international conference attendance
   d. age-related education

SHORT-ANSWER QUESTIONS

Define the following abbreviations.

1. *[LO 1.2]* A/R ____________________
2. *[LO 1.1]* EHR ____________________
3. *[LO 1.5]* EMR ____________________
4. *[LO 1.2]* HIE ____________________
5. *[LO 1.1]* HIT ____________________
6. *[LO 1.2]* HIPAA ____________________
7. *[LO 1.4]* QQP ____________________
8. *[LO 1.5]* PHR ____________________
9. *[LO 1.1]* PM ____________________
10. *[LO 1.2]* RCM ____________________

APPLYING YOUR KNOWLEDGE

Working with Documentation

1.1 *[LO 1.3]* Match the eight data points that are included in an ambulatory care medical record.

a. Georgina Warez ________
b. Saw this 27-year-old female patient on 10-1-2022 for a complaint of urinary tract problem. ________
c. Patient complains of frequency of urination, urgency, and burning sensation for about 3–5 days. She denies hematuria. She has slight suprapubic discomfort. She has been treated for bladder infection in the past. Her last menstrual period was 4 days ago. Upon examination, I confirmed a very vague tenderness over the suprapubic area. Flanks are clear. ________
d. Her laboratory results are: WBC 11,200. Urinalysis shows yellow, cloudy urine; specific gravity 1.015; 3–5 RBCs; 80–100 WBCs; and many bacteria. ________
e. Urinary tract infection. ________
f. Septra DS 1 b.i.d. was ordered X 10 days. ________
g. Repeat urinalysis after the 10-day medication regimen. ________
h. Grace Marotta, MD ________

1. Patient's name
2. Encounter date and reason
3. Appropriate history and physical examination

4. Review of all tests that were ordered
5. Diagnosis
6. Plan of care, or notes on procedures or treatments that were given
7. Instructions or recommendations that were given to the patient
8. Signature of the provider who saw the patient

Managing the Revenue Cycle

1.2 *[LO 1.2]* List the ten steps in the medical documentation and billing cycle.

Step 1:____________________

Step 2:____________________

Step 3:____________________

Step 4:____________________

Step 5:____________________

Step 6:____________________

Step 7:____________________

Step 8:____________________

Step 9:____________________

Step 10:____________________

1.3 *[LO 1.2]* Which documentation or billing step do you think each of the following tasks is related to?

_____ a. calculating what patients owe the practice after claims are paid

_____ b. checking off procedure codes on a form following the patient's examination

_____ c. calling the representative of a health plan to learn the patient's eligibility and benefits for an immunization to prevent swine flu

_____ d. calling a patient about an overdue bill

_____ e. sending an email message to a health plan concerning a claim that seems to be missing

_____ f. electronically transmitting a claim to a health plan

_____ g. reviewing a new patient's name and contact information before the visit

_____ h. scanning a patient's driver's license

_____ i. sending an email query to a physician who has entered a prostate cancer screening code on the encounter form for a female patient

_____ j. calculating the amount to be billed a health plan whose contract stipulates that it will pay 10 percent less than the amount customarily charged to patients

Working with Integrated PM/EHR Programs

1.4 *[LO 1.6]* Which program, a PM or an EHR, do you think would handle each of the following tasks?

_____ a. The medical assistant verifies and documents a patient's medications and allergies during an examination.

_____ b. A patient's payment of coinsurance is entered.

_____ c. A physician enters needed prescriptions and orders tests following a patient's examination.

_____ d. A biller sends a claim for the encounter to the patient's health plan.

_____ e. A payment from the health plan is received via EFT and checked.

chapter 2

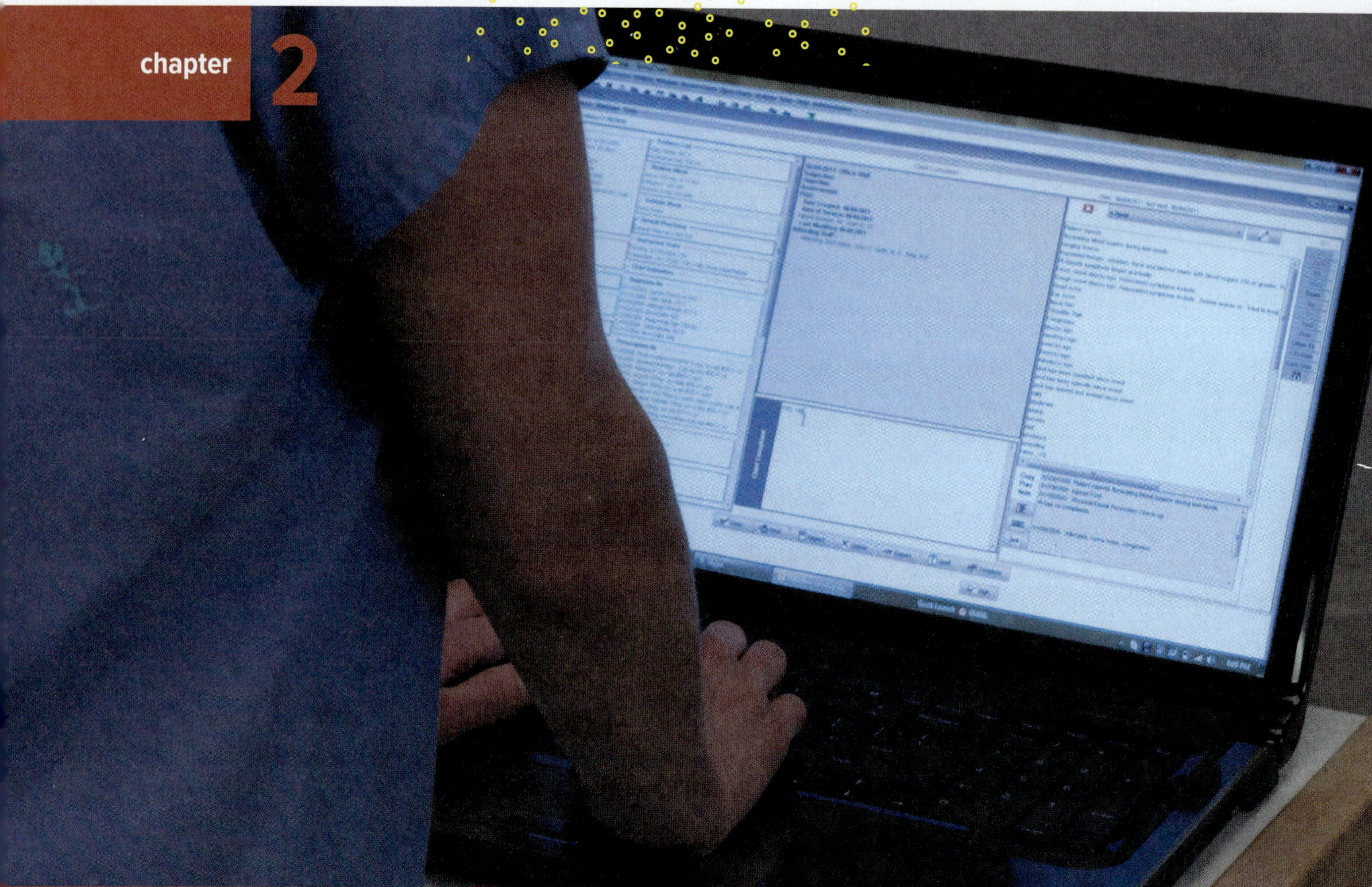

Understanding Electronic Health Records

LEARNING OUTCOMES

When you finish this chapter, you will be able to:

2.1 Explain the purpose of medical records.

2.2 Discuss the implementation and use of EHRs in health care.

2.3 Describe the functions of a practice management program.

2.4 Differentiate between the use of electronic health records in the inpatient and outpatient settings.

2.5 Explain how EHR data is captured and recorded.

2.6 Navigate an electronic health record: EHRclinic.

Should We Release This Record?

Taylor Hutchins is conducting a patient interview with Janine Bell. While reviewing medications, Mrs. Bell states that she was never prescribed a blood pressure medication and was never told that she has high blood pressure. Taylor responded by stating, "This is in your electronic health record, so the medication must have been prescribed to you. Maybe you didn't realize it at the time or maybe the pharmacy made a mistake." Upon Mrs. Bell's insistence that the medication was never prescribed to her, Taylor goes on to explain that one of the advantages of EHR use is improved accuracy in medical records and that Mrs. Bell must be mistaken.

What do you think most likely happened in this situation? As you read this chapter, consider the importance of documentation in electronic health records. Compare how EHRs are used differently from paper charts.

2.1 The Purpose and Use of Medical Records

Medical records, or charts, are created by physicians and other providers in physician practices, hospitals, surgery centers, clinics, and other health care facilities. They are created and shared to help make accurate diagnoses of patients' conditions and to trace the course of care.

A patient's medical record contains facts, findings, and observations about that patient's health history. It also contains communications with and about the patient in the health care setting. The medical record in the medical office begins with a patient's first contact and continues through all treatments and services. The record provides continuity and communication among physicians and other health care professionals who are involved in the patient's care. Patient medical records are also used in research and for education.

Patient medical records are legal documents. Physicians own the physical record (although patients own the information about themselves), and properly documented patient care is part of the physician's defense against accusations that patients were not treated correctly. Medical records should clearly state who performed what service and describe why, where, when, and how it was done. Physicians document the rationale behind their treatment decisions. This rationale is the basis for the concept of medical necessity–a clinically logical link between a patient's condition and the treatment provided.

Documentation means organizing a patient's health record in chronological order, using a systematic, logical, and consistent method. The patient's health history, examinations, tests, and results of treatments are all documented. Complete and comprehensive documentation is important to show that physicians have followed the medical standards of care that apply in their state.

Medical standards of care are state-specified performance measures for the delivery of health care by medical professionals. Health care providers are liable (legally responsible) for providing this level of care to their patients. The term *medical professional liability* describes this responsibility

THINKING IT THROUGH 2.1

Sally Darfure is sixty-four years old and has severe diabetes and high blood pressure. She requires regular blood tests to monitor the diabetes. Both her primary care physician and her endocrinologist (diabetes specialist) draw blood regularly. One provider uses electronic health records and the other does not.

- In your opinion, how could an EHR system help ensure continuity of care in this situation?
- Do you think Sally's insurance carrier will agree to pay regularly for separate blood work for both physicians?

of licensed health care professionals. Medical malpractice can result when a provider injures or harms a patient due to failure to follow the standards.

Regardless of whether providers are using paper or electronic health records, they follow generally recognized guidelines to document patient encounters. The initial examinations and assessments show the treatment plan for the patient. Progress reports document the patient's progress and response to the treatment plan. Discharge summaries are prepared during the patient's final visit for a particular treatment plan. If either the patient or the physician ends the relationship, the physician must still maintain the patient's medical record. The physician also sends the patient a letter that documents the situation and provides for continuity of care with the next provider.

The documentation of diagnoses and treatments is also used as proof of billed services. An unwritten law of medical insurance is that if it was not documented, it was not done, and if it was not done, it cannot be billed. Payers use documentation to decide whether reported services should be reimbursed.

2.2 Forces Driving EHR Evolution

Simply put, a medical record is the documentation of a single patient's medical history and care over the time spent in a health care facility or medical practice. Electronic health records (EHRs) automate the management of these medical records and clinical information about the practice's patients.

What's in a Name?

Since the idea of computer-based medical records came about, the records have been referred to by a number of different names. In the 1990s, they were known as electronic patient records (EPRs), computerized patient records (CPRs), and computerized medical records (CMRs). These terms gave way to the current usage, which includes electronic health records (EHRs), electronic medical records (EMRs), and personal health records (PHRs).

Although there is not universal agreement on definitions, the consensus is that **electronic medical records (EMRs)** are computerized records of one physician's encounters with a patient over time. They serve as the physician's legal record of patient care. While EMRs may contain information from external sources, including pharmacies and laboratories, the information in the EMR reflects treatment of a patient by a single physician.

electronic medical record (EMR) computerized record of one physician's encounters with a patient over time

Electronic health records, on the other hand, can include information from the EMRs of a number of different physicians as well as from pharmacies, laboratories, hospitals, insurance carriers, and so on. Information is added to the record by health care professionals working in a variety of settings, and the record can be accessed by professionals when needed.

Personal health records (PHRs) are private, secure electronic files that are created, maintained, and owned by the patient. The patient decides whether to share the contents with doctors or other health professionals. PHRs typically include current medications and dosages, health insurance information, immunization records, allergies, medical test results, past surgeries, family medical history, and more. Personal health records are created and stored on the Internet, but the files can easily be downloaded to a storage device such as a flash drive for portability. It is important to note that while EMRs and EHRs are considered legal medical records, PHRs are not because they are maintained by patients.

personal health record (PHR) private, secure electronic health care files that are created, maintained, and owned by the patient

Contents of EHRs in Ambulatory Care Settings

As shown in Table 2.1, the content of an EHR in the physician practice is similar to the content of the paper medical record or chart.

TABLE 2.1 Electronic Health Record Content

Patient identifying information	This demographic and insurance information is obtained when the patient first comes to the practice, and it is updated as needed.
History and physical	This section of the record contains information about the patient's past medical history, family medical problems, prior hospitalizations, current medications, and past surgeries. It also includes information from a physical examination.
Office visit notes	Office visit notes document the physician's findings during an examination, including observations of the patient's current medical problem, a diagnosis of the condition, and a plan for treatment. The notes also list physician orders. During each subsequent visit with the physician, notes about the patient's condition and response to treatment are added to the chart.
Laboratory tests and results	This portion of the patient record contains the results of all diagnostic procedures such as laboratory test results and pathology reports, including blood tests, X-rays, and biopsies.
Miscellaneous consents and releases	A number of miscellaneous forms are saved in the patient chart, such as release of information requests, Acknowledgment of Receipt of Notice of Privacy Practices, and consents for certain procedures.
Prescriptions	The patient chart contains a record of all medications prescribed by the physician as well as patient requests for refills.
External correspondence about patients	Correspondence to and from the patient or a third party, such as a consulting physician, is part of a patient record. Physicians receive requests to sign forms for patients, such as applications for disability benefits and proof of immunizations.

Functions and Uses

While paper and electronic health records serve many of the same purposes, the electronic record is much more than a computerized version of a paper record. The Institute of Medicine has suggested that an EHR should include eight core functions:

1. **Health information and data elements** This includes demographic information about the patient, such as address and phone number, as well as clinical information about the patient's past and present health concerns. An electronic health record must include information that enables health care providers to provide effective care to patients, such as signs and symptoms, a problem list, procedures, diagnoses, a medication list, allergies, diagnostic test and radiology results, and health maintenance.
2. **Results management** Providers must have access to current and past laboratory, radiology, and other test results performed by anyone involved in the treatment of the patient. These computerized results can be accessed by multiple providers when and where they are needed, which allows diagnosis and treatment decisions to be made more quickly.
3. **Order management** EHR programs must be able to send, receive, and store orders for medications, tests, and other services by any provider involved in treating the patient. Orders are then transmitted directly to the appropriate department for completion of the test or fulfillment of a prescription, which eliminates unnecessary delays and duplicate testing. The process of entering orders electronically is known as **computerized provider order entry,** or CPOE. CPOE has had an enormous impact on medication safety. Most medication errors occur during the process of prescribing and/or administering medication. Through computerized physician order entry of prescriptions, known as electronic, or **E-Prescribing (ERX),** many medication errors can be eliminated. Many systems automatically alert the physician to potential errors in dosages, drug interactions, drug diagnosis interactions, and drug-allergy problems.
4. **Decision support** As the practice of medicine becomes more complex, the amount of information available to physicians continues to grow. Hundreds of new studies are published on a daily basis. It is not possible for a physician to remember all this information or to be aware of all the latest, most effective treatments. The latest medical evidence is incorporated into care only 50 percent of the time.

   Electronic health records allow computer-based access to the latest clinical research, used for **clinical decision support (CDS),** while the physician is still in the examination room with the patient. The physician can also view the latest information on medications, including suggested doses, common side effects, and possible interactions.

   In addition, electronic record systems provide a variety of alerts and reminders that physicians can use to improve a patient's health. A physician can, for example, see a list of all women patients over forty years of age who have not had mammograms in the past year and can send them letters reminding them that they are due for this preventive screening.

computerized provider order entry (CPOE) a provider's use of computer software to enter medical orders (medication, lab, or radiology orders) directly from a computer or mobile device

E-Prescribing (ERX) a provider's ability to electronically send accurate and understandable prescriptions directly to a pharmacy from the point-of-care, such as the provider's practice during an office visit

clinical decision support (CDS) provides timely information to help inform decisions about a patient's care, including preventive care reminders, alerts about drug interactions, and so on

5. **Electronic communication and connectivity** Today a patient is typically treated by more than one provider in more than one facility. Physicians, nurses, medical assistants, referring doctors, testing facilities, and hospitals all need to communicate with one another to provide the safest and most effective care to patients. Health plans also need information from the health record to process claims for reimbursement. Electronic health record systems offer a number of mechanisms to facilitate these communications, including email and the Internet. **Interoperability** refers to the ability of two or more EHR systems or their components to communicate via information exchange. In interoperable systems, data is shared and used between these systems. Some examples of interoperability in EHR systems include communication with practice management systems for scheduling and patient demographic collection, electronic lab ordering, and E-Prescribing.

interoperability allows computer applications or software to share and exchange information

6. **Patient support** Electronic health records should offer patients access to appropriate educational materials on health topics and instructions for preparing for common medical tests. Patients on home health care should be able to use the EHRs to report to their physicians. Some EHR programs also offer tools that allow patients to access their medical records and to request appointments electronically through **patient portals.**

patient portal secure website that enables communication between patients and health care providers for tasks such as scheduling, completing registration forms, and making payments

7. **Administrative processes** The administrative area of health care also benefits from the use of EHRs. While most physician practices already use computers for billing and scheduling, an EHR streamlines the processes. Procedure and diagnosis codes entered by the physician in the EHR are transmitted electronically to the practice management program, where a coding specialist reviews them.
8. **Reporting and population management** Electronic health record programs also enhance reporting capabilities both for internal practice use and for external reporting requirements. This makes it easier for physician offices and health care organizations to comply with federal, state, and private reporting requirements.

Advantages of Electronic Health Records

EHR programs offer a number of advantages when compared to paper record-keeping systems. The most frequently cited advantages, supported by the core functions of an EHR, are increased patient safety, improved quality of care, and greater efficiency.

Safety

There is growing evidence that electronic record keeping can reduce medical errors and improve patient safety. Some of the factors that contribute to greater safety include the following:

- Medication and physician order errors due to illegible handwriting are eliminated.
- Providers receive instant electronic alerts about patient allergies and possible drug interactions.
- Physicians receive alerts when medications deemed unsafe have been pulled from the market.

- Medical records are not lost in the event of a natural disaster, such as a hurricane, or an intentional attack such as a terrorist bombing, provided that an electronic backup copy of the records is stored at a secure off-site location.
- Information is communicated in a timely manner in the event of an act of bioterrorism or the widespread outbreak of disease.

Quality

Quality health care is described as care that focuses on being safe, effective, patient-centered, timely, efficient, and equitable. Effective care is defined as "providing services based on scientific knowledge to those who could benefit and at the same time refraining from providing services to those not likely to benefit." With EHRs, physicians have access to evidence-based guidelines for diagnosing and treating conditions and to the latest clinical research and best practice guidelines.

Electronic health records also enhance the quality of health care in the following ways:

- Patients are contacted with reminders for preventive care screenings.
- Patients suffering from chronic diseases, such as diabetes, can monitor their conditions at home and report results via the Internet, saving them numerous visits to the doctor.
- Health care consumers can review data about the quality and performance of providers and facilities and can choose facilities and providers accordingly.
- Efficiency is managed by avoiding duplication of tests and services.
- Health providers can access electronic health records in real time, which promotes timely care and treatment.
- Patients are encouraged to participate in their own health care outcomes by accessing patient portals and communicating with health providers electronically.

Efficiency

The retrieval of information from an EHR is immediate, which greatly improves efficiency and can be critical in emergency situations. Compared to sorting through papers in a folder, an electronic search saves critical time when vital patient information is needed. Electronic health records also save valuable time by reducing the time it takes health care providers to enter information about patients. Providers who used paper medical records in the past would spend almost 40 percent of their time documenting their encounters with patients. With EHRs, physicians are finished entering notes when the patient leaves the examination room or shortly after. Nurses and medical assistants also record information directly into the computer, so there is no need to copy information to a paper chart.

Implementation Issues

Despite offering a number of significant advantages, the migration from paper to electronic records experienced a number of barriers, including cost, lack of standards, training and workflow issues, and privacy and security concerns.

- **Cost** An electronic health record system is estimated to cost approximately $33,000 per physician to install and roughly $8,400 per physician per year to maintain. These estimates include one-time costs associated with switching from paper to electronic records, such as scanning existing paper records into the new system and purchasing updated computers.
- **Lack of standards** A lack of **standards** for sharing digital information has been a major obstacle to EHR adoption. Without common standards, EHRs cannot share clinical information in a meaningful way, whether from one physician office to another or from a physician office to an inpatient facility such as a hospital. New standards have been created and are reviewed and maintained continually to ensure that EHRs are used meaningfully and appropriately.

standards statements of expected quality in the performance of a health care activity

- **Training and workflow issues** It often takes a significant amount of time for staff members to become proficient with new technology. Technology also alters the workflow in a physician office, which can require staff members to make adjustments. For example, in a practice using an EHR, there is no need to pull charts of patients with upcoming appointments. Papers such as referral letters, lab reports, and copies of prescriptions are not filed in folders, and charts do not have to be filed at the end of the day. While these improve efficiency, the job responsibilities and tasks of staff members must be analyzed and altered as necessary. This is a time-consuming process, and many people were resistant to change in the adoption and implementation of electronic health records.
- **Privacy and security risks** One of the greatest challenges to EHR implementation is protecting private information about a patient's past and present health. By its nature, information contained in an electronic health record is stored on a computer and exchanged with other providers and facilities. There is always a risk that hackers may break into computers or that security may be unintentionally breached. The frequent transfer of patient health information from one computer to another over a network, along with the number of people who have access to the record, increases the likelihood of the information's being obtained by an unauthorized party. A number of laws, including HIPAA, address the issue of patient privacy and the security of electronic patient information, as discussed in greater detail in Chapter 3.

2.3 Functions of a Practice Management Program

Practice management (PM) programs are the health information technology (HIT) applications that facilitate the day-to-day financial operations of a medical practice. PMs automate the medical billing cycle so staff members can record patient demographics, schedule appointments, maintain lists of payers, perform billing tasks, and generate reports.

practice management (PM) program program used to perform administrative and financial functions in a medical office

Initial Setup

Not all medical offices use the same PM, but most programs operate in a similar manner. Initially, the program is prepared for use by entering basic facts about the practice. Often a computer consultant or an accountant helps set up these records. Information about many aspects of the business is entered, including:

- **Patient data** Information about each patient, such as name, address, contact numbers, insurance coverage, and more
- **Provider data** Information about each provider, including facts about providers, referring providers, and outside providers such as labs
- **Health plan data** Details about the health plans used by the practice's patients
- **Transaction data** The dates of visits, the location of treatment, diagnosis and procedure codes, and payments made at the time of office visits

In addition, the program's security feature is set up to accommodate the requirements of the staff.

Daily Activities

Once the initial setup and data entry are complete, the PM is used to complete many of the daily tasks of a medical practice, including:

- Verifying insurance eligibility and benefits
- Organizing patient and payer information
- Generating and transmitting insurance claims
- Monitoring the status of claims
- Recording payments from payers
- Generating patients' statements, posting payments, and updating accounts
- Managing collections activities
- Creating financial and productivity reports

Focus on Health Care Claim Processing

One of the most important uses of a PM is to process health care claims, from creation to transmission, payer payment decisions, and payment posting.

Creating Electronic Claims

The PM collects required digital information from its various databases to create a claim file. This file can be printed, but in most cases it is sent electronically, using an Internet connection. This replaces the previous task of filling out paper claim forms and sending them in the mail.

Electronic Monitoring of Claim Status

The PM is used to follow up on the status of claims being adjudicated by health plans. If payer response is slow, the PM can be used to transmit electronic queries to locate the claim in the health plan's processing system and ensure prompt payment.

THINKING IT THROUGH 2.2

Autoposting—in which payments from health plans are automatically posted to patient accounts in a practice management program—takes less time than posting payments manually. However, some practices prefer to have a person post payments. Why do you think this is the case?

Receiving Electronic Payment Notification

Payer adjudication refers to making a decision about claim payment, such as whether the claim is paid, paid at a reduced rate, or denied. When the payer has adjudicated the claims, the PM receives a remittance advice (RA), which lists the amount that has been paid on each claim as well as codes that represent the reasons for nonpayment or partial payment. PMs are designed to receive RAs as electronic documents sent over the Internet. Such a document is sometimes called an electronic remittance advice (ERA).

Once the payment information has been reviewed and determined to be as expected, the data on the RA are entered in the PM and applied to each patient's account. While this process may be done manually by matching payments with individual patient transactions and then entering the payments in the program, many practices with PMs use a process called *autoposting.* In autoposting, the payment data are automatically posted to the correct patient accounts in the PM, and the medical biller performs an audit function, verifying that the payments are correct, rather than manually entering the information. Every date and procedure has to be carefully checked to uncover any errors or underpayments and to follow up with the health plan.

Handling Electronic Payments

Also contributing to improved cash flow is the PM's ability to handle electronic payments that are sent directly to the practice's bank accounts. This transaction is called an EFT, for electronic funds transfer, and it puts revenue in the bank much faster than does manually receiving and depositing paper checks.

2.4 Use of EHRs in the Inpatient Setting

Electronic health record use has become the standard for maintaining both inpatient and outpatient medical records. Although both types of EHRs serve the same function–to document a patient's health care–the types of data recorded vary. For example, inpatient EHRs focus on orders and medication management, whereas outpatient (ambulatory) EHRs require patient-centric capabilities, such as e-prescribing, clinical summaries, and patient portals, as discussed earlier in this chapter.

Elements of Inpatient and Outpatient EHRs

Hospital electronic health record programs are tailored to provide information relevant to a patient's hospital stay and treatment, whereas outpatient EHRs are designed for a long-term approach to patient care. As such, there are similarities and differences in the type of records and features used in inpatient and outpatient EHRs, as compared in Table 2.2.

TABLE 2.2 Comparison of Features in Inpatient and Outpatient EHRs

Inpatient	Outpatient
Manage health records and streamline day-to-day workflows	Help processes for outpatient care facilities and smaller practices
Offer interoperable architecture for seamless integration and exchange of patient information across departments	Allow providers to track a patient's medical records and long-term care without interacting within a hospital's complex web of departments
Integration of internal support departments such as labs, pharmacies, and radiology	Often communicate with external sources such as local pharmacies, labs, and radiology facilities
EHR certification focuses on orders and medication management—for example, medication orders are sent to an in-hospital pharmacy for dispensing	EHR certification centers around patient-centric functionality—for example, prescriptions are sent to a patient's pharmacy via e-prescribing functionality
Records include admissions notes, operative reports, and progress notes	Records include ambulatory encounters such as office visits, telephone calls, and written correspondence

Despite the differences between inpatient and outpatient EHRs, there are a number of similarities. Both must have high standards for electronic systems and security. They also provide interaction checks for drugs and allergies, privacy and security standards, and medication and allergy records. Additionally, certification for both inpatient and outpatient EHRs require the availability of clinical decision support (CDS) and the use of computerized provider order entry (CPOE).

Inpatient Electronic Health Records

The term *inpatient* refers to a patient who needs to be admitted to a hospital or other type of facility to receive treatment for at least one night. Inpatient EHR systems are designed to manage inpatient data and are commonly used by hospitals, made up of groups of various departments and systems.

The Master Patient Index (MPI)

Master Patient Index (MPI) a database that links patient records from multiple financial and administrative source systems

Hospitals manage their data through the use of a **Master Patient Index (MPI),** sometimes referred to as a patient registry. The purpose of the MPI is to store demographic information for every patient who receives care from a hospital facility. Through the MPI, records can be accurately matched and linked by using patients' unique identifiers. This practice prevents a hospital organization from creating multiple accounts for one patient.
Benefits of using a Master Patient Index (MPI) include:

- Maintaining a central registry of patients, including their demographics, for accurate identification and timely retrieval of health records
- Updating information in real time, ensuring that the most current health information is available
- Eliminating duplicate patient registration, promoting efficiency and accuracy
- Improving patient safety by reducing the risk of errors
- Supporting the delivery of cost-effective and timely services

Use of EHR Data by Hospitals

While each hospital EHR system varies somewhat in how data is collected and used, they typically perform similar functions, such as:

- Supporting quality improvement
- Monitoring patient safety
- Measuring organizational performance
- Identifying high-risk patients
- Measuring unit performance
- Informing strategic planning
- Assessing adherence to guidelines
- Creating individual provider profiles

2.5 Recording Data in the EHR

Using the EHR

Documents in electronic health records may be created in a variety of ways, but they are ultimately viewed on a computer screen. For example, one general practice uses a number of medical-history-taking templates for gathering and recording "consistent history and physical information from patients." The computer-based templates range in focus from abdominal pain to depression, with from ten to twenty questions each. The on-screen templates are filled out in the exam rooms. Responsible providers then sign the entries, using e-signature technology that verifies the identity of the signer.

Advantages of Documenting in the EHR

EHRs offer both patients and providers significant advantages:

- *Immediate access to health information:* The EHR is simultaneously accessible from computers in the office and at other sites such as hospitals. An EHR database can save time when vital patient information is needed. Once information is updated in a patient record, it is available to all who need access, whether across the hall or across town.
- *Computerized physician order entry (CPOE) management:* Physicians can enter orders for prescriptions, tests, and other services at any time. This information is then transmitted to the staff for implementation or directly to pharmacies linked to the practice.
- *Clinical decision support (CDS):* An EHR system can provide access to the latest medical research on approved medical websites to help in medical decision making.
- *Automated alerts and reminders:* The system can provide medical alerts and reminders for office staff to ensure that patients are scheduled for regular screenings and other preventive practices. Alerts can also be created to identify patient safety issues, such as possible drug interactions.
- *Electronic communication and connectivity:* An EHR system can provide a means of secure and easily accessible communication between physicians and staff and in some offices between physicians and patients.

- *Patient support:* Most EHR programs allow patients to access their medical records and request appointments through patient portals. These programs also offer patient education on health topics and instructions on preparing for common medical tests, such as an HDL cholesterol test.
- *Administration and reporting:* The EHR may include administrative tools, including reporting systems that enable medical practices to comply with federal and state reporting requirements.
- *Error reduction:* An EHR can decrease medical errors that result from illegible chart notes because notes are entered electronically on a computer or a handheld device. Nevertheless, the accuracy of the information in the EHR is only as good as the accuracy of the person entering the data; it is still possible to click the wrong button or enter the wrong letter.

2.6 Getting Started with EHRs: Introduction to EHRclinic

An Internet search for practice management and electronic health record software programs would show you hundreds of results. There are a number of PM and EHR programs available, and some that even combine the two types of software. Medical practices and health care organizations function differently, so it is important that they find the PM and EHR systems that meet their unique needs. For example, some practices may need more comprehensive billing programs, while other practices need the capacity to accommodate a large number of patients. A practice should carefully research its needs, budget, and future goals when comparing PM and EHR systems for potential adoption.

Selecting PM and EHR Software

When choosing PM and EHR software systems, a practice should consider the following:

- **Software design** Is the software intuitive and easy to navigate? Consider the software's interface, including the colors, shapes, placement, and form of information.
- **Cost** How much does the system cost to implement and run? Consider software, hardware, support, training, upgrading, and maintenance.
- **Ease of use** How easy will it be for staff to learn and use the new software? Consider implementation, minimal training to start, and support provided by the vendor.
- **Individual needs** Does this software fit with the practice's needs and workflows? Consider daily operations, standard operating procedures, patient flow, customization, and staffing availability.
- **Long-term goals** What are the long-term goals of the practice? Consider growth potential, future projections, and anticipated changes in the operational framework.

EHRclinic

Although many PM and EHR software systems are available for use in health care facilities, we will be using *EHRclinic* for the purpose of this worktext.

About EHRclinic

EHRclinic is a PMEHR solution for students to learn hands-on practice management and electronic health record skills in a simulated environment. You will find reference to EHRclinic exercises integrated within most chapters, and your instructor may assign some or all of them to you in Connect.

Each exercise also has a corresponding step document that can be downloaded at www.mhhe.com/pmehr2. These are step-by-step directions, including a scenario and tips, that can be used to assist you with exercise completion.

EHRclinic Exercise Modes

There are three modes available for each EHRclinic exercise:

1. **Demo Mode** In Demo Mode, you will watch a recording of each exercise as it is completed. As shown in Figure 2.1, audio can be toggled on or off and the path (corresponding steps) can be shown or hidden. Click the *Help* icon in the upper right corner for more information about Demo Mode.
2. **Practice Mode** In Practice Mode, you will complete each exercise with guidance. As shown in Figure 2.1, audio can be toggled on or off, and the path (corresponding steps) can be shown or hidden. Click the *Help* icon in the upper right corner for more information about Practice Mode.
3. **Assessment Mode** In Assessment Mode, you will demonstrate mastery of the exercise by completing it on your own and inputting the data provided. In this mode, you may use the exercise steps as a guide, but you can make and correct mistakes before submitting the exercise. Assessment Mode grades the exercise based on the required data and not on the steps taken. As shown in Figure 2.2, the exercise data can be shown or hidden, but the exercise steps are not available within the exercise. Click the *Help* icon in the upper right corner for more information about Assessment Mode.

Overview of EHRclinic

EHRclinic functions with two main components: the practice menu and the practice dashboard with administrative tools.

Practice Menu The practice menu, shown in Figure 2.3, runs along the left side of the screen and contains the following menu items:

- **Schedules**
  - Make, cancel, and reschedule appointments
  - Check patients in
  - Manage the recall list (reminders to follow up with patients, also known as *tickler files*)

Figure 2.1 EHRclinic Demo and Practice Mode Menu

Figure 2.2 EHRclinic Assessment Mode Menu

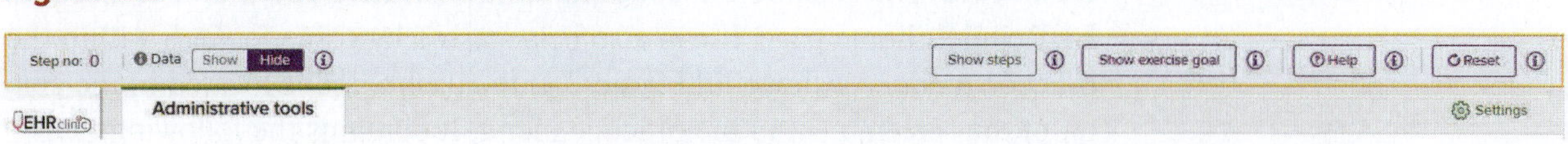

Figure 2.3 EHRclinic Practice Menu

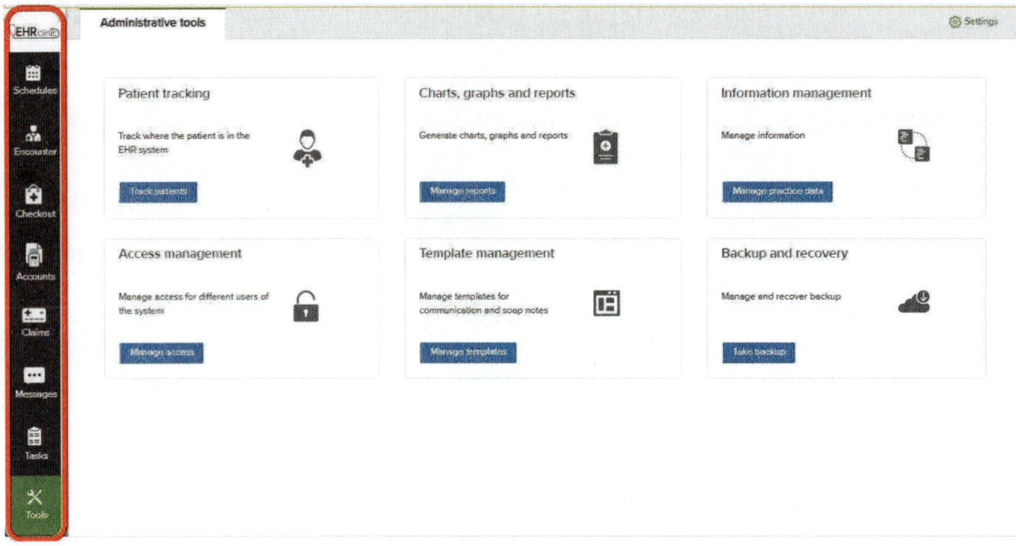

- **Encounter**
  - Record patients' vital signs
  - Document patient intake
  - Initiate and complete patient encounters (office visits)
  - Follow up providers' orders
- **Checkout**
  - Charge capture
  - Review patient insurance information
  - Perform code linkage to prepare for billing
- **Accounts**
  - Review patient accounts and ledgers
  - Add payments and adjustments
  - Create patient statements
- **Claims**
  - Generate patient claims
  - Review electronic remittance advices
- **Messages**
  - Manage incoming patient and nonpatient messages
  - Facilitate internal messages
  - Record messages in patients' charts
  - Manage email messages
- **Tasks**
  - Manage practice task lists
  - Create new tasks for providers and staff
- **Tools**
  - Manage administrative tools
  - Access the practice dashboard

Dashboard The dashboard contains administrative tools and is used as EHRclinic's home page. It can also be accessed by going to *Tools* within the practice menu. As shown in Figure 2.4, the dashboard is located in the center of the screen, next to the practice menu. It contains the following tools:

Figure 2.4 EHRclinic Dashboard (Administrative Tools)

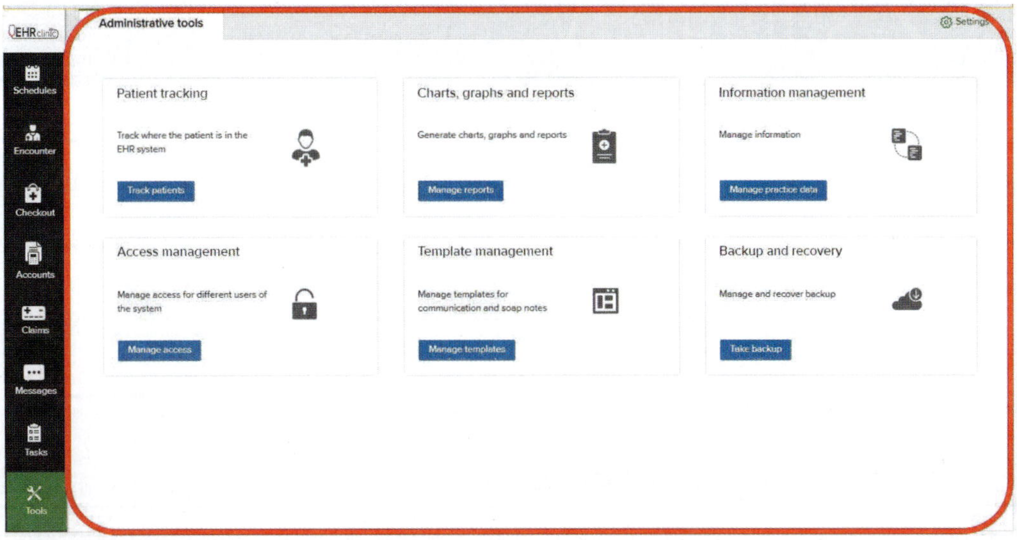

- **Track patients**
  - Shows the patient tracker
  - Indicates a patient's progress throughout an encounter
- **Manage reports**
  - Access patient charts
  - Review patient graphs (labs, vital signs, growth charts)
  - Run financial, analysis, statement, and aging reports
- **Manage practice data**
  - Access patient lists and information
  - Edit patient demographics
  - Add and edit patient insurance information
  - Manage provider and staff information
  - Maintain practice databases (ICD, CPT, insurance carriers, drugs, patient education, practice information)
- **Manage access**
  - Assign access levels to providers and staff
  - Manage practice and software error logs
- **Manage templates**
  - Create new templates for messages, letters, and SOAP notes
  - Manage existing templates
- **Backup**
  - Back up practice data
  - Restore backup files

EXERCISE 2.1

Navigate an EHR

As a new employee at Trilogy Family Care Center, you have been asked to explore EHRclinic and review a patient's chart. You will also set up your personal preferences.

Your instructor may assign this exercise to you in Connect. Exercise steps and EHRclinic Help Guides can be downloaded at www.mhhe.com/pmehr2.

chapter 2 summary

KEY TERMS

clinical decision support (CDS)
computerized provider order entry (CPOE)
E-Prescribing (ERX)
electronic medical record (EMR)
interoperability
Master Patient Index (MPI)
patient portal
personal health record (PHR)
practice management (PM)
program
standards

LEARNING OUTCOME	KEY CONCEPTS/EXAMPLES
2.1 Explain the purpose of medical records.	Legal uses of patients' medical records, which contain the complete, chronological, and comprehensive documentation of their health history and status, include the following: - Documenting the rationale behind treatment decisions - Providing continuity and communication among physicians and other health care professionals involved in the patient's care - Verifying billing - Preparing and supporting health care claims - Conducting research - Furthering education
2.2 Discuss the implementation and use of EHRs in health care.	Computer-based medical record naming over time, including the differentiation between electronic health records and electronic medical records. Contents of EHRs to include the following: - Patient identifying information - History and physical - Office visit notes - Laboratory tests - Miscellaneous consents and releases - Prescriptions - External correspondence Functions and uses of EHRs include: - Health information and data elements - Results management - Order management, including E-Prescribing - Decision support, including clinical decision support (CDS) - Electronic communication and connectivity, including interoperability - Patient support

	- Administrative processes - Reporting and population management Safety, quality, and efficiency are advantages to EHRs. Conversely, cost, lack of standards, workflow issues, and privacy and security risks are considered potential implementation issues.
2.3 Describe the functions of a practice management program.	Practice management (PM) programs are health information technology programs that facilitate the day-to-day financial operations of a medical practice. Included in PM functions are management of daily activities and health care insurance claim processing.
2.4 Differentiate between the use of electronic health records in the inpatient and outpatient settings.	Electronic health record use varies between inpatient and outpatient health care facilities, although there are similarities, including drug/allergy interaction checks, privacy and security standards, availability of clinical decision support (CDS), and the use of computerized provider order entry (CPOE). The Master Patient Index (MPI) is sometimes referred to as a patient registry, and it is used to store demographic information for every patient receiving care from a hospital facility. The goals of maintaining the MPI database include ensuring efficient processes and preventing the duplication of patient records.
2.5 Explain how EHR data is captured and recorded.	EHRs are created in a variety of ways but ultimately viewed on a computer screen. Documentation within an EHR includes the following advantages: - Immediate access to health information - Computerized physician order entry (CPOE) - Automated alerts and reminders - Electronic communication and connectivity - Patient support - Administration and reporting - Error reduction
2.6 Navigate an electronic health record: EHRclinic.	Selection of PM and EHR software for practices and health care facilities should be done with the following considerations: - Software design - Cost - Ease of use - Individual practice needs - Long-term goals Overview of EHRclinic, including exercise modes, the practice menu, and the EHRclinic dashboard.

chapter 2 review

MATCHING QUESTIONS

Match the key terms with their definitions.

_____ 1. *[LO 2.2]* computerized provider order entry

_____ 2. *[LO 2.2]* clinical decision support

_____ 3. *[LO 2.2]* patient portal

_____ 4. *[LO 2.2]* personal health record

_____ 5. *[LO 2.4]* Master Patient Index

_____ 6. *[LO 2.2]* standards

_____ 7. *[LO 2.3]* practice management program

_____ 8. *[LO 2.2]* electronic medical record

_____ 9. *[LO 2.2]* interoperability

_____ 10. *[LO 2.2]* E-Prescribing

a. Private, secure electronic health files that are owned and maintained by the patient.

b. A provider's use of computer software to enter medical orders directly from a computer or mobile device.

c. A database that links patient records from multiple financial and administrative source systems.

d. Statements of expected quality in the performance of a health care activity.

e. Provides timely information to providers, such as preventive care reminders and alerts about drug interactions.

f. Allows computer applications or software to share and exchange information.

g. Secure website that enables communication between patients and their providers.

h. Program used to perform administrative and financial functions in a medical office.

i. Provider's ability to electronically send an accurate and understandable prescription directly to a pharmacy from the point of care.

j. Computerized record of one physician's encounters with a patient over time.

MULTIPLE-CHOICE QUESTIONS

Select the letter that best completes the statement or answers the question.

1. *[LO 2.1]* State-specified performance measures for the delivery of health care by medical professionals are known as medical _________.
   a. ethics
   b. etiquette standards
   c. morals
   d. standards of care

2. *[LO 2.1]* Organizing a patient's health record in chronological order is known as _________.
   a. coding
   b. documentation
   c. interoperability
   d. record retention

3. *[LO 2.2]* A provider uses computer records for ongoing documentation of his encounters with patients, although his software system does not incorporate data from all sources that provide treatment for his patients. What type of medical record system does this provider use?
   a. Computerized patient record
   b. Electronic health record
   c. Electronic medical record
   d. Personal health record

4. *[LO 2.2]* Who is responsible for the creation, maintenance, and ownership of a PHR?
   a. Health care facility
   b. Insurance carrier
   c. Patient
   d. Provider

5. *[LO 2.2]* Which of the following is an example of a provider's use of CDS?
   a. Chart alerts to identify patients who are due for vaccines
   b. Electronic prescription submission
   c. Inputting an order for a radiology test
   d. Documenting an electronic telephone encounter

6. *[LO 2.3]* What processes are automated by practice management programs?
   a. Clinical
   b. Inpatient
   c. Medical billing cycle
   d. Staff management

7. *[LO 2.3]* An insurance carrier determines that a claim should be denied due to an error during the ________ process.
   a. accounts receivable
   b. adjudication
   c. audit
   d. autoposting

8. *[LO 2.4]* Which of the following is an EHR feature for inpatient processes?
   a. Communicates with external sources such as local pharmacies and labs
   b. EHR certification centers around patient-centric functionality
   c. Records include ambulatory encounters
   d. Records include operative reports and progress notes

9. *[LO 2.4]* A major benefit of using a Master Patient Index is to ________.
   a. avoid duplication of patient records
   b. facilitate storage of electronic records
   c. record procedures
   d. record transactions

10. *[LO 2.5]* An EHR system can provide access to the latest medical research on approved medical websites to help with medical ________.
   a. alerts
   b. billing procedures
   c. data collection
   d. decision making

SHORT-ANSWER QUESTIONS

Define the following abbreviations.

1. *[LO 2.2]* EHR ______________________
2. *[LO 2.2]* EMR ______________________
3. *[LO 2.3]* PM ______________________
4. *[LO 2.2]* CMR ______________________
5. *[LO 2.2]* PHR ______________________
6. *[LO 2.2]* CPR ______________________
7. *[LO 2.4]* MPI ______________________
8. *[LO 2.2]* CDS ______________________
9. *[LO 2.2]* ERX ______________________
10. *[LO 2.4]* CPOE ______________________

APPLYING YOUR KNOWLEDGE

Understanding PM and EHR Programs

2.1 *[LO 2.4]* How does the focus of EHR certification between inpatient and outpatient medical facilities differ?

2.2 *[LO 2.3]* Explain how practice management systems help with each of the following functions of health care claim processing.

a. Creating electronic claims
b. Electronic monitoring of claim status
c. Receiving electronic payment notification

2.3 *[LO 2.1]* What is the purpose of documentation in medical records?

____

____

2.4 *[LO 2.4]* Which element of an EHR–patient identifying information, history and physical, office visit notes, laboratory tests/results, prescriptions, or external correspondence–is represented by each of the following examples?

a. A patient provided the practice with an insurance card and driver's license. __________
b. An electronic telephone encounter was documented after the patient called with a question about lab work. __________
c. A patient's chest X-ray report was sent from the radiology department. __________
d. A provider documents a patient's follow-up for hypertension. __________
e. A medical assistant records the patient's description of his mother's diagnosis of diabetes. __________
f. A provider communicates with a pharmacy to refill a patient's asthma medications. __________

chapter 3

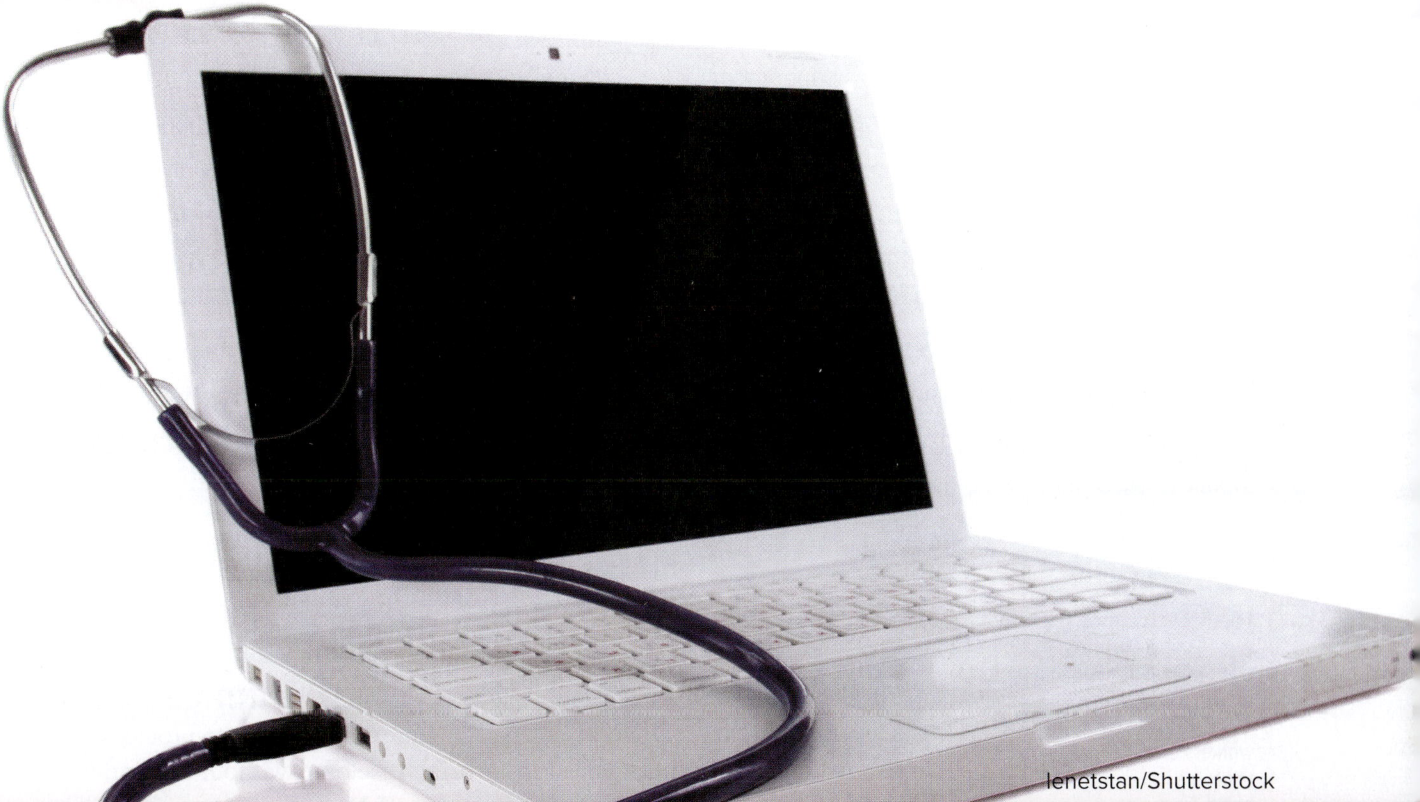

lenetstan/Shutterstock

Privacy and Security of Health Records

LEARNING OUTCOMES

When you finish this chapter, you will be able to:

3.1 Explain HIPAA and its regulations

3.2 Discuss HIPAA transactions and code sets

3.3 Describe HIPAA unique identifiers

3.4 Describe the HIPAA Privacy Rule

3.5 Describe the HIPAA Security Rule

3.6 Discuss all policies and procedures related to privacy and security of health records

3.7 Describe compliance plans

3.8 Explain breach notification requirements

Reason to Worry?

Today the staff is meeting with Tiffany Patel, the consultant who is helping the Trilogy Family Care Center make a smooth transition from paper records to electronic records. A major portion of the meeting is devoted to understanding the impact of the change on office workflow—the order in which tasks are completed. Ms. Patel explains that workflow in an electronic office differs from workflow in a paper-based office. She provides several examples. "When you have an integrated PM and EHR, you no longer need paper encounter forms, or superbills," she explains. "Also, there is no need to enter office visit charges manually, since the charges flow electronically from the EHR to the PM." As Ms. Patel continues to describe some of the upcoming changes, Joseph Sanchez, the practice's coder, and Chris Yakamoto, the billing specialist, begin sending text messages back and forth. "With all the changes, u think we'll still have jobs in 6 months?" Chris wrote. Joseph replied, "Not sure. Have 2 wait & see I guess."

What do you think made Chris and Joseph nervous about their job security? As you read this chapter, think about how the jobs of coders and billing specialists will be different in an office with an integrated PM/EHR.

Health Insurance Portability and Accountability Act of 1996 (HIPAA) legislation that protects patient's private health information, ensures health care coverage when workers change or lose jobs, and uncovers fraud and abuse in the health care system

US Department of Health and Human Services (HHS) government agency that mandates laws to enhance the health and well-being of all Americans, by providing for effective health and human services and by fostering sound, sustained advances in the sciences underlying medicine, public health, and social services; the agency that has mandated the HIPAA Privacy Rule to implement the requirements of HIPAA

HIPAA Privacy Rule law that regulates the use and disclosure of patients' protected health information

Health Information Technology for Economic and Clinical Health (HITECH) Act provisions in the American Recovery and Reinvestment Act (ARRA) of 2009 that extend and reinforce HIPAA and contain new breach notification requirements for covered entities and business associates, guidance on ways to encrypt or destroy PHI to prevent a breach, requirements for informing individuals when a breach occurs, higher monetary penalties for HIPAA violations, and stronger enforcement of the Privacy and Security Rules

3.1 Understanding HIPAA

The Health Insurance Portability and Accountability Act (HIPAA) of 1996 is a federal law that required the creation of national standards to protect sensitive patient health information from being disclosed without the patient's consent or knowledge. The **US Department of Health and Human Services (HHS)** issued the **HIPAA Privacy Rule** to implement the requirements of HIPAA. A major provision of HIPAA is the Administrative Simplification.

There are three parts of HIPAA's Administrative Simplification provisions:

1. HIPAA Electronic Transaction and Code Set Standards Requirements
2. HIPAA Privacy Requirements
3. HIPAA Security Requirements

Implementing HIPAA has changed administrative, financial, and case management policies and procedures. There are now strict requirements for the transfer of electronic health care data, such as for billing and payment; new patient rights regarding personal health information, including the right to access this information and to limit its disclosure; and broad new security rules that health care organizations must put in place to safeguard the confidentiality of patients' medical information.

The American Recovery and Reinvestment Act (ARRA) of 2009, enacted February 17, 2009, and known as Public Law 111-5, extends and reinforces HIPAA. The major provision relating to privacy and security standards is Title XIII–the **Health Information Technology for Economic and Clinical Health (HITECH) Act.** As the health care industry in the United States moves toward widespread use of EHRs and the electronic transmission of health information, the HITECH Act increases protection for patients' privacy by implementing new breach notification requirements, higher monetary penalties for HIPAA violations, and greater enforcement of the Privacy and Security Rules.

3.2 HIPAA Transaction and Code Sets

The **HIPAA Transaction and Code Set Standards** require standardization in health care e-commerce. The standards require the provider to submit information electronically, always in the same format. Every payer must accept the standardized format and standard codes. This submission is known as a transaction. A **transaction** is an electronic exchange of information between two parties to carry out financial or administrative activities related to health care.

HIPAA standards for electronic transactions are described as X12 transactions. HIPAA has approved standards for transmitting any medical data electronically. The following are the standards that covered entities must adhere to when conducting business and patient treatment:

- Claims or encounters: X12 837P, version 5010 for physicians, and X12 847I, version 5010A2 for hospitals (formally known as the paper CMS-1500, UB-04, and ADA dental claim forms)
- Claim status inquiry and response: X12 276, X12 277
- Eligibility inquiry and response: X12 270, X12 271
- Enrollment and disenrollment in a health plan: X12 834
- Referral certification and authorization: X12 278
- Payment and remittance advice: X12 835
- Health plan premium payments: X12 820
- Coordination of benefits (COB): X12 837; uses the same number as the health care claim because it sends a claim to both the primary and the secondary health care plans
- Health care claim attachment (Patient Information Transaction): X12 275
- First Report of Injury: X12 148 (workers' comp)

HIPAA Transaction and Code Set Standards HIPAA -mandated standardization in health care e-commerce, the standard requires the provider to submit information electronically, always in the same format

transaction an electronic exchange of information between two parties to carry out financial or administrative activities related to health care

Under HIPAA, HHS adopted specific code sets for diagnoses and procedures used in all transactions. A code set is any group of codes used for encoding data elements, such as medical concepts, medical diagnosis, or medical procedure codes. Medical data code sets used in the health care industry include coding systems for diseases, impairments, other health-related problems, and their manifestations. They also include actions taken to diagnose, treat, or manage diseases, injuries, and impairments; and any substances, equipment, supplies, or other items used to perform these actions. The following are HIPAA code sets for data elements in the administrative and financial health care transaction standards:

- **Diagnosis coding** for diseases, injuries, impairments, and other health-related problems.
    - *International Classification of Diseases, 10th edition, Clinical Modification (ICD-10-CM)*
- **Procedural coding** to prevent, diagnose, treat, or manage diseases, injuries, and impairments.
    - *International Classification of Diseases, 10th edition, Procedure Coding System (ICD-10-PCS);* inpatient hospital services
    - *Code on Dental Procedures and Nomenclature (CDT);* dental services
    - *Current Procedural Terminology (CPT);* physicians' services

- **Other hospital-related services** used for other services not found in the CPT manual, drugs, and durable medical equipment.
    - *Healthcare Common Procedure Coding System (HCPCS)*
- **Drug codes** in FDA's list of unique identifier numbers for drugs
    - *National Drug Code (NDC) Directory*

Implementing transactions and code set rules is a major business process reengineering effort that involves complex and expensive undertakings for an office or hospital.

3.3 HIPAA Unique Identifiers

HIPAA National Identifiers HIPAA-mandated identification systems for employers, health care providers, health plans, and patients; national provider system and employer system are in place; health plan and patient systems have not been created

National Provider Identifier (NPI) under HIPAA, system for identifying all health care providers using unique ten-digit identifiers

The HIPAA National Identifier standards mandate using certain identifying numbers in HIPAA transactions. There are **HIPAA National Identifiers** for employers, health care providers, health plans, and patients.

Identifiers are numbers of predetermined length and structure, such as Social Security numbers. They are important because the unique numbers can be used in electronic transactions. The new unique numbers can replace the many numbers that are currently used. Two identifiers have been set up–for employers and for providers–and two are to be established in the future–for patients and for health plans.

Employer Identification Number

The *Employer Identification Number (EIN)* issued by the Internal Revenue Service has been the HIPAA standard for the identification of employers in electronic transactions since July 30, 2002. The EIN is used when employers enroll or disenroll employees in a health plan (X12 834) or make premium payments to plans on behalf of their employees (X12 820).

National Provider Identifier

The **National Provider Identifier (NPI)** is the standard for the identification of providers when filing claims and other transactions. The NPI replaced other identifying numbers that were in use, such as the UPIN for Medicare and the numbers assigned by each payer to the provider, on May 23, 2008. The older numbers are known as *legacy numbers.*

The NPI has nine numbers and a check digit, for a total of ten numbers. The numbers are assigned by the federal government to individual providers, such as physicians, nurses, and pharmacists, and also to provider organizations such as hospitals, clinics, and pharmacies. CMS maintains the NPIs as they are assigned in the NPPES (National Plan and Provider Enumerator System), a database of all assigned numbers. Once assigned, an NPI will not change; it remains with the provider regardless of job or location changes.

BILLING TIP

Physician and Group NPIs

If a physician is in a group practice, both the individual doctor and the group have NPIs.

All health care providers who transmit health information electronically must obtain NPIs, even if they use business associates to prepare the transactions. Most health plans, including Medicare, Medicaid, and private payers, and all clearinghouses must accept and use NPIs in HIPAA transactions. This includes small plans as well as larger ones.

3.4 HIPAA Privacy Rule

The first part of the Administrative Simplification provisions includes the HIPAA Standards for Privacy of Individually Identifiable Health Information rule, known as the **HIPAA Privacy Rule.** Enacted on April 14, 2003, it provides protection for individually identifiable health information and grants certain rights to individuals in regard to their medical records. It was the first comprehensive federal protection for the privacy of health information. Before that, an individual's personal health information and medical records were governed by a patchwork of federal and state laws. Some state laws were strict, but others were not.

HIPAA Privacy Rule law that regulates the use and disclosure of patients' protected health information

protected health information (PHI) individually identifiable health information transmitted or maintained by electronic media or in any other form or medium

The Privacy Rule says that a covered entity must:

- Have a set of privacy practices that are appropriate for its health care services
- Notify patients about their privacy rights and how their information can be used or disclosed
- Train employees so that they understand the privacy practices
- Appoint a privacy official responsible for seeing that the privacy practices are adopted and followed
- Safeguard patients' records

The HIPAA Privacy Rule covers the use and disclosure of patients' **protected health information (PHI).** PHI is defined as individually identifiable health information that is transmitted or maintained by electronic media, such as over the Internet, or that is transmitted or maintained in any other form or medium. Covered entities must follow HIPAA regulations for the protection of health information. However, not all of a patient's information is subject to the law. Table 3.1 lists the information that meets the definition of PHI.

The Privacy Rule applies to PHI in any form, whether it is communicated verbally, written or printed on paper, or maintained in an electronic format.

Minimum Necessary Standard

When using or disclosing health information, a covered entity must try to limit the information to the minimum amount of PHI necessary for the intended purpose. The *minimum necessary standard* means using reasonable safeguards to protect PHI from being accidentally released to those not needing the information during an appropriate use or disclosure. For example, a medical insurance specialist would not disclose a patient's history of cancer on a workers' compensation claim for a broken wrist. Only the information the recipient needs to know is given. Similarly, a medical assistant would not hand over medical supplies and a prescription to someone who was not a family member or a legally appointed representative of the patient.

TABLE 3.1	Information Considered Protected Health Information (PHI)
Name	
Address (including street address, city, county, ZIP code)	
Names of relatives and employers	
Birth date	
Telephone numbers	
Fax number	
Email address	
Social Security number	
Medical record number	
Health plan beneficiary number	
Account number	
Certificate or license number	
Serial number of any vehicle or other device	
Website address	
Fingerprints or voiceprints	
Photographic images	

Designated Record Set

The covered entity must release a designated record set only, not all information. For purposes of the HIPAA Privacy Rule, a *record* is any item, collection, or grouping of information that includes PHI and is maintained by a covered entity. The HIPAA term for a group of records is *designated record set (DRS).* For a provider, the designated record set is the medical and billing records the provider maintains. It does not include appointment and surgery schedules, requests for lab tests, and birth and death records. It also does not include mental health information, psychotherapy notes, and genetic information, which are protected by more stringent release guidelines. For a health plan, the designated record set includes enrollment information, payment information, claim decisions, and the medical management systems of the plan.

Notice of Privacy Practices and Acknowledgment

Notice of Privacy Practices (NPP) a HIPAA-mandated document stating the privacy policies and procedures of a covered entity

To comply with the Privacy Rule, covered entities, including medical offices as well as other providers and health plans, must give each patient an explanation of privacy practices at the patient's first contact or encounter. To satisfy this requirement, a medical office gives the patient a copy of the office's **Notice of Privacy Practices (NPP)** (see Figure 3.1). The notice explains how patients' PHI may be used and describes the patients' rights. The NPP is usually a paper form that is handed to the patient; in the case of

Figure 3.1 Example of a Notice of Privacy Practices

Family Care Clinic

NOTICE OF PRIVACY PRACTICE

THIS NOTICE DESCRIBES HOW MEDICAL INFORMATION ABOUT YOU MAY BE USED AND DISCLOSED AND HOW YOU CAN GET ACCESS TO THIS INFORMATION. PLEASE REVIEW CAREFULLY.

WHY ARE YOU GETTING THIS NOTICE?
Family Care Clinic is required by federal and state law to maintain the privacy of your health information. The use and disclosure of your health information is governed by regulations under the Health Insurance Portability and Accountability Act of 1996 (HIPAA) and the requirements of applicable state law. For health information covered by HIPAA, we are required to provide you with this notice and will abide by this notice with respect to such health information. If you have questions about this notice, please contact out Privacy Officer at 877-555-1313. We will ask you to sign an "acknowledgment" indicating that you have been provided with this notice.

WHAT HEALTH INFORMATION IS PROTECTED?
We are committed to protecting the privacy of Information we gather about you while providing health-related services. Some examples of protected health information are:

- Information indicating that you are a patient receiving treatment or other health-related services from our physicians or staff;
- Information about your health condition (such as a disease you may have);
- Information about health care products or services you have received or may receive in the future (such as an operation); or
- Information about your health care benefits under an insurance plan (such as whether a prescription is covered);

When combined with:

- Demographic information (such as your name, address, or insurance status);
- Unique numbers that may identify you (such as your Social Security number, your phone number, or your driver's license number); and
- Other types of information that may identify who you are.

SUMMARY OF THIS NOTICE

This summary includes references to paragraphs throughout this notice that you may read for additional information.

1. Written Authorization Requirement
We may use your health information or share it with others in order to treat your condition, obtain payment for that treatment, and run our business operations. We generally need your written authorization for other uses and disclosures of your health information, unless an exception described in notice applies.

2. Authorizing Transfer of Your Records
Your may request that we transfer your records to another person or organization by completing a written authorization form. This form will specify what information is being released, to whom, and for what purpose. The authorization will have an expiration date.

3. Canceling Your Written Authorization
If you provide us with written authorization, you may revoke, or cancel, it at any time, except to the extent that we have already relied upon it. To revoke a written authorization, please write to the doctor's office where you initially gave your authorization.

4. Exception to Written Authorization Requirement
There are some situations in which we do not need your written authorization before using your health information or sharing it with others. They include:

Treatment, Payment, and Operations
As mentioned above, we may use your health information or share it with others in order to treat your condition, obtain payment for that treatment, and run our business operations.

Family and Friends
If you do not object, we will share information about your health with family and friends involved in your care.

Research
Although we will generally try to obtain your written authorization before using your health information for research purposes, there may be certain situations in which we are not required to obtain your written authorization.

De-identified Information
We may use or disclose your health information if we have removed any information that might identify you. When all identifying information is removed, we say that the health information is "completely de-identified." We may also use and disclose "partially de-identified" information if the person who will receive it agrees in writing to protect your privacy when using the information.

Incidental Disclosures
We may inadvertently use or disclose your health information despite having taken all reasonable precautions to protect the privacy and confidentiality of your health information.

Emergencies or Public Need
We may use or disclose your health information in an emergency or for important public health needs. For example, we may share your information with public health officials at the state or city health departments who are authorized to investigate and control the spread of diseases.

5. How to Access Your Health Information
You generally have the right to inspect and get copies of your health information.

6. How to Correct Your Health Information
You have the right to request that we amend your health information if you believe it is inaccurate or incomplete.

7. How to Identify Others Who Have Received Your Health Information
You have the right to receive an "accounting of disclosures." This is a report that identifies certain persons or organizations to which we have disclosed your health information. All disclosures are made according to the protections described in this Notice of Privacy Practices. Many routine disclosures we make (for treatment, payment, or business operations, among others) will not be included in this report. However, it will identify any nonroutine disclosures of your information.

8. How to Request Additional Privacy Protections
You have the right to request further restrictions on the way we use your health information or share it with others. However, we are not required to agree to the restriction you request. If we do agree with your request, we will be bound by our agreement.

9. How to Request Alternative Communications
You have the right to request that we contact you in a way that is more confidential for you, such as at home instead of at work. We will try to accommodate all reasonable requests.

10. How Someone May Act on Your Behalf
You have the right to name a personal representative who may act on your behalf to control the privacy of your health information. Parents and guardians will generally have the right to control the privacy of health information about minors unless the minors are permitted by law to act on their own behalf.

11. How to Learn About Special Protections for HIV, Alcohol and Substance Abuse, Mental Health, and Genetic Information
Special privacy protections apply to HIV-related information, alcohol and substance abuse treatment information, mental health information, psychotherapy notes, and genetic information.

12. How to Obtain a Copy of This Notice
If you have not already received one, you have the right to a paper copy of this notice. You may request a paper copy at any time, even if you have previously agreed to receive this notice electronically. You can request a copy of the privacy notice directly from your doctor's office. You may also obtain a copy of this notice from our website or by requesting a copy at your next visit.

13. How to Obtain a Copy of Revised Notice
We may change our privacy practices from time to time. If we do, we will revise this notice so you will have an accurate summary of our practices. You will be able to obtain your own copy of the revised notice by accessing our website or by calling your doctor's office. You may also ask for one at the time of your next visit. The effective date of the notice is noted in the top right corner of each page. We are required to abide by the terms of the notice that is currently in effect.

14. How to File a Complaint
If you believe your privacy rights have been violated, you may file a complaint with us or with the federal Office for Civil Rights. To file a complaint with us, please contact our Privacy Officer.

No one will retaliate or take action against you for filling a complaint.

a provider conducting business electronically, this information may be received as an electronic file. A patient must be given a copy of the NPP at the time of the first encounter and at least once every three years thereafter.

For compliance purposes, covered entities keep track of when patients receive the form. The office must make a good-faith effort to obtain a patient's acknowledgment of having received and read the NPP. This is accomplished through a form known as the **Acknowledgment of Receipt of Notice of Privacy Practices** (see Figure 3.2). This form states that the patient has read the privacy practices and understands how the provider intends to protect the patient's rights to privacy under HIPAA. Like the NPP, the acknowledgment can be a paper form or an electronic file.

Acknowledgment of Receipt of Notice of Privacy Practices form accompanying a covered entity's Notice of Privacy Practices; covered entities must make a good-faith effort to have patients sign it

release of information (ROI) process followed by employees of covered entities when releasing patient information

> **TIP**
>
> NPPs on the Website
>
> If a covered entity has a website that describes its services and benefits, it must also put its NPP on the site.

Disclosure for Treatment, Payment, and Health Care Operations (TPO)

Members of the physician practice health care team follow a **release of information (ROI)** process to access PHI, prepare it for transmission, and send it to an individual or entity that has permission under HIPAA to obtain it. The Privacy Rule recognizes that medical offices and payers must be able to exchange PHI in the normal course of business. *Use of PHI* means sharing or analysis within the entity that holds the information. *Disclosure* means the release, transfer, provision of access to, or divulging of PHI outside the entity holding the information.

Acknowledgment of Receipt of Notice of Privacy Practices

I understand that the providers of Family Care Clinic may share my health information for treatment, billing, and health care operations. I have been given a copy of the organization's Notice of Privacy Practices that describes how my health information is used and shared. I understand that Family Care Clinic has the right to change this notice at any time. I may obtain a current copy by contacting the practice's office or by visiting the website at www.xxx.com

My signature below constitutes my acknowledgment that I have been provided with a copy of the Notice of Privacy Practices.

____

Signature of Patient or Legal Representative   Date

If signed by legal representative,
relationship to patient: ________________________

Figure 3.2 Example of an Acknowledgment of Receipt of Notice of Privacy Practices

The rule says that there are three everyday situations in which PHI can be used and disclosed by providers without the patient's permission. These situations are **treatment, payment, and health care operations (TPO):**

treatment, payment, and health care operations (TPO) under HIPAA, three conditions under which patients' protected health information may be released without their consent

- *Treatment* means providing and coordinating a patient's medical care. Physicians and other medical staff can discuss the patient's case in the office and with other physicians. Laboratory or X-ray technicians may call to obtain clarification of unreadable requests. This information can be provided by the physician or another medical staff member.
- *Payment* refers to the exchange of information with health plans. Medical office staff members can take the required information from patients' records and prepare health care claims that are transmitted to health plans.
- *Health care operations* are the general business management functions needed to run the office. They include such activities as tracking and measuring adherence to quality standards, staff training, and business planning.

Release by Any Method

Information for TPO can be released by using any method of communication, including in writing, verbally, by fax, or by email.

PHI Release to Individuals Acting on a Patient's Behalf

A member of the physician practice health care team or another employee of a covered entity may release PHI to a family member, a relative, a friend, or another individual who asks for information on behalf of the patient. The covered entity must have reasonable assurance that the person has been identified by the patient as being involved in his or her care. The covered entity can release this information if the patient does not object. Informal permission can be obtained by asking the patient. If the patient is not present or is incapacitated, the covered entity can make the disclosure if doing so is in the best interests of the patient.

EXAMPLES

A health plan discloses relevant PHI to a beneficiary's daughter who has called to assist her hospitalized elderly mother with a payment issue.

A pharmacist dispenses filled prescriptions to a son who is picking up the items for his mother.

Release of Information for Purposes Other than TPO

For the provider to use or disclose PHI other than for treatment, payment, or operations (TPO), the patient must sign an authorization to release the information. For example, a patient who wishes a provider to disclose PHI to a life insurance company must authorize this action. This is an example of a general authorization. Information about alcohol or drug abuse, sexually transmitted infections (STIs) (except in the case of public health issues in some states) or human immunodeficiency virus (HIV), and behavioral or mental health services may not be released without a specific authorization from the patient.

Authorization Document

The authorization document must be easy to understand and must include the following information:

- A description of the information to be used or disclosed
- The name or other specific identification of the persons authorized to use or disclose the information
- The name of the persons or group to whom the covered entity may make the use or disclosure
- A description of each purpose of the requested use or disclosure
- An expiration date
- The signature of the individual (or authorized representative) and the date

In addition, the rule states that a valid authorization must include:

- A statement of the individual's right to revoke the authorization in writing
- A statement about whether the covered entity is able to base treatment, payment, enrollment, or eligibility for benefits on the authorization
- A statement that information used or disclosed after the authorization may be disclosed again by the recipient and may no longer be protected by the rule

TIP

PHI and Release of Information Document

A patient release of information document is not needed when PHI is shared for TPO under HIPAA. However, state law may require authorization to release data, so many practices continue to ask patients to sign releases.

Uses or disclosures for which the covered entity has received specific authorization from the patient do not have to follow the minimum necessary standard.

Accounting for Disclosures

Patients have the right to an accounting of disclosures of their PHI. The medical office keeps a disclosure log for each patient so that authorized disclosures can be listed. When a patient's PHI is accidentally disclosed, the disclosure should also be documented in the individual's medical record, since the individual did not authorize it and it was not a permitted disclosure. An example is faxing a discharge summary to the wrong physician's office.

Exceptions to Disclosure Standards

The rules for use and disclosure do not apply to the release of PHI in certain circumstances, including such public interest purposes as public health, law

THINKING IT THROUGH 3.1

- A physician consults with another physician about a patient's condition by email. Has the HIPAA Privacy Rule been followed?
- Two nurses are having a confidential conversation about a patient's condition in the hospital hallway directly outside the visitor waiting room for that floor. Someone visiting another patient accidentally overhears their conversation. Has the HIPAA Privacy Rule been followed?
- On July 13, 2022, Angelo Diaz requests City Medical, the office of his primary care physician, for an accounting of disclosures of his electronic PHI for the last year. The receptionist provides him with a printout. Angelo notices that the printout does not include TPO disclosures. The receptionist says that the office has never been responsible for tracking TPO disclosures. Is the receptionist correct? Should the office be able to provide Angelo Diaz with TPO disclosures for the last year?

enforcement, research, workers' compensation cases, and national security situations. Even in such cases, however, other conditions may need to be met before PHI can be released. For example, if the provider receives a judicial order requiring a patient's PHI for use as evidence in a court of law, the provider may release it without the patient's approval.

De-identified Health Information There are no restrictions on the use or disclosure of de-identified health information. *De-identified health information* is information that neither identifies nor provides a reasonable basis for identifying an individual. For example, for information to be de-identified, the following identifiers must be removed from patient data: names, medical record numbers, health plan beneficiary numbers, device identifiers (such as pacemakers), and biometric identifiers, such as fingerprints and voiceprints.

State Statutes Some state statutes are more stringent than HIPAA specifications with regard to the use and disclosure of PHI. Areas in which state statutes may differ from HIPAA include the following:

- Designated record set
- Psychotherapy notes
- Rights of inmates
- Information compiled for civil, criminal, or administrative court cases

When a state law and the federal HIPAA provision both cover a particular situation, the law that is the strictest–the one with the toughest provisions–is followed. Each practice's privacy official reviews state laws and develops policies and procedures accordingly.

Patients' Rights

The HIPAA Privacy Rule also provides significant rights to patients, including the right to:

- Receive a written notice of information practices
- Ask to access, inspect, and obtain a copy of their PHI
- Request an accounting of most disclosures of their health information

- Request amendment of records (meaning to fix incorrect information, but not to change or delete items because the patient does not agree with the data)
- Receive communications from providers through an alternate means, such as in a closed envelope rather than on a postcard
- File a complaint about a violation with the organization or with the Office for Civil Rights (OCR) in the Department of Health and Human Services
- Request restrictions on uses or disclosures of their PHI

In addition, the HITECH Act contains these new provisions:

- **Accounting of disclosures** Individuals are permitted to ask for an accounting of the disclosures of their electronic PHI, including TPO, over the preceding three years. Previously, individuals could request an accounting over the preceding six years, but TPO was not part of the disclosures.
- **Restricting access to some PHI** When an individual asks a covered entity not to release PHI to a health plan for purposes of carrying out payment or health care operations (not for treatment purposes), and the individual has paid the provider in full for the out-of-pocket expenses associated with the service, the covered entity must comply with the patient's request to restrict release of the PHI. This is a change to the previous HIPAA rule, under which a covered entity was permitted to deny the patient's request.

3.5 HIPAA Security Rule

HIPAA Security Rule law that requires covered entities to establish administrative, physical, and technical safeguards to protect the confidentiality, integrity, and availability of health information

The **HIPAA Security Rule,** the second part of the Administrative Simplification provisions, was enacted in 2005 specifically to protect health information on computer networks, the Internet, and electronic storage media. The security requirements indicate the administrative, technical, and physical safeguards that are required to protect the privacy of patients' electronic health information against unintended disclosure through breach of security.

While the HIPAA Privacy Rule requires covered entities to protect PHI in any form—paper, electronic, or otherwise—the HIPAA Security Rule focuses specifically on electronic health information. Electronic protected health information (ePHI) is PHI that is created, received, maintained, or transmitted in electronic form. The regulations apply to information stored on physical devices such as computers, USB flash drives, CDs, and magnetic tapes as well as to information located on computer networks or sent or received over the Internet.

The goals of the HIPAA security standards (see Figure 3.3) are to ensure:

- The confidentiality of ePHI, so that the information is shared only among authorized individuals or organizations
- The integrity of ePHI, so that the information is not changed in any way during storage or transmission and that it is authentic and complete and can be relied on to be sufficiently accurate for its purpose
- The availability of ePHI, so that the systems responsible for delivering, storing, and processing data are accessible when needed in both routine and emergency situations

Figure 3.3 Security Goals

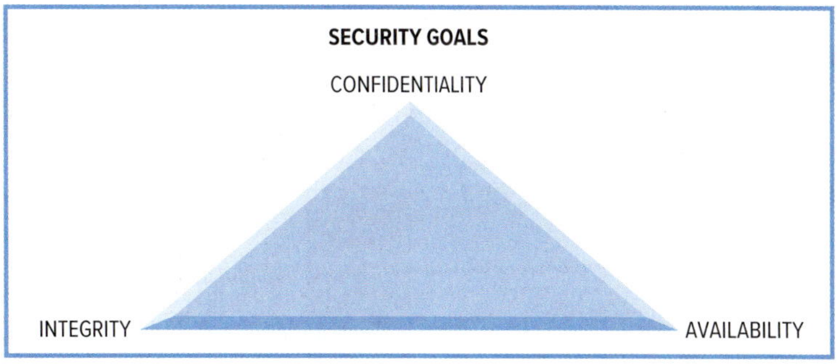

The HIPAA security standards do not state specific actions that covered entities must take to protect ePHI. The rule is intentionally flexible, recognizing that security policies and procedures vary according to the size of the organization and the nature of the work performed. For example, the policies and procedures required in a two-physician practice are different from those needed in a large city hospital. Each covered entity must determine which security measures and specific technologies are reasonable and appropriate for implementation in its organization.

The security standards contain requirements for three types of safeguards to prevent security breaches: administrative, physical, and technical.

Administrative Safeguards

Administrative safeguards are the administrative actions that a covered entity must perform, or train staff to do, to carry out security requirements. These actions include implementing office policies and procedures to prevent, detect, contain, and correct security violations. The management of security is assigned to one individual who conducts a risk assessment of the current level of data security. Once that assessment is complete, security policies and procedures are developed or modified to meet current needs.

Examples of administrative safeguards include the creation of a sanction policy that states the consequences of violations of security policies and procedures by employees, agents, and contractors; a backup plan for recovering from a security incident that jeopardizes critical data; a disaster recovery plan; and an emergency mode operation plan. Security training is provided to educate staff members on the policies and to raise awareness of security and privacy issues.

Physical Safeguards

Physical safeguards are mechanisms to protect electronic systems, equipment, and data from threats, environmental hazards, and unauthorized intrusion. These include devices that limit physical access to facilities housing protected information, such as reinforced doors, locks, and identification badge readers. Physical security also includes maintaining appropriate controls of files that are retained, stored, or scheduled for destruction.

Technical Safeguards

Technical safeguards are the technology and related policies and procedures used to protect electronic data and control access to it. They include the use of firewalls, intrusion detection systems, access control, and antivirus software.

Firewalls

A firewall examines traffic entering and leaving a computer network, using defined rules to determine whether to allow it to continue toward its destination. Packet filtering is a process in which a firewall examines each piece of information traveling into or out of the network. The firewall acts as a gatekeeper, deciding who has legitimate access to a network and what data should be allowed in and out. Firewalls can log attempted intrusions and report them to appropriate security personnel.

TIP

Record Retention

According to the American Health Information Management Association (AHIMA), transactional and billing records must be retained for at least ten years. Medical histories should be retained indefinitely.

Intrusion Detection Systems

An intrusion detection system (IDS) provides constant surveillance of the network. Unlike a firewall, an IDS monitors and analyzes packet data streams, searching for unauthorized activity. If such activity is suspected, the suspicious user's access to the network is immediately terminated.

Access Control

User authentication procedures are necessary to confirm the claimed identity of all users who access the data. In this context, authentication confirms that the user is the person he or she claims to be. In contrast, authorization is the process of determining whether an identified person has been granted access rights to information. Authorization procedures are needed to ensure that only appropriate users view the information.

username name that an individual uses for identification purposes when logging onto a computer or an application

A unique **username** is given to each practice employee to provide identification to access a computer, network, or application. A username can also be referred to as an account name, user ID, or log-in. In most cases, usernames are generated by the practice, typically following a format designated by the practice. A practice's username parameters might be the first initial of an employee's first name, the first five letters of the employee's last name, and a number.

EXAMPLES

Practices can designate their own parameters for generating usernames, or the PM/EHR may have username specifications. In either case, the parameters are consistent among all employees.

For example, a practice's username parameters might be the first initial of an employee's first name, the first five letters of the employee's last name, and a number.

Following are some employee usernames that would be created with these specifications:

- Amber Harthwaite - aharth01
- Alexander Harthorn - aharth02

Notice that these examples contain identical first initials and first five letters of the last name. The numbers 01 and 02 are used to ensure that the usernames are unique.

Passwords are specific codes that are required for gaining access to information on a computer or network. The code is known by the user, but it is not known to others. This very basic user authentication system is used in most health care organizations, since it is easy to implement. Used successfully, a password utilization program can keep unauthorized users from successfully logging onto a system or network. Password logging programs can track all successful and failed log-in attempts, which can be useful in detecting possible break-in attempts.

password confidential authentication information

TIP

Creating Strong Passwords

Password security is an important measure to maintain the integrity of an individual's access to protected information. A strong password is one that is unique, difficult for others to guess, and easy for users to remember.

Some tips for effective password use and creation include:

- Avoid using simplistic terms or plain dictionary words because these can be hacked with the use of hacking tools.
- Use a phrase or combination of words that is meaningful to you but would be difficult for others to guess.
- Use a combination of upper- and lowercase letters, numbers, and characters.
- Use different variations of passwords for multiple accounts.
- Never share passwords or write them down in areas that can be accessed by others.
- Use secure password managers to store multiple passwords.
- Change passwords often. Many PM/EHR systems automatically remind users to change passwords within a specific time frame, such as every 45 or 60 days.

EXAMPLES

Jonah Portillo is a new medical coder at Trilogy Family Care Center. His supervisor, Elrene, is setting up his access to EHRclinic, the practice's PM/EHR system.

Elrene informs Jonah that his username is *jporti01* and provides him with a temporary password. Jonah must now create a new password so he can access EHRclinic.

At first, Jonah considers using his beloved dog's name, Jackson, as his password because it would be easy to remember. He thought that adding a number to it would make it more secure, so *Jackson1* became his new password.

After giving it some thought, Jonah realized that *Jackson1* is not a very secure password because everyone knows how much he loves his dog. He decided to change his password to something equally memorable but difficult for others to guess.

His new password became *JacksonIsTheBest2022!*. Formatting the password as a phrase and using a variety of upper- and lowercase letters with a special character was a great strategy. He also added the year that Jackson was born to provide an extra layer of password security. This new password would be much more difficult to hack!

THINKING IT THROUGH 3.2

A medical assistant at a small medical practice took home an office laptop to work on one of the office's brochures over the weekend. The laptop, which contained clinical and billing information for the practice, was left unattended at a coffee shop and was stolen. Both the clinical data and the billing database were protected by passwords. An encryption program was also used to protect the data. What types of safeguards do these represent? Do you think these security methods will be enough to block a breach in the security of patients' information? Do you think it was a good idea for the medical assistant to take the laptop home?

Much more sophisticated systems, including biometric methods, are being used to identify people who need to gain access to information. Biometric devices use some measurable feature of an individual to authenticate the person's identity. They can use such physical characteristics as fingerprints, facial features, or retinal patterns to confirm identity. Because they are based on unique physical characteristics, they cannot be forged, stolen, or duplicated.

access levels security option that determines the areas of the program a user can access, and whether the user has rights to enter or edit data

encryption process of converting electronic information into an unreadable format before it is distributed

Role-based authorization limits access to patient information based on the user's role in an organization. Once **access levels** have been assigned, each user is given a key to the designated databases. The user must enter an ID and a key to see files to which he or she has been granted access rights. Role-based authorization meets the HIPAA standard of releasing only the minimum amount of information necessary to provide care. In a medical office, for example, a billing specialist requires access to more areas in an electronic health record than does a medical assistant. Technology permits the system to prevent the user from viewing or modifying any part of the record that is not directly related to his or her job, which is discussed in greater detail in Chapter 18.

Encryption is the process of converting data into an unreadable format before it is distributed. To read a message, the recipient must have a key that deciphers the information. For example, encryption can protect the privacy of restricted data that are stored on a laptop computer even if the computer is stolen. Similarly, it can protect data that are transmitted over a network even if that network is accessed by an unauthorized third party. These techniques also make it possible to determine whether the information has been altered in any way.

Audit trails are records that show who has accessed a computer or a network and what operations were performed. At a minimum, an audit trail should contain the following information:

- Type of event
- Date and time of occurrence
- User ID associated with the event
- Program, command, or method used to initiate the event
- Patient and data elements that were changed

The log is reviewed on a regular basis to detect irregularities. If an error or a suspicious entry has been made, the program lists the name of the person and the date the information was entered.

Most applications, including PM/EHR systems, have an **auto log-off** feature. Although it is a best practice to log out of a system before leaving the computer, there are times in which a program is inactive for a period of time. After this time frame, the system will automatically log the user off to prevent others from being able to access records through that user's account.

auto log-off feature of PM/EHR systems that automatically logs a user out of the program after a period of inactivity

Health Care Fraud and Abuse Control Program government program to uncover misuse of funds in federal health care programs; run by the Office of the Inspector General

False Claims Act prohibits submitting a fraudulent claim or making a false statement or representation in connection with a claim; encourages reporting suspected fraud and abuse by protecting and rewarding people involved in qui tam (whistleblower) cases

Antivirus Software

Antivirus software scans a system for known viruses. After detection, the software attempts to remove the virus from the system and, in some cases, fix any problems the virus created. Antivirus tools cannot detect and eliminate all viruses. New viruses are continually being developed, and antivirus software must be regularly updated to maintain its effectiveness.

3.6 Policies and Procedures

Almost everyone involved in the delivery of health care is trustworthy and is devoted to patients' welfare. However, some people are not. Health care fraud and abuse laws help control cheating in the health care system. Are the laws really necessary? The evidence says that they are. During 2019, the federal government recovered an estimated $3 billion in fraud-related judgments and settlements. This loss directly affects patients, taxpayers, and government through higher health care costs, insurance premiums, and taxes. Health care fraud also may hurt patients, possibly subjecting some of them to unnecessary or unsafe procedures or making them victims of identity theft. Allied health employees are trained to be alert for health care fraud and abuse and to know which agencies are responsible for watching for them and acting when they are suspected.

The Health Care Fraud and Abuse Control Program

HIPAA created the **Health Care Fraud and Abuse Control Program** to uncover and prosecute fraud and abuse. The HHS Office of the Inspector General (OIG) has the task of detecting health care fraud and abuse and enforcing all laws relating to them. OIG works with the U.S. Department of Justice (DOJ), which includes the Federal Bureau of Investigation (FBI), under the direction of the U.S. attorney general to prosecute those suspected of medical fraud and abuse.

Federal False Claims Act and State Laws

The federal **False Claims Act** (FCA, 31 USC § 3729) prohibits submitting a fraudulent claim or making a false statement or representation in connection with a claim. It also encourages reporting suspected fraud and abuse by protecting and rewarding people involved in *qui tam* (whistleblower) cases. The person who makes the accusation of suspected fraud is called the *relator.* Relators are generally current or former employees of insurance companies or medical practices, program beneficiaries, and independent contractors. Under the law, the relator is protected against employer retaliation. If the fraud investigation results in the payment of a fine to the federal government, the whistleblower may be entitled to 15 to 25 percent of the amount paid.

> **TIP**
>
> **Extending Federal Laws to Private Payers**
>
> HIPAA created a new category of crimes that apply to billing transactions with private payers in addition to Medicare and Medicaid billing. These offenses include health care fraud, making false statements, theft and embezzlement, obstruction of criminal investigations, and money laundering.

At present, twenty states also have passed versions of the federal False Claims Act. These laws allow private individuals to bring actions alone or to work with state attorneys general against any person who knowingly causes the state to pay a false claim. The state laws generally provide for civil penalties and damages related to the cost of any losses sustained because of the false claim.

OIG Enforcement Actions for Fraud, False Claims, and Substandard Care: Case Examples

Seven Miami-area residents were sentenced in a Medicare infusion fraud scheme. The employees, who worked at an infusion clinic, were ordered to pay $19.8 million in restitution and were sentenced to prison terms ranging from thirty-seven to ninety-seven months. In their guilty pleas, they admitted to activities that included manipulating patients' blood samples to generate false medical records, ordering and administering medications to treat conditions that were falsely documented with fraudulent test results, and billing Medicare for services that were medically unnecessary or never provided.

Pfizer Inc. entered into a $1 billion civil False Claims Act settlement with the United States in connection with marketing and promotion practices associated with the anti-inflammatory drug Bextra and several other drugs. The settlement agreement includes a comprehensive five-year corporate integrity agreement between Pfizer and OIG. Pfizer and its subsidiary Pharmacia & Upjohn agreed to pay a total of $2.3 billion in this case, the largest health care fraud settlement in history, to resolve both the civil and criminal liability arising from the illegal promotion of certain pharmaceutical products.

Emmanuel Bernabe, the president and board chair of Pleasant Care Corporation, agreed to be permanently excluded from federal health care programs following an investigation of substandard care at nursing homes formerly operated by the corporation. OIG alleged that Bernabe, through his management and oversight of Pleasant Care, caused services to be furnished to Pleasant Care residents that substantially departed from the professional standard of care. For example, Pleasant Care failed to maintain adequate staffing levels, properly administer medication, provide adequate hydration and nutrition, and prevent accidents.

Additional Laws

Additional laws relating to health care fraud and abuse control include:

- An antikickback statute that makes it illegal to knowingly offer incentives to induce referrals for services that are paid for by government health care programs. Many financial actions are considered to be illegal incentives, including direct payments to other physicians and routine waivers of coinsurance and deductibles.

- Self-referral prohibitions (called Stark rules) that make it illegal for physicians or members of their immediate families to have financial relationships with clinics to which they refer their patients, such as radiology service clinics and clinical laboratories. (Note that there are many legal exceptions to this prohibition under various business structures.)
- The Sarbanes-Oxley Act of 2002 that requires publicly traded corporations to attest that their financial management is sound. These provisions apply to for-profit health care companies. The act includes whistleblower protection so that employees can report wrongdoing without fear of retaliation.

Definition of Fraud and Abuse

fraud intentional act of deception to take financial advantage of another person

abuse actions that improperly use another person's resources

Fraud is an act of deception undertaken with the intention of taking financial advantage of another person. Fraudulent acts are intentional; the individual expects an illegal or unauthorized benefit to result. For example, misrepresenting professional credentials and forging another person's signature on a check are fraudulent. Pretending to be a physician and treating patients without a valid medical license is also fraudulent.

Claims fraud occurs when health care providers or others falsely report charges to payers. A provider may bill for services that were not performed, overcharge for services, or fail to provide complete services under a contract. A patient may exaggerate an injury to get a settlement from an insurance company or may ask a medical insurance specialist to change a date on a chart so that a service is covered by a health plan.

In federal law, **abuse** is an action that misuses money that the government has allocated, such as Medicare funds. Abuse is illegal because taxpayers' dollars are misspent. An example of abuse is an ambulance service that billed Medicare for transporting a patient to the hospital when the patient did not need ambulance service. This abuse–billing for services that were not medically necessary–resulted in improper payment of the ambulance company. Abuse is not necessarily intentional. It may be the result of ignorance of a billing rule or of inaccurate coding.

Examples of Fraudulent and Abusive Acts

A number of billing practices are fraudulent or abusive. Investigators reviewing physicians' billing work look for patterns like these:

- Intentionally billing for services that were not performed or documented

EXAMPLES

A lab bills Medicare for two tests when only one was done.

A physician asks a coder to report a physical examination when the physician actually talked to the patient on the telephone.

- Reporting services at a higher level than was carried out

EXAMPLE

After a patient visit for a flu shot, the provider bills the encounter as a comprehensive physical examination plus a vaccination.

- Performing and billing for procedures that are not related to the patient's condition and therefore are not medically necessary

EXAMPLE

After reading an article about Lyme disease, a patient is worried about having worked in her garden over the summer, and she requests a Lyme disease diagnostic test. Although no symptoms or signs have been reported, the physician orders and bills for the *Borrelia burgdorferi* (Lyme disease) confirmatory immunoblot test.

Medicaid Fraud: A Case Example

Keven Wayne Louderback, a Springfield insurance broker, pleaded guilty to twelve felony counts related to Medicaid fraud. (Medicaid is the federal/state health insurance program for low-income beneficiaries.) According to Missouri Attorney General Chris Koster, Louderback misappropriated more than $700,000 from Medicaid by furnishing applications with false information to a Missouri Medicaid program that pays for private health insurance premiums for certain individuals with high medical costs. Louderback represented the monthly insurance premium rates as greater than they actually were and pocketed the overpayment. He also offered kickbacks to get people to enroll in an insurance program, fraudulently misstated an insurance company's rate, and forged documents to set out the false rate. Louderback pleaded guilty to five counts of Medicaid fraud, one count of offering a kickback to receive a Medicaid payment, four counts of insurance fraud, and two counts of forgery.

TIP

Fraud Versus Abuse

To bill when the task was not done is fraud; to bill when it was not necessary is abuse. Remember the rule: If a service was not documented, in the view of the payer it was not done and cannot be billed. To bill for undocumented services is fraudulent.

Excluded Parties

Employees, physicians, and contractors who have been found guilty of fraud may be excluded from being able to work for government programs. An OIG exclusion has national scope, and Congress has established a civil monetary penalty for institutions that knowingly hire excluded parties. OIG maintains the List of Excluded Individual/Entities (LEIE), a database that provides the public, health care providers, patients, and others with information about parties excluded from participation in Medicare, Medicaid, and federal health care programs. The list is available on OIG's website for the exclusion program.

3.7 Compliance Plans

Because of the risk of fraud and abuse liability, medical practices must be sure that billing rules are followed by all staff members. In addition to responsibility for their own actions, physicians are liable for the professional actions of employees they supervise. This responsibility is a result of the law of *respondeat superior,* which states that an employer is responsible for an employee's actions. Physicians are held to this doctrine, so they can be charged for the fraudulent behavior of any staff member.

A wise slogan is that "the best defense is a good offense." For this reason, medical practices write and implement compliance plans to uncover compliance problems and correct them to avoid risking liability. A **compliance plan** is a process for finding, correcting, and preventing illegal medical office practices. It is a written document prepared by a compliance officer and committee that sets up the steps needed to (1) audit and monitor compliance with government regulations, especially in the area of coding and billing, (2) have policies and procedures that are consistent, (3) provide for ongoing staff training and communication, and (4) respond to and correct errors.

compliance plan a process for finding, correcting, and preventing illegal medical office practices. It is a written document prepared by a compliance officer and committee that sets up the steps needed to (1) audit and monitor compliance with government regulations, especially in the area of coding and billing, (2) have policies and procedures that are consistent, (3) provide for ongoing staff training and communication, and (4) respond to and correct errors

The goals of the compliance plan are to:

- Prevent fraud and abuse through a formal process to identify, investigate, fix, and prevent repeat violations relating to reimbursement for health care services
- Ensure compliance with applicable federal, state, and local laws, including employment and environmental laws as well as antifraud laws
- Help defend the practice if it is investigated or prosecuted for fraud by substantiating the desire to behave compliantly and thus reduce any fines or criminal prosecution

Having a compliance plan demonstrates to outside investigators that the practice has made honest, ongoing attempts to find and fix weak areas.

Compliance plans cover more than just coding and billing. They also cover all areas of government regulation of medical practices, such as Equal Employment Opportunity (EEO) regulations (for example, hiring and promotion policies) and Occupational Safety and Health Administration (OSHA) regulations (for example, fire safety and handling of hazardous materials such as blood-borne pathogens).

Parts of a Compliance Plan

Generally, according to OIG, a voluntary plan should contain seven elements:

1. Consistent written policies and procedures
2. Appointment of a compliance officer and committee
3. Training plans

4. Communication guidelines
5. Disciplinary systems
6. Auditing and monitoring
7. Responding to and correcting errors

> **TIP**
>
> **Have It in Writing!**
>
> Do not code or bill services that are not supported by documentation, even if instructed to do so by a physician. Instead, report this kind of situation to the practice's compliance officer.

Following OIG's guidance can help in the defense against a false claims accusation. Having a plan in place shows that efforts are made to understand the rules and correct errors. This indicates to OIG that the problems may not add up to a pattern or practice of abuse, but may simply be errors.

Compliance Officer and Committee

To establish the plan and follow up on its provisions, most medical practices appoint a compliance officer who is in charge of the ongoing work. The compliance officer may be one of the practice's physicians, the practice manager, or the billing manager. A compliance committee is also usually established to oversee the program.

Ongoing Training

Physician Training

Part of the compliance plan is a commitment to keep physicians trained in pertinent coding and regulatory matters. Often the medical insurance specialist or medical coder is assigned the task of briefing physicians on changed codes or medical necessity regulations. The following guidelines are helpful in conducting physician training classes:

- Keep the presentation as brief and straightforward as possible.
- In a multispecialty practice, issues should be discussed by specialty; all physicians do not need to know changed rules on dermatology, for example.
- Use actual examples, and stick to the facts when presenting material.
- Explain the benefits of coding compliance to the physicians, and listen to their feedback to improve job performance.
- Set up a way to address additional changes during the year, such as in an office newsletter or at compliance meetings.

Staff Training

An important part of the compliance plan is a commitment to train medical office staff members who are involved with coding and billing. Ongoing training also requires having the current annual updates, reading health plans' bulletins and periodicals, and researching changed regulations. Compliance officers often conduct refresher classes in proper coding and billing techniques.

THINKING IT THROUGH 3.3

As a member of the administrative staff for the practice, why would ongoing training be important to you?

Code of Conduct

The practice's compliance plan emphasizes the procedures that are to be followed to meet existing documentation, coding, and medical necessity requirements. It also has a code of conduct for the members of the practice, which covers:

- Procedures for ensuring compliance with laws relating to referral arrangements
- Provisions for discussing compliance during employees' performance reviews and for disciplinary action against employees, if needed
- Mechanisms to encourage employees to report compliance concerns directly to the compliance officer to reduce the risk of whistleblower actions

Promoting ethical behavior in the practice's daily operations can also reduce employee dissatisfaction and turnover by showing employees that the practice has a strong commitment to honest, ethical conduct.

Audits

The HIPAA Security Rule requires covered entities to conduct four types of audits. Three are periodic, and one is annual. The three periodic audits are an information systems activity review, user log-in monitoring, and an audit log review (from computer systems and databases to review the storage, use, and disclosure of PHI). The annual audit, called an *evaluation,* is more commonly known as a compliance audit.

Documentation

Documentation is a primary requirement for demonstrating HIPAA compliance. Common documentation includes:

- Retaining written or electronic results of risk analysis
- Documenting the results of an audit
- Developing and implementing comprehensive privacy and security policies and procedures
- Documenting staff training and security incident threats

3.8 Breach Notification Requirements

The **HIPAA Breach Notification Rule,** 45 CFR §§ 164.400-414, requires HIPAA covered entities and their business associates to provide notification following a breach of unsecured protected health information. A **breach** is an impermissible use or disclosure under the Privacy Rule that compromises the security or

HIPAA Breach Notification Rule law that requires HIPAA covered entities and their business associates to provide notification following a breach of unsecured protected health information

breach under the HIPAA Privacy Rule, impermissible use or disclosure that compromises the security or privacy of PHI that could pose a significant risk of financial, reputational, or other harm to the affected person

privacy of PHI in a way that could pose a significant risk of financial, reputational, or other harm to the affected person. To prevent breaches of health information, the HIPAA Breach Notification Rule requires keeping patients' protected health information secure by making it unusable, unreadable, or indecipherable to unauthorized individuals using specified technologies and methods. The Department of Health and Human Services has released guidance on specific technologies and methods that can make it impossible for unauthorized individuals to use, read, or decipher this information.

Following the discovery of a breach of unsecured PHI, a covered entity must notify each person whose unsecured PHI has been, or is reasonably believed to have been, inappropriately accessed, acquired, or disclosed. Following the discovery of a breach by a business associate, the business associate must notify the covered entity of the breach and of the identity of those whose unsecured PHI has been, or is reasonably believed to have been, breached. The act requires the notifications to be made without unreasonable delay, but in no case later than sixty calendar days after discovery of the breach. An exception may be made to the deadline only when a law enforcement official determines that notification would impede a criminal investigation or cause damage to national security. The Breach Notification Rule specifies the following:

- Notice to patients of breaches "without reasonable delay" within sixty days
- Notice to covered entities by business associates when the business associates discover a breach
- Notice to "prominent media outlets" on breaches involving more than five hundred individuals
- Notice to "next of kin" on breaches involving patients who are deceased
- Notice to the secretary of HHS about breaches involving 500 or more individuals without reasonable delay
- Annual notice to the secretary of HHS about breaches of "unsecured PHI" involving fewer than five hundred individuals that pose a significant financial risk or other harm to the individuals, such as to their reputations

breach notification document used by a covered entity to notify individuals of a breach in their protected health information required under the new HITECH breach notification rules

The document notifying an individual of a breach, called the **breach notification** form, must include (1) a brief description of what happened, including the date of the breach and the date of the discovery of the breach, if known; (2) a description of the types of unsecured PHI that were involved in the breach (such as full name, Social Security number, date of birth, home address, account number, or disability code); (3) the steps individuals should take to protect themselves from potential harm resulting from the breach; (4) a brief description of what the covered entity is doing to investigate the breach, to mitigate losses, and to protect against further breaches; and (5) contact procedures for individuals who have questions or want additional information, including a toll-free telephone number, an email address, a website, or a postal address.

In addition, the rule requires the secretary of HHS to annually prepare and submit to Congress a report regarding the breaches about which the secretary was notified and all enforcement actions taken. This means that a covered entity must maintain a log of breaches involving fewer than 500 individuals and submit it to HHS annually. HHS must post the report on the HHS public website. It is hoped that the negative publicity of public posting will act as a deterrent, offering greater incentives for covered entities and business associates to prevent breaches.

Threats in Connection with EHRs

While a nationwide health information network in which each person has an electronic health record would bring many benefits–such as the increased use of information technology to cut costs, improve patient safety, and provide the best possible care–a large network also places large amounts of protected health information at greater risk. The use of portable computing and storage devices for moving the data from place to place adds to this risk.

Sharing Clinical Data Through Networks

More personal health information is being created, accessed, and maintained on computers than ever before. In an electronic health record system, personal health information is entered and stored in a computer database. The database then connects to other databases in health information networks, making it possible to share information with authorized providers, hospitals, pharmacies, laboratories, and others. The larger the network, the greater the risk, so while a health information network brings the most benefits, it also presents the greatest privacy and security challenges.

Portable Computers and Storage Devices

In the past, personal health information did not commonly leave a physician office or hospital facility. Desktop computers, bulky paper files, and large backup tapes made it difficult to move data from one place to another. In large part, the locks on office doors were safeguards against intruders.

Today, hardware and data are portable and leave medical offices and hospital buildings regularly, increasing the possibility that they will be lost or stolen. One of the benefits of electronic health records is being able to access information when and where it is needed. Many health care professionals use laptop computers, personal digital assistants (PDAs), and smart cell phones to access and store data. Laptops are popular because they can be moved from one location to another, such as from a physician's desk to an examining room. It is not uncommon for employees to carry laptops to and from work.

USB flash drives and other removable storage devices are smaller and are becoming less expensive. They function like hard drives, and people require little instruction in using them to store data. Such small storage devices, including CDs and DVDs, easily fit in a briefcase. Although the portability of electronic data offers many benefits, the widespread use of portable hardware and small storage devices makes it more difficult to control access to a person's health information.

HITECH Provisions: Addressing Inadequacies in Privacy Standards

HIPAA is not a universal law; that is, it does not apply to every person or organization. It was designed to provide protection for personal health information that was exchanged by certain groups and individuals in certain electronic transactions. Since HIPAA was enacted in 1996, the field of health information technology has changed dramatically. Increasingly, an individual's personal health information is accessed, maintained, and exchanged by groups that may not be covered under current HIPAA privacy laws. The HITECH Act, enacted as part of the American Recovery and Reinvestment Act of 2009, tries to address this inadequacy in a number of ways. One way is by making business associates subject to the same privacy and security requirements as covered entities. Before the HITECH Act, only covered entities could be penalized for violations of the Privacy and Security Rules. Under HITECH, a much wider range of businesses must comply.

Overseas Business Associates

Overseas companies in India and other countries currently provide services to health care providers and organizations in the United States, including coding, transcription processing, and claim management. Some of these tasks cannot be completed without access to protected health information. Some companies in developing countries lack security systems that protect sensitive health data. Previously, offshore vendors did not have to comply directly with HIPAA security and privacy legislation. However, under HITECH, an overseas vendor that signs a business associate agreement with a U.S. covered entity is now required to abide by HIPAA.

Personal Health Records

Many organizations, including employers, health plans, and providers, offer personal health records (PHRs) to individuals. Companies including Walmart, Intel, BP, Pitney Bowes, and Allied Materials have joined together to provide personal health record systems for their 2.5 million employees. Commercial software vendors are offering PHRs to individuals at no charge or for a fee. Previously, as business associates, PHR vendors were not directly required to comply with HIPAA. As a result, many of the PHRs offered were not covered by the Privacy Rule, leaving protected health information subject to release without a patient's consent or authorization.

Under HITECH, as business associates, PHR vendors and third-party partners supporting PHR hosting or management are now required to comply with the HIPAA Privacy and Security Rules, as well as with the new breach notification rules. Vendors using PHRs must notify patients and the Federal Trade Commission (FTC) of any breach caused by their products or services. The FTC is required to publish notification requirements for PHR vendors and third-party providers and to inform HHS if it is notified of a breach.

Private Sector Electronic Networks

While the federal government continues its work on developing a strategy for the creation of a national health information network (NHIN), businesses and organizations in the private sector (not associated with the government) have created new models of health information networks for sharing information. For example, health information exchanges (HIEs) have been created at the state, regional, and community levels. A health information exchange enables health care information to be exchanged electronically across organizations and retain its meaning. A regional health information organization (RHIO) is a type of HIE in which a group of health care entities in a geographic area exchange health information over an electronic network

THINKING IT THROUGH 3.4

Health plans, employers, and the government are encouraging patients to create personal health records (PHRs). If a provider is using an EHR system, a patient can ask the provider to send data to his or her PHR. Because patients control the data in their PHRs, depending on the PHRs used, they may be able to add to or delete physician or hospital data. Why do you think physicians are advocating for safeguards to be added to PHRs so that patients cannot alter the information?

for the purpose of improving the delivery of health care. Participants may include health care providers, clinics, hospitals, laboratories, pharmacies, health plans, mental health agencies, and local health departments.

Previously, while some of these providers, such as health care providers and health plans, were subject to HIPAA privacy laws, the overall organizations were not. Under HITECH, organizations such as HIEs and RHIOs that provide data transmission of PHI and require access to that information are now categorized as business associates and are therefore required to comply with HIPAA Privacy and Security Rules. Also, business agreements need to be executed between RHIO or HIE participants and the organization managing the RHIO or HIE.

chapter 3 summary

KEY TERMS

abuse
access levels
Acknowledgment of Receipt of Notice of Privacy Practices
auto log-off
breach
breach notification
compliance plan
encryption
False Claims Act
fraud
Health Care Fraud and Abuse Control Program
Health Information Technology for Economic and Clinical Health (HITECH) Act
Health Insurance Portability and Accountability Act (HIPAA)
HIPAA Breach Notification Rule
HIPAA National Identifiers
HIPAA Privacy Rule
HIPAA Security Rule
HIPAA Transaction and Code Set Standards
National Provider Identifier (NPI)
Notice of Privacy Practices (NPP)
password
protected health information (PHI)
release of information (ROI)
transaction
treatment, payment, and health care operations (TPO)
U.S. Department of Health and Human Services (HHS)
username

LEARNING OUTCOME	KEY CONCEPTS/EXAMPLES
3.1 Explain HIPAA and its regulations.	HIPAA is a federal law that required the creation of national standards to protect sensitive patient health information from being disclosed without the patient's consent or knowledge. The U.S. Department of Health and Human Services (HHS) issued the HIPAA Privacy Rule to implement the requirements of HIPAA. A major provision of HIPAA is the Administrative Simplification: • HIPAA Electronic Transaction and Code Set Standards Requirements • HIPAA Privacy Requirements • HIPAA Security Requirements
3.2 Discuss HIPAA transactions and code sets.	HIPAA Transaction and Code Set Standards require standardization in health care. This requires the provider to submit information electronically and always in the same format. Transactions are electronic exchanges of information between two parties to carry out financial or administrative activities related to health care. Medical data code sets used in the health care industry include coding systems: • Diagnosis coding • Procedural coding • Other hospital-related services • Drug codes

<table>
<tr><th>LEARNING OUTCOME</th><th>KEY CONCEPTS/EXAMPLES</th></tr>
<tr><td>3.3 Describe HIPAA unique identifiers.</td><td>HIPAA establishes and requires unique identifiers for employers and providers. Identifiers are numbers of predetermined length to be used in electronic transactions. Employer Identification Number (EIN) and National Provider Identifier (NPI) are the two required identifiers.</td></tr>
<tr><td>3.4 Describe the HIPAA Privacy Rule.</td><td>HIPAA Privacy Rule standards address the use and disclosure of individuals' health information, known as protected health information (PHI). PHI is an identifiable piece of health information that is transmitted or maintained by electronic media. Those who transmit information for health care are known as covered entities. Examples are:
• Health care providers
• Health plans
• Health care clearinghouses
• Business associates</td></tr>
<tr><td>3.5 Describe the HIPAA Security Rule.</td><td>The HIPAA Security Rule protects a subset of information. The subset is a patient's health information (PHI). The rule states that covered entities must do the following:
• Ensure the confidentiality, integrity, and availability of all electronic protected health information.
• Detect and safeguard against anticipated threats to the security of the information.
• Protect against anticipated impermissible uses or disclosures.
• Certify compliance by their workforce.</td></tr>
<tr><td>3.6 Discuss all policies and procedures related to privacy and security of health records.</td><td>• HIPAA created the Health Care Fraud and Abuse Control Program to uncover and prosecute fraud and abuse. The HHS Office of the Inspector General (OIG) has the task of detecting health care fraud and abuse and enforcing all laws relating to them.
• The federal False Claims Act (FCA, 31 USC § 3729) prohibits submitting a fraudulent claim or making a false statement or representation in connection with a claim.
• Fraud is an act of deception undertaken with the intention of taking financial advantage of another person. Fraudulent acts are intentional; the individual expects an illegal or unauthorized benefit to result.
• Abuse is an action that misuses money that the government has allocated, such as Medicare funds. Abuse is illegal because taxpayers' dollars are misspent.</td></tr>
<tr><td>3.7 Describe compliance plans.</td><td>A compliance plan is a process for finding, correcting, and preventing illegal medical office practices. It is a written document prepared by a compliance officer and committee that sets up the steps needed to:
• Audit and monitor compliance with government regulations, especially in the area of coding and billing
• Have policies and procedures that are consistent
• Provide for ongoing staff training and communication
• Respond to and correct errors</td></tr>
</table>

LEARNING OUTCOME	KEY CONCEPTS/EXAMPLES
3.8 Explain breach notification requirements.	• The **HIPAA Breach Notification Rule,** 45 CFR §§ 164.400-414, requires HIPAA covered entities and their business associates to provide notification following a breach of unsecured protected health information. A breach is an impermissible use or disclosure under the Privacy Rule that compromises the security or privacy of PHI in a way that could pose a significant risk of financial, reputational, or other harm to the affected person. • Following the discovery of a breach of unsecured PHI, a covered entity must notify each person whose unsecured PHI has been, or is reasonably believed to have been, inappropriately accessed, acquired, or disclosed. • Following the discovery of a breach by a business associate, the business associate must notify the covered entity of the breach and of the identity of those whose unsecured PHI has been, or is reasonably believed to have been, breached.

chapter 3 review

Match the key terms with their definitions.

_____ 1. *[LO 3.3]* National Provider Identifier (NPI)

_____ 2. *[LO 3.1]* U.S. Department of Health and Human Services (HHS)

_____ 3. *[LO 3.2]* transaction

_____ 4. *[LO 3.6]* abuse

_____ 5. *[LO 3.8]* breach

_____ 6. *[LO 3.7]* compliance plan

_____ 7. *[LO 3.4]* HIPAA Privacy Rule

_____ 8. *[LO 3.8]* breach notification

_____ 9. *[LO 3.5]* HIPAA Security Rule

_____ 10. *[LO 3.4]* release of information

a. Actions that improperly use another person's resources.

b. Agency that mandates laws to enhance the health and well-being of all Americans by providing for effective health and human services and by fostering sound, sustained advances in the sciences underlying medicine, public health, and social services; this agency has mandated the HIPAA Privacy Rule to implement the requirements of HIPAA.

c. The impermissible use or disclosure of a patient's PHI under the Privacy Rule due to a compromise in privacy or security that could pose a significant risk to the individual involved.

d. Law that requires covered entities to establish safeguards to protect the confidentiality, integrity, and availability of health information.

e. An electronic exchange of information between two parties to carry out financial or administrative activities related to health care.

f. Under HIPAA, system for identifying all health care providers using unique ten-digit identifiers.

g. A process for finding, correcting, and preventing illegal medical office practices.

h. A process followed by employees of covered entities when releasing patient information.

i. A document used by a covered entity to notify individuals of a breach in their PHI.

j. Law that regulates the use and disclosure of patients' protected health information.

MULTIPLE-CHOICE QUESTIONS

Select the letter that best completes the statement or answers the question.

1. *[LO 3.2]* Which of the following is NOT a HIPAA code set for data elements in the administrative and financial health care transaction standards?
   a. diagnosis coding
   b. procedural coding
   c. drug code
   d. clinical code

2. *[LO 3.1]* The HIPAA Administrative Simplification provisions contain all of the following parts EXCEPT the ________.
   a. Privacy Rule
   b. Security Rule
   c. breach notification rule
   d. Electronic Health Care Transaction and Code Set standards

3. *[LO 3.1]* The HITECH Act provides all of the following EXCEPT ________.
   a. new breach notification requirements
   b. funding for experimental procedures
   c. higher monetary penalties for HIPAA violations
   d. greater privacy and security enforcement

4. *[LO 3.4]* The ________ is used to protect PHI from being accidentally released to those not needing the information during an appropriate use or disclosure.
   a. minimum necessary standard
   b. designated record set
   c. National Provider Identifier (NPI)
   d. maximum security standard

5. *[LO 3.4]* Individuals are permitted to ask for an accounting of the disclosures of their electronic protected health information, including TPO disclosures, over the preceding ________ years.
   a. two
   b. three
   c. five
   d. six

6. *[LO 3.5]* HIPAA security requirements state the administrative, technical, and ________ safeguards that are required to protect patients' electronic health information.
   a. personal
   b. clinical
   c. economic
   d. physical

7. *[LO 3.5]* ________ is the process of converting data into an unreadable format before it is distributed.
   a. Password
   b. Physical data
   c. Encryption
   d. PHI

8. *[LO 3.6]* Intentionally billing for services that were not performed or documented is an example of:
   a. abuse
   b. hacker
   c. fraud
   d. compliance

9. *[LO 3.2]* The ________ codes used in the United States are based on the *International Classification of Diseases* (ICD).
   a. diagnosis
   b. treatment
   c. procedure
   d. transaction

10. *[LO 3.7]* A compliance plan will have documentation requirements, a code of conduct, and a(n):
    a. audit plan
    b. coding plan
    c. breach plan
    d. fraud plan

SHORT-ANSWER QUESTIONS

Define the following abbreviations.

1. *[LO 3.3]* NPI ________________
2. *[LO 3.2]* ICD ________________
3. *[LO 3.4]* PHI ________________
4. *[LO 3.4]* NPP ________________
5. *[LO 3.4]* TPO ________________
6. *[LO 3.1]* HIPAA ________________
7. *[LO 3.1]* EIN ________________
8. *[LO 3.1]* HITECH ________________
9. *[LO 3.2]* CPT ________________
10. *[LO 3.2]* HCPCS ________________

APPLYING YOUR KNOWLEDGE

Working with HIPAA

3.1 *[LO 3.5, 3.8]* How is the HITECH breach notification rule an extension of the HIPAA Security Rule?

3.2 *[LO 3.4]* Based on your knowledge of the HIPAA Privacy Rule, do you think each of the following actions is compliant?

a. A medical insurance specialist does not disclose a patient's history of an eating disorder on a workers' compensation claim for a broken leg. Only the information the recipient needs to know is given.__________

b. A medical assistant faxes appropriate patient X-ray results before a scheduled surgery.__________

c. Unsupervised maintenance and housekeeping personnel are allowed into record storage and processing areas.__________

3.3 *[LO 3.8]* Identity theft occurs when a criminal uses another person's personal information to take on that person's identity. Any online transaction, such as online banking, increases an individual's risk of identity theft. In some cases, identity theft occurs when someone's medical information is stolen and misused. What are a number of ways in which a person's identity, such as a Social Security number in a medical record, could be stolen?

____

____

3.4 *[LO 3.4]* Which technology safeguard–administrative, physical, or technical–is represented by each of the following policies?

a. Each individual authorized to work with patient records has a unique password. __________

b. Access to the hospital's record storage area requires electronic fingerprinting. __________

c. Medical claims sent from the provider to the clearinghouse are encrypted. __________

d. Paper files scheduled for destruction are kept securely in an off-site location. __________

e. A provider's sanction policy states the consequences for violations of security policies and procedures by employees. __________

f. A medical office revises the data backup procedure that is used as part of normal business activities. __________

Composing a Breach Notification Letter

3.5 *[LO 3.8]* The following case describes an incident in which an office laptop containing personal health information for 2000 patients was stolen.

Case

On November 18, 2023, City Medical discovers that a laptop is missing from its office. Officials suspect that at least one new employee is behind the theft and that it occurred sometime after office hours the previous night. The unsecured PHI involved in the breach includes partial medical records of approximately two thousand patients input over the past year, containing the patients' names, addresses, dates of birth, clinical data, and about nine hundred Social Security numbers. Although the data are encrypted, Britney Blackwell, the compliance officer at City Medical, expresses concern that the employee suspected of stealing the laptop may be able to obtain help in exposing the information. City Medical is therefore offering credit protection monitoring free of charge for one year to all patients involved. Corecheck, a company that provides identity-theft protection services, will provide the monitoring. The toll-free number for Corecheck is 800-707-1000. City Medical has reported the theft to authorities and is doing everything it can to track down the missing laptop and the suspected employee. City Medical has also hired a company to perform thorough background checks of all employees in the future and is reviewing its policies with regard to technical safeguards. City Medical's toll-free number for any questions or concerns regarding the loss of personal information is 800-888-2909.

Based on the following template, compose a breach notification letter to be sent to all patients of City Medical whose data have been compromised. City Medical's address is 5001 Avenue K, Oakland, CA 94601. The letter is sent two days after the breach is discovered. The slanted brackets indicate where you are to supply the missing information.

Assume that the first patient to whom the letter is sent is:
Beverly Abbington
667 Oak Street
Oakland, CA 94601

<Letterhead of the organization, including address>

<Date of letter>

<Patient name>

<Patient address>

Dear <Patient name>:

This letter is to inform you that your personal health information on record with <Name of medical practice> was recently compromised. We first became aware of this breach on <Date>. We are notifying you and all others involved so that you can help ensure that this information is not used inappropriately.

<Provide the following details: (1) a brief description of what happened, including the date of the breach and the date of the discovery of the breach; (2) a description of the types of unsecured PHI that were involved in the breach; (3) the steps individuals should take to protect themselves from potential harm resulting from the breach; (4) a brief description of what the covered entity involved is doing to investigate the breach and to protect against any further breaches; (5) a toll-free telephone number or website for individuals to ask questions or learn additional information.>

<Name of medical practice> apologizes for any negative consequences this situation has brought about. We are hopeful that we can <name most likely solution to recovering the lost data>. Representatives are available twenty-four hours at our toll-free number to answer any questions you have. <Name of credit protection monitoring company> will help you in contacting the major credit bureaus to place a fraud alert on your credit report, order credit reports, and continue to monitor the reports. <Name of credit protection monitoring company> will also provide you with links to websites that offer information on what to do when personal information is compromised.

Sincerely,

<Name and title of appropriate contact person>

part two

Documenting Patient Encounters

chapter 4

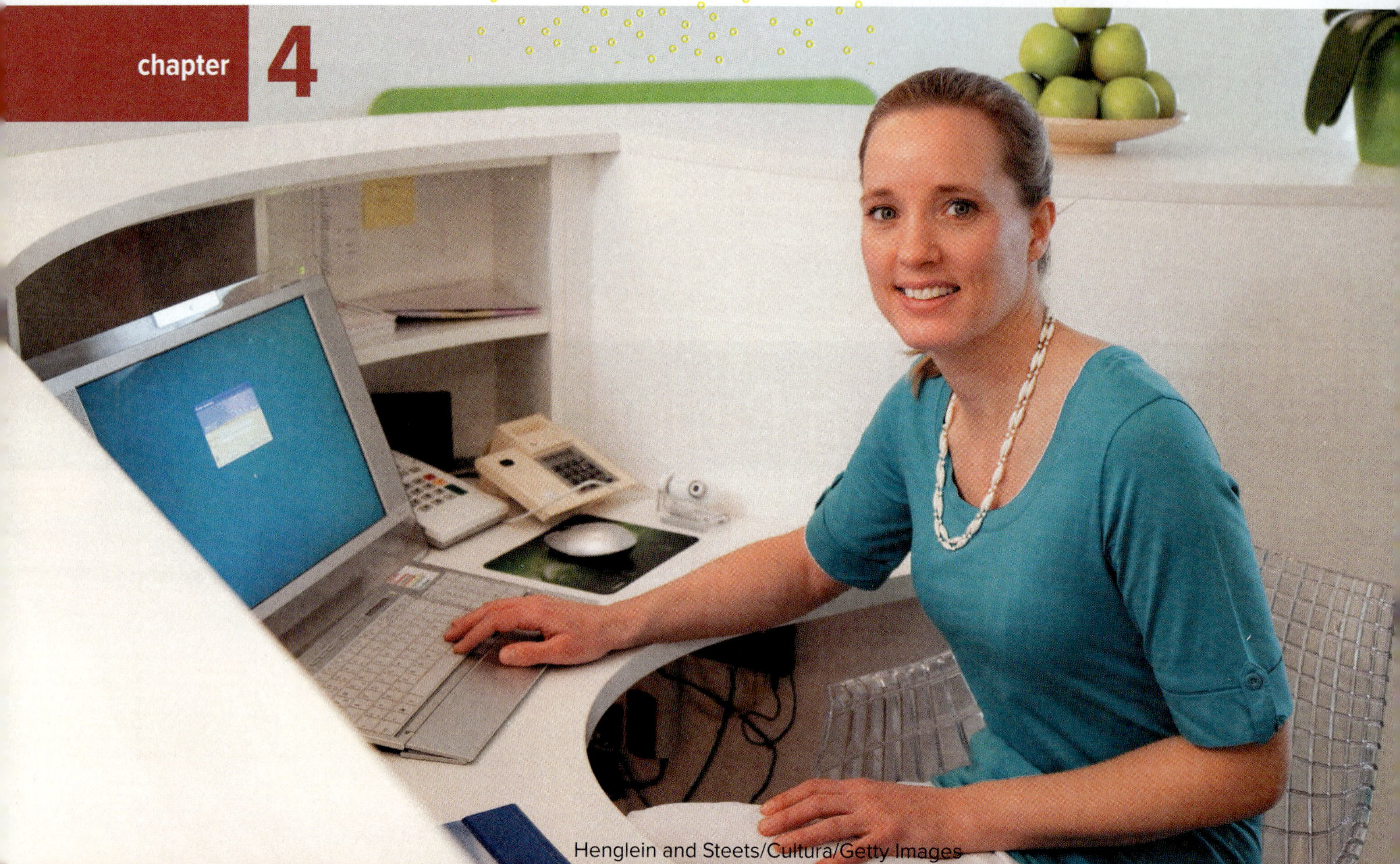

Henglein and Steets/Cultura/Getty Images

Scheduling

LEARNING OUTCOMES

When you finish this chapter, you will be able to:

4.1 Describe the primary methods used to schedule appointments.

4.2 Differentiate between new and established patients.

4.3 List the three categories of information new patients provide during telephone preregistration and demonstrate use of the patient scheduler.

4.4 Identify the information that needs to be verified for established patients when making an appointment.

4.5 Describe covered and noncovered services under medical insurance policies.

4.6 List the three main points to verify with the payer regarding a patient's benefits prior to a visit.

4.7 Explain when a preauthorization number or referral document is required for a patient's encounter.

Making Changes

As the receptionist, Laurie Harcourt does most of the scheduling for the Trilogy Family Care Center. The first call to the office this morning is from Mrs. Jones, who is very upset because she needs to reschedule her appointment again. "You know, I had a little accident and my daughter made me stop driving. Honestly, I don't blame her, but I hate having to depend on her to get me where I need to go." Laurie reassures Mrs. Jones that it's easy to reschedule her appointment on the computer. "Making changes to the schedule is getting easier and easier. In fact, patients can often reschedule their appointments using our new website."

In this chapter, you will learn to navigate the scheduler with confidence. In the example given above: How does ease of scheduling serve the office staff? How does it serve the patient?

4.1 Scheduling Methods

The first step in a patient encounter occurs when the patient contacts the medical office to make an appointment. If the appointment will be for the patient's first visit to the practice, this initial contact is the patient's first impression of the medical office. Registration staff help make this a good impression by having a caring attitude and being attentive to the patient's needs.

Creating a Schedule Matrix

Before patient appointments can be made, a practice must establish and maintain a *schedule matrix*. The **schedule matrix** is the framework that gives schedulers the parameters for scheduling appointments for each **provider,** such as:

- Provider start times (when the first patient can be scheduled in a day)
- Provider end times (when the last patient can be scheduled in a day)
- Lunch breaks
- Meeting breaks
- Vacation hours
- Administrative time
- Hospital rounds

schedule matrix schedule framework that provides parameters for scheduling appointments, such as blocking schedule times for office closures, meetings, or lunch

provider person or entity that supplies medical or health services and bills for or is paid for the services in the normal course of business; may be a professional member of the health care team, such as a physician, or a facility, such as a hospital or skilled nursing home

Imagine if these times were not blocked on the schedule! Schedulers would continually schedule patients at times when the provider is not available. To prevent scheduling issues, a designated person in the office is typically assigned to maintain the schedule matrix for long-term schedule blocks (opening, closing, lunch) and short-term or immediate blocks (emergencies, meetings). Figure 4.1 depicts an example of a schedule matrix with blocks in place for a meeting and lunch. This tells the scheduler that the provider is not available for appointments during those times.

Figure 4.1 Example of Schedule Matrix with Breaks

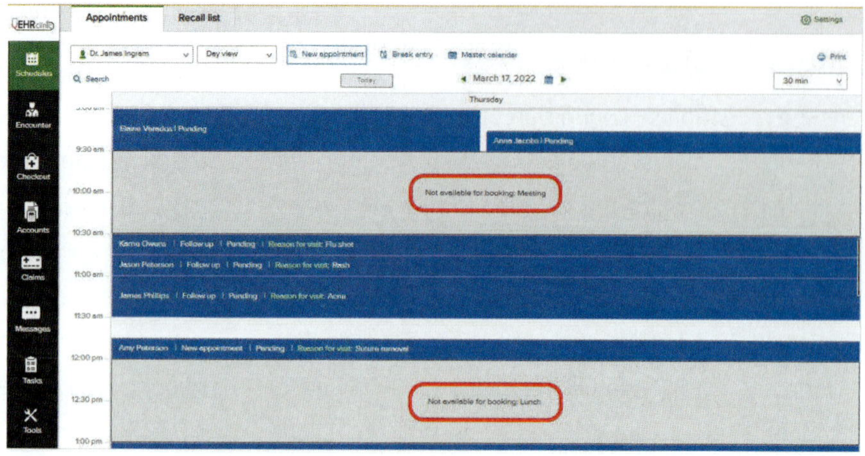

> ## TIP
> ### When Should a Schedule Matrix be Created?
> Consider that the purpose of the schedule matrix is to set parameters for each provider's schedule. Often, providers can schedule up to six months in advance, so it is necessary to have the schedule matrix built out at least that far. Start and end times, as well as lunches and standing meetings, can be added ahead of time to avoid having patients inappropriately scheduled. Other schedule breaks can be added whenever necessary.

EXERCISE 4.1

Maintain the Schedule Matrix

EHRclinic

You have been asked to assist the office manager at Trilogy Family Care Center with setting up a new provider's schedule matrix. You will be adding lunch, meeting, and hospital round breaks to build the new schedule.

Your instructor may assign this exercise to you in Connect. Exercise steps and EHRclinic Help Guides can be downloaded at www.mhhe.com/pmehr2.

EXERCISE 4.2

Schedule a Provider Meeting

EHRclinic

Once the schedule matrix has been built, you will be adding a staff meeting that is scheduled for every Friday afternoon from 4:00 to 5:00.

Your instructor may assign this exercise to you in Connect. Exercise steps and EHRclinic Help Guides can be downloaded at www.mhhe.com/pmehr2.

> ## EHRclinic TIP
> EHRclinic
> ### Managing Time in Schedules
> In breaks and patient schedules, time designations and durations can be set by using the increase and decrease buttons or by clicking directly on the hour or minute number and selecting a time increment.

Making Appointments via Telephone or Online

Although scheduling appointments online is becoming more common, patients often use the traditional method of telephoning to contact the office. The medical office keeps the electronic scheduling program open so that it is easy to access when a patient calls to make an appointment. The scheduling program is usually a separate but integrated part of the practice management or EHR program. It houses a calendar that can be set to display a provider's schedule for the day, the week, or the month (see Figure 4.2).

When a patient calls to schedule a new appointment, the receptionist or other member of the front desk staff views the scheduling program, selects a provider, and has instant access to an electronic calendar displaying the provider's schedule. The staff member then selects the open time slot on the calendar that best suits the patient, and the program blocks off that slot with the patient's name. If a patient calls to cancel or reschedule an appointment, the scheduler's search feature can be used to locate the original appointment and reschedule or cancel it in a matter of seconds.

More and more practices are using the Internet to communicate with their patients. Patient portals are websites that enable communication between patients and health care providers. The portals are designed to benefit both patients and health care providers by increasing efficiency and productivity. Using a secure user name and password, a patient can perform a variety of tasks, such as:

- Request an appointment
- Review lab results
- Review an account and make payments
- Request a prescription refill
- Complete registration forms
- Send secure messages to the provider

The patient portal is also used by providers to communicate with patients. For example, appointment reminders, test results, and messages

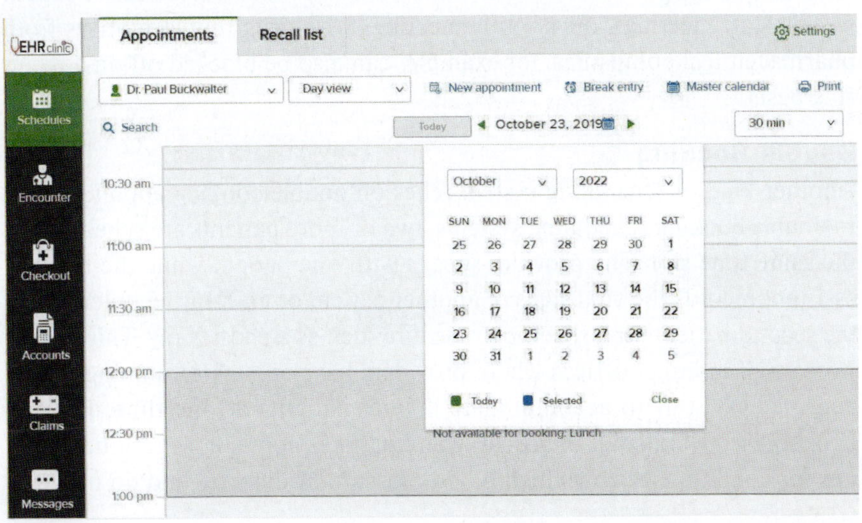

Figure 4.2 Sample Screen from Scheduling Program

can be sent to patients via the patient portal. If a practice has a patient portal, patients may have the option of making appointments online. They can view an electronic calendar showing available openings and select a time slot. Making appointments online reduces the amount of time the front desk staff spend scheduling, since appointments are initially made without their assistance. This information is transmitted to the office, and if it is approved by the scheduling system, the patient receives an email confirmation.

Scheduling Systems

Electronic schedulers can be set up to accommodate various types of scheduling systems. Examples of scheduling systems include open-hours scheduling, stream scheduling, double-booking, and wave scheduling. A good scheduling system maintains a consistent flow of patients to providers with a minimum amount of waiting time for patients. Depending on the type of facility, different scheduling systems work best.

Open Hours

In urgent care clinics and many walk-in clinics, patients may not have the option of making appointments. It is understood that they will be seen within a given window of time, say between the hours of 10:00 A.M. and 2:00 P.M., on a first-come, first-served basis—except in the case of an emergency. In this setting, the scheduler is set up using an open-hours scheduling system. The hours when a given provider is available to see patients is blocked off, and patients are added to the schedule as they arrive. Although the provider may have a steady stream of patients, the waiting time is often long because there are no prearranged appointments.

Stream Scheduling

Small medical practices commonly use a stream scheduling system, designed to give the provider a steady stream of patients throughout the day at regular, blocked-off intervals. The intervals are usually fifteen minutes long but can vary by practice. If an appointment, such as a physical exam, requires more than fifteen minutes, additional fifteen-minute slots are blocked off. Stream scheduling is used in the EHRclinic exercises in this text. Each patient is given a specific amount of time for an appointment based on the estimated length of time for the procedure. Time for lunch, weekly staff meetings, or monthly meetings with drug representatives from pharmaceutical companies, for example, can also be blocked off on a recurring basis.

Double-Booking

Another kind of scheduling system relies on double-booking appointments. In double-booking scheduling systems, two or more patients are scheduled in the same time slot. The provider speaks with one patient while the medical assistant records the vital signs of another patient or an X-ray technician sees the second patient for a specific procedure such as a chest X-ray. This system works well in larger offices where providers have enough examining rooms and medical staff to accommodate several patients at one time. Double-booking also works well in offices where patients come in for routine check-ups for conditions such as high blood pressure or diabetes and do not have

THINKING IT THROUGH 4.1

Why is it important to have both verbal and computer skills when scheduling patient appointments?

to see the physician each time. Consideration should be given to patients' chief complaints when double-booking appointments. For example, a routine physical exam can be double-booked with a patient who is complaining of a sore throat. It would not be ideal to book two lengthy or complicated appointments at once.

Wave Scheduling

In wave scheduling, patients are scheduled in waves at the beginning of each hour, with the rest of the hour left open. The patient who arrives first or has the most serious condition is usually seen first. Ideally, each member of the group for that hour is taken care of by the end of the hour, when the next wave arrives. Wave scheduling, like double-booking, is designed in part to accommodate patients who arrive late or do not show up (no-shows). Both types of scheduling also require a facility and staff that can accommodate several patients simultaneously. Otherwise, patients may become frustrated when they are not taken in the usual order and have to wait for stretches of time.

Regardless of the scheduling system used, every system should be evaluated regularly to make sure the average waiting time for patients is acceptable and to analyze whether medical staff and equipment are being used in the most efficient way. Electronic schedulers can be customized to accommodate any scheduling system a practice desires. In addition, electronic schedulers usually come with various reporting capabilities for analyzing the medical office's scheduling practices in order to help improve overall efficiency in scheduling.

4.2 New Versus Established Patients

When scheduling a patient appointment, it is important to determine whether the patient is new to the practice or is returning. Different information will be gathered in each case, and, for some procedures, different codes will be assigned. A **new patient (NP)** is someone who has not received any services from the provider (or another provider of the same specialty who is a member of the same practice) within the past three years. A returning patient is called an **established patient (EP).** This patient has seen the provider (or another provider in the practice who has the same specialty) within the past three years.

New patients complete many forms before their first appointment. Established patients review and update the information that is already on file about them. Figure 4.3 illustrates how to decide which category—new or established—fits the patient. Some of this information may be obtained over the phone while the patient is scheduling the appointment or online if the practice has a secure website. The process of gathering new patient information before an appointment is known as **preregistration.**

new patient (NP) a patient who has not received professional services from a provider (or another provider with the same specialty in the same practice) within the past three years

established patient (EP) patient who has received professional services from a provider (or another provider with the same specialty in the same practice) within the past three years

preregistration the process of gathering basic contact, insurance, and reason for visit information before a new patient comes into the office for an encounter

THINKING IT THROUGH 4.2

If a returning patient telephones to make an appointment for her young daughter who has not yet been seen by any of the practice's providers, is the daughter listed as a new or an established patient? Explain your answer.

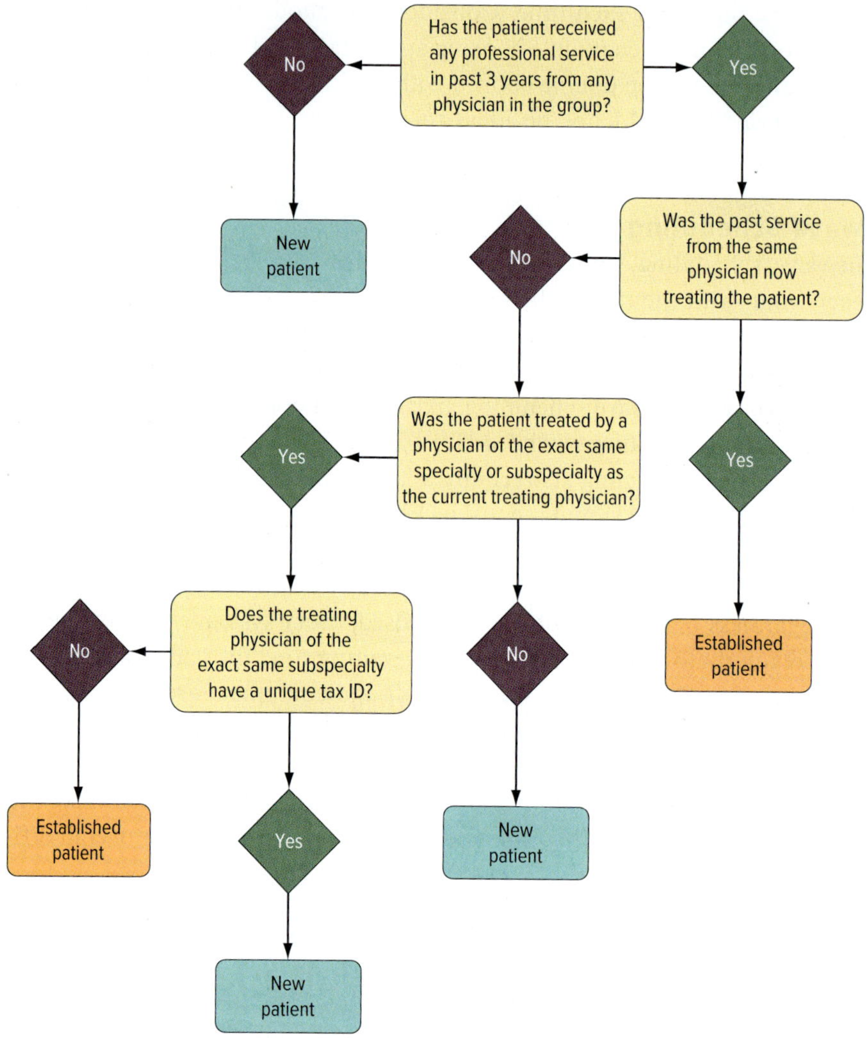

Figure 4.3 Decision Tree for New Versus Established Patients

4.3 Preregistration for New Patients

During preregistration, new patients usually provide three types of information: patient demographics, basic insurance information, and the reason for the visit, also known as the chief complaint.

Gathering Patient Demographics

demographics various identifying characteristics of an individual, such as a patient's name, date of birth, address, telephone number, and gender

Basic identifying information about the patient, known as patient **demographics,** is obtained first. Patient demographics include the person's:

- Name
- Address
- Gender

THINKING IT THROUGH 4.3

During preregistration, why is it important for the physician practice's health care team to be knowledgeable about the practice's participation with different insurance carriers?

- Date of birth
- Home, work, and cell telephone numbers
- Email address

Additional details about the patient, such as marital status, Social Security number, and a contact person, are normally obtained during registration at the time of the appointment.

As the new patient is being added to the system, the EHR will automatically generate a unique chart number. This number identifies the patient's account and does not change. Often, the **chart number** is used to find patient information in the EHR and to identify patients for billing, documents, orders, and files.

chart number unique alphanumeric code that identifies a patient

participating (PAR) provider a provider who agrees to provide medical services to a payer's policyholders according to the terms of the plan's contract

nonparticipating (nonPAR) provider a provider who chooses not to join a particular government or other health plan

Gathering Insurance Information

If the patient has health insurance, basic information about the insurance is also gathered during preregistration, including the:

- Name of the patient's health plan
- Plan member's identification number
- Name of the policyholder, who may be the patient, a spouse, a divorced spouse, a guardian, or another relation
- Name of the guarantor, which is the individual who agrees to accept financial responsibility for a patient (often the policyholder)
- Type of plan, and whether a copay is required
- Name of the referring physician, if the patient was referred by another physician

Before deciding to make an appointment, a new patient may need information about provider participation in a health insurance plan. Members of the medical administrative team need to know which plans their providers participate in. In most managed care insurance plans, patients are required to use network physicians to avoid paying higher charges. For this reason, patients check whether the provider is a **participating (PAR) provider** in their health plan. When patients see **nonparticipating (nonPAR) providers,** they must pay more–a higher copayment, greater coinsurance, or both–so a patient may choose not to make an appointment because of the additional expense.

Recording the Reason for the Visit

When scheduling a patient's appointment, in addition to gathering personal and insurance information, it is important to establish the reason for the patient's visit. The reason for the visit will determine the length of time required for the appointment. A complete physical exam for a new patient may require forty-five minutes or an hour, whereas a follow-up visit for a bladder infection may require only fifteen minutes. Many providers require that new patients come in for a complete physical before they will provide other routine services. In most electronic schedulers, the length of time required for a procedure can be set up in the practice management program's database along with the procedure code and description.

TIP

Documenting Appointments

As is true of other aspects of a patient visit, it is important to document appointments carefully and consistently. The practice should keep a permanent record of all appointments, including cancellations, walk-ins, emergencies, and no-shows. If a legal issue arises—for example, if a provider is accused of neglect—the record of appointments can be used to prove that a patient was or was not seen, how many times a patient canceled an appointment or did not show up, and whether the patient or the practice attempted to reschedule. Traditionally, a paper sign-in sheet was used for this purpose. Today, electronic schedulers are designed to keep track of all appointments and changes made to them.

EXERCISE 4.3 **Schedule a New Patient**

EHRclinic

A patient calls to schedule an appointment for a complete physical exam, and she states that she has never been seen by the provider. Create a new patient registration in EHRclinic, record her insurance information, and schedule the appointment.

Your instructor may assign this exercise to you in Connect. Exercise steps and EHRclinic Help Guides can be downloaded at www.mhhe.com/pmehr2.

4.4 Appointments for Established Patients

As discussed earlier in this chapter, an established patient is one who has been seen by a provider within a practice within the past three years. Because established patients have a recent history with the practice, front desk staff will have some information on file, although it is still important to confirm its accuracy.

Scheduling Appointments for Established Patients

When an established patient contacts the office for an appointment, the members of the front desk staff verify that the information they have on file for the patient is still correct. In particular, it is important to note changes to demographics, such as a patient's address or phone number. If the electronic scheduling program is integrated with the practice management program, simple changes to a patient's address are usually made in the scheduler and are automatically carried over to the practice management program. More detailed changes, such as changes to a patient's health plan or employment, need to be made in the practice management program.

The front desk staff member also inquires about the reason for the visit so that the correct amount of time can be blocked off for the encounter. The office may want to know whether the patient is carrying a balance on his or her account. Most practice management programs contain reports that will identify patients with upcoming appointments who have overdue balances. Patients are increasingly paying for a greater percentage of their health care bills. Medical practices, in response, have had to assume a greater role in monitoring and collecting overdue amounts from patients. A patient who is late in paying can be reminded of the amount due while on the phone or via an email message and can be asked to take care of it during the upcoming visit.

EXERCISE 4.4

Schedule an Established Patient

EHRclinic

A patient calls to schedule an appointment and confirms being seen by a provider at Trilogy Family Care Center within the last three years. Schedule an appointment for this established patient.

Your instructor may assign this exercise to you in Connect. Exercise steps and EHRclinic Help Guides can be downloaded at www.mhhe.com/pmehr2.

Booking Follow-Up and Repeating Appointments

Some patients need either follow-up or repeating appointments. Follow-up appointments are scheduled at a certain time in the future. For example, suppose a physician would like a patient to return for a checkup in three weeks. Repeating appointments occur at the same time for a limited period of time. For example, a patient may need an appointment once a month for three months to monitor the effectiveness of a new medication.

EXERCISE 4.5

Add Patients to the Schedule

EHRclinic

You are working at the front desk at Trilogy Family Care Center. Several patients are checking out and need to schedule follow-up appointments. Schedule future appointments for these patients.

Your instructor may assign this exercise to you in Connect. Exercise steps and EHRclinic Help Guides can be downloaded at www.mhhe.com/pmehr2.

EXERCISE 4.6

Schedule a Recurring Appointment

EHRclinic

A patient who is checking out needs to be seen for blood pressure checks every Friday for the next four weeks. Schedule the recurring appointments for this patient.

Your instructor may assign this exercise to you in Connect. Exercise steps and EHRclinic Help Guides can be downloaded at www.mhhe.com/pmehr2.

Rescheduling, Canceling, and No-Show Appointments

Both new and established patients often schedule appointments and later need to reschedule or cancel them. This occurs for a variety of reasons, such as a scheduling conflict or the issue the appointment was made for has resolved.

Rescheduling an appointment refers to a patient who contacts the office to change the date and/or time of an existing appointment. When an appointment is canceled, on the other hand, a new appointment is not made in its place at the same time.

It is important that patients are encouraged to call in advance if they need to reschedule or cancel their appointments. This opens the appointment on the provider's schedule so it can be booked by another patient. If a patient does not call to reschedule or cancel and does not arrive to a scheduled appointment, it is called a *no-show.* No-show appointments should be documented in the patient's chart for liability and tracking purposes. This identifies that a patient did not arrive for scheduled medical care or treatment, and it also identifies a pattern of behavior if it occurs repeatedly.

EXERCISE 4.7

Cancel a Patient's Appointment

EHRclinic

A patient calls to say that she has a schedule conflict and is unable to keep her appointment. She will call back to schedule a new one. Cancel this patient's appointment in EHRclinic.

Your instructor may assign this exercise to you in Connect. Exercise steps and EHRclinic Help Guides can be downloaded at www.mhhe.com/pmehr2.

EXERCISE 4.8

Reschedule a Patient's Appointment

EHRclinic

A patient calls to say that he would like to change his appointment day and time. Reschedule this patient's appointment in EHRclinic.

Your instructor may assign this exercise to you in Connect. Exercise steps and EHRclinic Help Guides can be downloaded at www.mhhe.com/pmehr2.

EXERCISE 4.9

Chart a No-Show

EHRclinic

A patient does not show for his appointment, and he did not call to cancel or reschedule. Document this patient's no-show appointment in EHRclinic.

Your instructor may assign this exercise to you in Connect. Exercise steps and EHRclinic Help Guides can be downloaded at www.mhhe.com/pmehr2.

Creating a Patient Recall List

Medical offices often must keep track of patients who need to return for future appointments. Some offices schedule future appointments when the patient is leaving the office. For example, if a patient has just seen a physician and needs to return for a follow-up appointment in six weeks, the

Figure 4.4 Sample Recall List

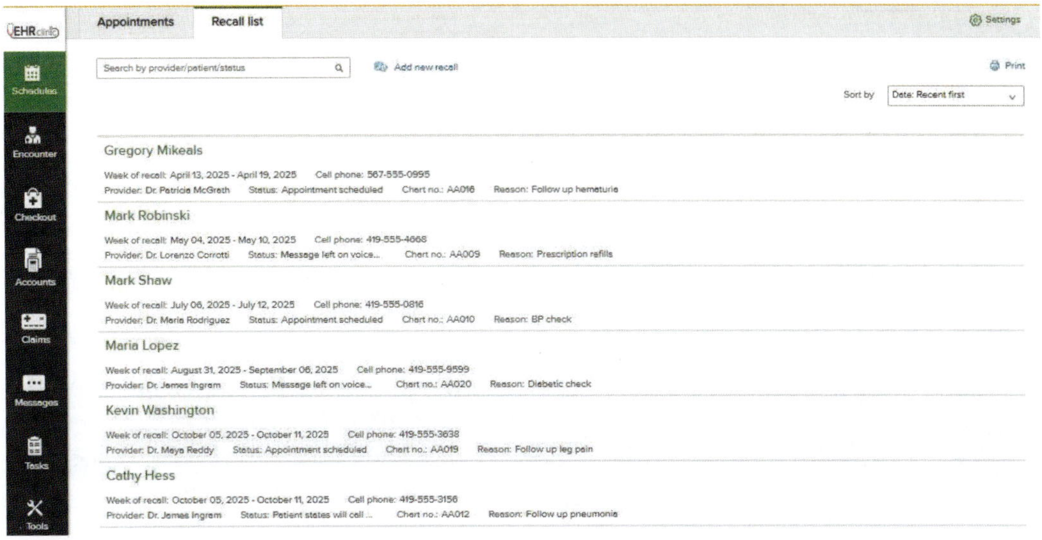

appointment is usually made before the patient leaves the office. However, when the appointment is needed further in the future, such as one year later, it is not always practical to set up the appointment. It is difficult for the patient and the physician to know their schedules a year in advance. For this reason, many offices keep a list of patients who need to be contacted for future appointments, commonly referred to as a *recall list*. As shown in Figure 4.4, the recall list reminds schedulers to contact patients, at which time the status can be updated for documentation.

EXERCISE 4.10

Maintain the Patient Recall List

EHRclinic

Your office manager has asked you to contact patients who are on the recall list and add some new patients for reminders about future appointments. Update the patient recall list with this information.

Your instructor may assign this exercise to you in Connect. Exercise steps and EHRclinic Help Guides can be downloaded at www.mhhe.com/pmehr2.

Printing Schedules

While provider schedules can be viewed from within the PM or EHR system, most medical offices still print schedules on a daily basis. In EHRclinic, schedules can be printed for individual providers or as a group schedule from the Master Calendar (see Figure 4.5)

EXERCISE 4.11

Print the Provider's Schedule

EHRclinic

Dr. Williams called the practice this morning and said that she will not be in due to a family emergency. Block her available time slots and print the provider's list-view schedule and the master practice schedule so today's appointments can be rescheduled with another provider or with Dr. Williams for another day.

Your instructor may assign this exercise to you in Connect. Exercise steps and EHRclinic Help Guides can be downloaded at www.mhhe.com/pmehr2.

Figure 4.5 Printing Schedules in EHRclinic

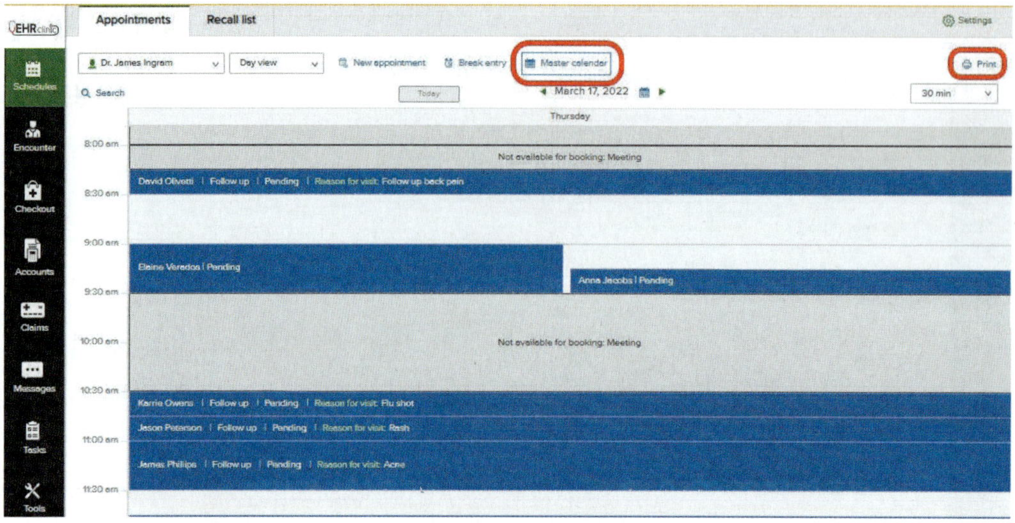

4.5 Insurance Basics

To be paid for services, medical practices need to establish financial responsibility for each visit. Although some patients pay the costs of medical care directly, the costs of most medical services are covered, in part or in full, by medical insurance. Data from the U.S. Census Bureau reports that 92% of people in the United States (about 326 million people) have some sort of health insurance through either their employers, direct-purchase, or government programs.

The first step in establishing financial responsibility for insured patients is to verify the patient's eligibility. This is done by obtaining answers to questions such as:

- Has the policyholder paid the latest premium?
- What are the billing rules of the plan?
- What is the patient responsible for paying?
- What services are covered under the plan, and what medical conditions establish medical necessity for these services?
- What services are not covered?

Knowing the answers to these questions is essential in order to correctly bill payers for patients' covered services. This knowledge is also needed to determine what patients are responsible for so that they can be asked to pay their bills when benefits do not apply. To be able to answer questions about patients' benefits, the medical administrative team needs to be familiar with the basic terminology of medical insurance policies, what a standard set of health care benefits normally includes, and the types of insurance plans available.

medical insurance financial plan that covers the cost of hospital and medical care

policyholder person who buys an insurance plan; the insured, subscriber, or guarantor

health plan an individual or group plan that either provides or pays for the cost of medical care; includes group health plans, health insurance issuers, health maintenance organizations, Medicare Part A and B, Medicaid, TRICARE, and other government and nongovernment plans

payer health plan or program

premium money the insured pays to a health plan for a health care policy; usually paid monthly

benefits the amount of money a health plan pays for services covered in an insurance policy

Medical Insurance Policies

What is medical insurance? **Medical insurance** (health insurance) is a written policy between an individual or entity, called the **policyholder,** and a **health plan**—an insurance company or government program that is the **payer.** The policyholder pays a specified amount of money, usually monthly, called a **premium.** In exchange, the payer provides **benefits**—defined by America's Health Insurance Plans (AHIP) as payments for covered medical services—for a specific period of time.

THINKING IT THROUGH 4.4

Imagine a telephone call with an established patient prior to the use of electronic schedulers. A traditional paper calendar is being used to set up an appointment. Now picture a contemporary office. How has using a computer changed the amount of information documented before a patient visit?

There are actually three participants in the medical insurance relationship. The patient (policyholder) is the first party, and the physician is the second party. Legally, a patient–physician contract is created when a physician agrees to treat a patient who is seeking medical services. Through this unwritten contract, the patient is legally responsible for paying for services. The patient may have a policy with a health plan, the third party, that agrees to carry some of the risk of paying for those services and therefore is called a third-party payer.

The major types of third-party payers are:

- *Private payers:* Nationwide insurance companies that dominate the national market offer all types of health plans. They include such companies as WellPoint, UnitedHealth Group, Aetna, Kaiser Permanente, and the member companies of the Blue Cross and Blue Shield Association.
- *Self-funded health plans:* These are health plans set up by employers that assume the risk of paying directly for medical services.
- *Government-sponsored health care programs:* Four major government-sponsored health care programs offer benefits for which various groups in the population are eligible.
    - Medicare is a 100 percent federally funded health plan that covers people who are sixty-five and over and those who are disabled or have permanent kidney failure (end-stage renal disease, or ESRD).
    - Medicaid, a federal program that is jointly funded by the federal and state governments, covers low-income people who cannot afford medical care. Each state administers its own Medicaid program, determining the program's qualifications and benefits under broad federal guidelines.
    - TRICARE, a Department of Defense program, covers medical expenses for active-duty members. known as **sponsors,** of the uniformed services and their spouses, children, and other dependents; retired military personnel and their dependents; and family members of deceased active-duty personnel.
    - CHAMPVA, the Civilian Health and Medical Program of the Department of Veterans Affairs, covers veterans with permanent service-related disabilities and their dependents. It also covers surviving spouses and dependent children of veterans who died from service-related disabilities.

sponsor in TRICARE, the active-duty service member

schedule of benefits list of the medical expenses that a health plan covers

Health Care Benefits

Although most plans contain standard benefits for inpatient and outpatient care, the amount the patient owes for different services varies depending on the type of plan. The medical insurance policy for each health plan contains a **schedule of benefits** that summarizes the payments that may be made for medically necessary medical services. Figure 4.6 illustrates the range of benefits included in a popular managed care plan.

Standard Benefits

This is a preferred provider organization (PPO) plan. That means members can receive the highest level of benefits when they use any of the more than 5,000 physicians and other health care professionals in this network. When members receive covered in-network services, they simply pay a copayment. Members can also receive care from providers that are not part of the network, however benefits are often lower and covered claims are subject to deductible, coinsurance and charges above the maximum allowable amount. Referrals are not needed from a Primary Care Physician to receive care from a specialist.

PREVENTIVE CARE	In-Network	Out-of-Network
Well child care		
Birth through 12 years	OV Copayment	Deductible & Coinsurance
All others	OV Copayment	Deductible & Coinsurance
Periodic, routine health examinations	OV Copayment	Deductible & Coinsurance
Routine eye exams	OV Copayment	Deductible & Coinsurance
Routine OB/GYN visits	OV Copayment	Deductible & Coinsurance
Mammography	No Charge	Deductible & Coinsurance
Hearing Screening	OV Copayment	Deductible & Coinsurance
MEDICAL CARE	**In-Network**	**Out-of-Network**
PCP office visits	OV Copayment	Deductible & Coinsurance
Specialist office visits	OV Copayment	Deductible & Coinsurance
Outpatient mental health & substance abuse – *prior authorization required*	OV Copayment	Deductible & Coinsurance
Maternity care – *initial visit subject to copayment, no charge thereafter*	OV Copayment	Deductible & Coinsurance
Diagnostic lab, x-ray and testing	No Charge	Deductible & Coinsurance
High-cost outpatient diagnostics – *prior authorization required. The following are subject to copayment: MRI, MRA, CAT, CTA, PET, SPECT scans*	No Charge OR $200 Copayment	Deductible & Coinsurance Deductible & Coinsurance
Allergy Services		
Office visits/testing	OV Copayment	Deductible & Coinsurance
Injections – *90 visits in 3 years*	$25 Copayment	Deductible & Coinsurance
HOSPITAL CARE – Prior authorization required	**In-Network**	**Out-of-Network**
Semi-private room *(General/Medical/Surgical/Maternity)*	HSP Copayment	Deductible & Coinsurance
Skilled nursing facility – *up to 120 days per calendar year*	HSP Copayment	Deductible & Coinsurance
Rehabilitative services – *up to 60 days per calendar year*	No Charge	Deductible & Coinsurance
Outpatient surgery – *in a hospital or surgi-center*	OS Copayment	Deductible & Coinsurance
EMERGENCY CARE	**In-Network**	**Out-of-Network**
Walk-in centers	OV Copayment	Deductible & Coinsurance
Urgent care centers – *at participating centers only*	UR Copayment	Not Covered
Emergency care – *copayment waived if admitted*	ER Copayment	ER Copayment
Ambulance	No Charge	No Charge
OTHER HEALTH CARE	**In-Network**	**Out-of-Network**
Outpatient rehabilitative services – *30 visits maximum for PT, OT, and ST per year, 20 visit maximum for Chiro, per year*	OV Copayment	Deductible & Coinsurance
Durable medical equipment/Prosthetic devices – *Unlimited maximum per calendar year*	No Charge OR 20%	Deductible & Coinsurance
Infertility Services (diagnosis and treatment)	Not Covered	Not Covered
Home Health Care	No Charge	$50 Deductible & 20% Coinsurance

KEY: Office Visit (OV) Copayment; Hospital (HSP) Copayment; Emergency Room (ER) Copayment; Outpatient Surgery (OS) Copayment; Urgent Care (UR) Copayment

PREVENTIVE CARE SCHEDULES

Well Child Care (including immunizations)
- 6 exams, birth to age 1
- 6 exams, ages 1–5
- 1 exam every 2 years, ages 6–10
- 1 exam every year, ages 11–21

Adult Exams
- 1 exam every 5 years, ages 22–29
- 1 exam every 3 years, ages 30–39
- 1 exam every 2 years, ages 40–49
- 1 exam every year, ages 50+

Mammography
- 1 baseline screening, ages 35–39
- 1 screening per year, ages 40+

Vision Exams
- 1 exam every 2 calendar years

Hearing Exams
- 1 exam per calendar year

OB/GYN Exams
- 1 exam per calendar year

Figure 4.6 Example of Range of Benefits for a Popular Plan

The payer's definition of *medical necessity* is the key to coverage and payment. A medically necessary service is reasonable and is consistent with generally accepted professional medical standards for the diagnosis or treatment of illness or injury. Payers scrutinize the need for medical procedures, examining each bill to make sure it meets their medical necessity guidelines.

The provider of the service must also meet the payer's professional standards. Providers include physicians, nurse-practitioners, physician assistants, therapists, hospitals, laboratories, long-term care facilities, and suppliers such as pharmacies and medical supply companies.

Covered Services

Covered services are listed on the schedule of benefits. They may include primary care, emergency care, medical specialists' services, and surgery. Coverage of some services is mandated by state or federal law; coverage of others is optional. Some policies provide benefits only for loss resulting from illnesses or diseases, while others also cover accidents or injuries. The policies of many managed care plans, such as the one illustrated in Figure 4.6, also cover **preventive medical services,** such as annual physical examinations, pediatric and adolescent immunizations, prenatal care, and routine screening procedures. Not all services that are covered have the same benefits; for example, a policy may pay a smaller proportion of the charges for vision or hearing services. Many services are also limited in frequency. A payer may cover just three physical therapy treatments for a condition, or a certain screening test every five years, not every year. In the example shown in Figure 4.6, the outpatient rehabilitative services for physical, occupational, and speech therapy are limited to thirty visits per year.

covered services medical procedures and treatments that are included as benefits under an insured's health plan

preventive medical services care that is provided to keep patients healthy or to prevent illness, such as routine checkups and screening tests

noncovered services medical procedures that are not included in a plan's benefits

preexisting condition illness or disorder of a beneficiary that existed before the effective date of insurance coverage

Noncovered Services

The medical insurance policy also describes **noncovered services**–those for which it does not pay. Such excluded services may include all or some of the following:

- Most medical policies do not cover dental services, eye examinations or eyeglasses, employment-related injuries, cosmetic procedures, infertility services, or experimental procedures.
- Policies may exclude specific items such as vocational rehabilitation or surgical treatment of obesity.
- Some policies do not have prescription drug benefits.

In the past, if a new policyholder had a medical condition that was diagnosed before the policy took effect–known as a **preexisting condition**–medical services to treat it were often not covered. Under the Affordable Care Act, insurers can no longer deny health coverage for people with preexisting conditions, subject them to waiting periods, or charge more for them.

Types of Health Care Plans

All health plans are based on one of the two essential types of insurance, indemnity and managed care. Knowing which type of plan a patient has is an indicator of the type of benefits the patient has, as well as of how much the plan is likely to pay for covered services. Chapter 12 explains health care plans in detail and the different methods of reimbursement used by each. This section introduces the different types of plans as they relate to understanding a patient's basic set of benefits.

Figure 4.7 Trends in Health Plan Enrollment

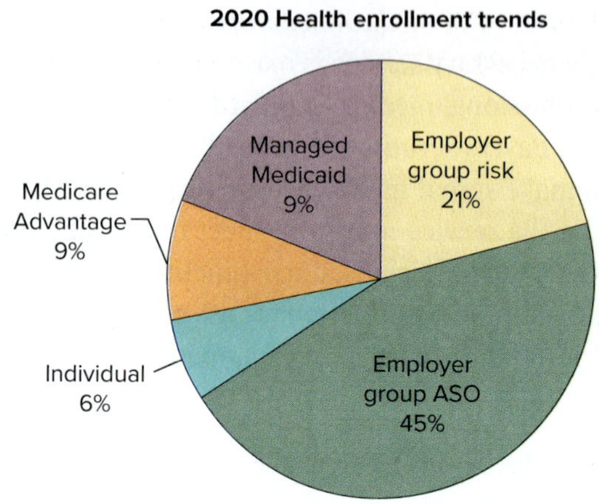

indemnity plan type of medical insurance that reimburses a policyholder for medical services under the terms of its schedule of benefits

deductible an amount that an insured person must pay, usually on an annual basis, for health care services before a health plan's payment begins

coinsurance the portion of charges that an insured person must pay for health care services after payment of the deductible amount; usually stated as a percentage

Indemnity

Indemnity is protection against loss. Under an **indemnity plan,** the payer indemnifies the policyholder against the costs of medical services and procedures as listed on the benefits schedule. Patients choose the providers they wish to see. The physician usually sends the health care claim–the formal insurance claim that reports data about the patient and the services provided by the physician–to the payer on behalf of the patient. Figure 4.7 shows the enrollment trends for the different types of health plans.

> **TIP**
>
> **Filing Claims for Patients**
>
> The provider usually bills the insurance company for patients. Patients are generally more satisfied with their medical encounters when billing is done for them, and the provider receives payment more quickly.

Conditions for Payment Four conditions must be met before the insurance company will make a payment on a claim processed by an indemnity plan:

1. The medical charge must be for medically necessary services that are covered by the insured's health plan.
2. The patient's payment of the premium–the periodic payment the patient is required to make to keep the policy in effect–must be up-to-date. Unless the premium is current, the patient is not eligible for benefits, and the insurance company will not make any payment.
3. If it is part of the policy, the **deductible**–the amount that the insured pays on covered services before benefits begin–must have been paid. Deductibles range widely, usually between two hundred dollars and thousands of dollars annually. Higher deductibles generally mean lower premiums.
4. Any **coinsurance**–the percentage of each claim that the insured pays–that is due must be taken into account. The coinsurance rate, such as 80-20, states the health plan's percentage of the charge, followed by

the insured's percentage. This means that the plan pays 80 percent of the covered amount and the patient pays 20 percent after the premiums and deductibles are paid. The formula is as follows:

Charge − Deductible − Coinsurance = Health plan payment

Example An indemnity policy states that the deductible is the first $200 in covered annual medical fees and that the coinsurance rate is 80–20. A patient whose first medical charge of the year was $2,000 would owe $560:

EXAMPLE

Charge	$2,000
Patient owes the deductible	200
Balance	1,800
Patient also owes coinsurance (20 percent of the balance)	360
Total balance due from patient	$200 + $360 = $ 560

In this case, the patient must pay an **out-of-pocket** expense of $560 this year before benefits begin. The health plan will pay $1,440, or 80 percent of the balance, after the deductible has been met:

out-of-pocket expenses the insured must pay before benefits begin (deductible) or as a portion of cost-sharing (coinsurance)

managed care system that combines the financing and delivery of appropriate, cost-effective health care services to its members

EXAMPLE

Charge	$2,000
Patient payment (deductible and 20% coinsurance)	− 560
Health plan payment	$1,440

If the patient has already met the annual deductible, the patient's benefits apply to the charge, as in this example:

EXAMPLE

Charge	$2,000
Patient coinsurance (20 percent)	400
Health plan payment (80 percent)	$1,600

Fee-for-Service Payment Approach Indemnity plans usually reimburse medical costs on a *fee-for-service* basis. The fee-for-service payment method is retroactive; the fee is paid after the patient receives services from the physician (see Figure 4.8).

Managed Care

The other type of insurance plan available is a managed care plan. **Managed care** offers a more restricted choice of (and access to) providers and treatments in exchange for lower premiums, deductibles, and other charges than

Figure 4.8 Payment Under Fee-for-Service

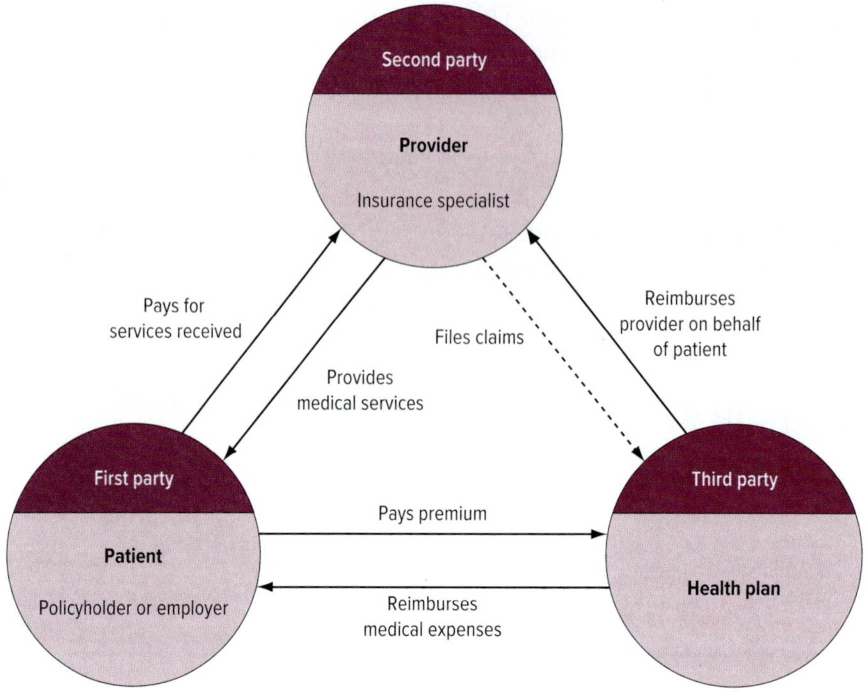

does traditional indemnity insurance. This approach to insurance combines the financing and management of health care with the delivery of services. A managed care organization (MCO) establishes links between provider, patient, and payer. Instead of only the patient having a policy with the health plan, the provider also has an agreement with the MCO. This arrangement gives the MCO more control over what services the provider performs and the fees for the services.

Managed care plans, first introduced in California in 1929, are now the predominant type of insurance. Over 90 percent of all insured employees are enrolled in some type of managed care plan, and thousands of different plans are offered. The basic types are health maintenance organizations (HMOs), point-of-service (POS) plans, preferred provider organizations (PPOs), and consumer-driven health plans (CDHPs).

In addition to ensuring correct billing and reimbursement for the services provided, being familiar with the different types of managed care plans is the best way to help patients obtain the highest level of care they are entitled to under their current plan. Descriptions of the four different types of managed care follow.

Health Maintenance Organizations

A health maintenance organization (HMO) combines coverage of medical costs and delivery of health care for a prepaid premium. In an effort to control costs and provide affordable insurance coverage options, most health insurance carriers offer some types of HMO options.

> **TIP**
>
> **Participation as a Provider**
>
> *Participation* means that a provider has contracted with a health plan to provide services to the plan's beneficiaries. Participation brings benefits, such as more patients, as well as contractual duties and, usually, reduced fees.

The HMO creates a network of physicians, hospitals, and other providers by employing them or negotiating contracts with them. The HMO then enrolls members in a health plan under which they use the services of those network providers. In most states, HMOs are licensed and are legally required to provide certain services to members and their dependents. Preventive care as appropriate for each age group is often required, such as immunizations and well-baby checkups for infants and screening mammograms for women.

Capitation in HMOs Capitation (from *capit,* Latin for *head*) is a fixed prepayment to a medical provider for all necessary contracted services provided to each patient who is a plan member (see Figure 4.9). The capitated rate is a prospective payment–it is determined before the patient visit, and it covers a specific period of time. The health plan makes the payment whether the patient receives many or no medical services during the specified period.

In capitation, the physician agrees to share the risk that an insured person will use more services than the fee covers. The physician also shares in the

EXAMPLE

A family physician has a contract for a capitated payment of \$40 a month for each of a hundred patients in a plan. This \$4,000 monthly fee (\$40 × 100 patients = \$4,000) covers all office visits from all the patients. If half of the patients see the physician once during a given month, the provider in effect receives \$80 for each visit (\$4,000 divided by 50 visits). If, however, half of the patients see the physician four times in a month, the average fee is \$4,000 divided by 200 visits, or \$20 for each visit.

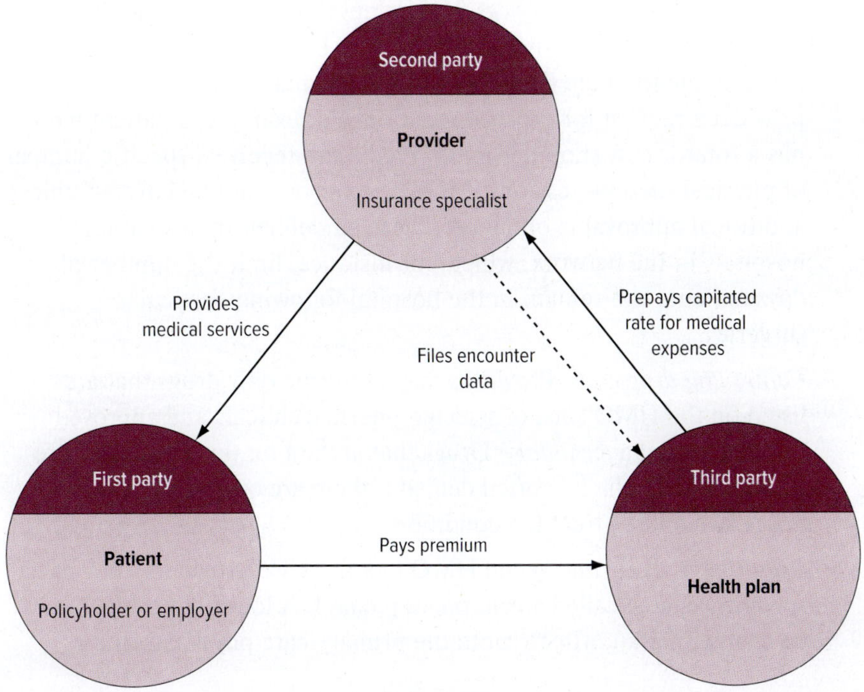

Figure 4.9 Payment Under Capitation

prospect that an insured person will use fewer services. In fee-for-service, the more patients the provider sees, the more charges the health plan reimburses. In capitation, the payment remains the same, and the provider risks receiving lower per-visit revenue.

A patient is enrolled in a capitated health plan for a specific time period, such as a month, a quarter, or a year. The capitated rate, which is called *per member per month (PMPM),* is usually based on the health-related characteristics of the enrollees, such as age and gender. The health plan analyzes these factors and sets a rate based on its prediction of the amount of health care each person will need. The capitated rate of prepayment covers only services listed on the schedule of benefits for the plan. The provider may bill the patient for any other services.

Medical Management Practices in HMOs Health maintenance organizations seek to control rising medical costs and at the same time improve health care. An HMO uses the following cost-containment methods:

- *Restricting patients' choice of providers:* After enrolling in an HMO, members must receive services from the network of physicians, hospitals, and other providers who are employed by or under contract to the HMO. Visits to **out-of-network** providers are not covered, except for emergency care or urgent health problems that arise when the member is temporarily away from the geographical service area.
- *Requiring preauthorization for services:* HMOs often require **preauthorization** (also called *precertification* or *prior authorization*) before the patient receives many types of services. Services that are not preauthorized are not covered. Preauthorization is almost always needed for nonemergency hospital admission, and it is usually required within a certain number of days after an emergency admission. It is also usually required for outpatient behavioral health care, including mental health care and substance abuse services.
- *Controlling the use of services:* HMOs develop medical necessity guidelines for the use of medical services. The HMO holds the provider accountable for a questionable service and may deny a patient's or provider's request for preauthorization. For example, a patient who has a rotator cuff shoulder injury repair can receive a specific number of physical therapy sessions. More sessions will not be covered unless additional approval is obtained. These guidelines are also applied to hospitals in the network, which, for instance, limit the number of days patients can remain in the hospital following particular surgeries.
- *Controlling drug costs:* Providers may prescribe only drugs that are listed on the HMO's list of selected pharmaceuticals and approved dosages, called a *formulary.* Drugs that are not on the list require preauthorization, which is often denied if there are other cost-effective drugs available to treat the condition.
- *Requiring cost-sharing:* When HMO members see providers, they pay a specified charge called a **copayment (copay).** A lower copayment may be charged for an office visit to the primary care physician, and a

out-of-network a provider that does not have a participation agreement with a plan; using an out-of-network provider is more expensive for the plan's enrollees

preauthorization prior authorization from a payer for services to be provided; if preauthorization is not received, the charge is usually not covered

copayment (copay) an amount that a health plan requires a beneficiary to pay at the time of service for each health care encounter

higher copayment may be required for a visit to the office of a specialist or for the use of emergency department services.

One other cost-control method is now used less frequently but was a major feature of early HMOs. This required a patient to select a primary care physician (PCP)—also called a *gatekeeper*—from the HMO's list of general or family practitioners, internists, and pediatricians. A PCP coordinates patients' overall care to ensure that all services are, in the PCP's judgment, necessary. In gatekeeper plans, an HMO member needs a medical referral from the PCP before seeing a specialist or a consultant and for hospital admission. Members who visit providers without referrals are directly responsible for the total cost of the services.

TIP

Open-Access Plans

Many HMOs have switched from gatekeeper plans that require referrals to all specialists to plans that permit members to visit any specialists in the network without referrals. Even if referrals are required for specialists, patients can usually see OB-GYN specialists without referrals.

Historically, the first HMOs used all these cost-containment methods and reduced operating costs. However, both physicians and patients became dissatisfied with the policies. Physicians working under managed care contracts complained that they were not allowed to order needed treatments and tests. Patients often reported that needed referrals were denied. In response, the medical management practices of HMOs increasingly emphasize the quality of health care as well as the cost of its delivery.

Point-of-Service Plans

Many patients dislike HMO rules that restrict their access to physicians. In order to better compete for membership, a point-of-service (POS) plan, also called an open HMO, reduces restrictions and allows members to choose providers who are not in the HMO's network. Over 20 percent of employees covered by employers' health care plans are enrolled in this type of plan.

Members must pay additional fees that are set by the plan when they use out-of-network providers. Typically, 20 to 30 percent of the charge for out-of-network service must be paid by the patient, and the deductible can be very high. The HMO pays out-of-network providers on a fee-for-service basis.

Preferred Provider Organizations

A preferred provider organization (PPO) is another health care delivery system that manages care. PPOs are the most popular type of insurance plan. They create a network of physicians, hospitals, and other providers with whom they have negotiated discounts from the usual fees. For example, a PPO might sign a contract with a practice stating that the fee for a brief appointment will be $60, although the practice's physicians usually charge

$80. In exchange for accepting lower fees, providers–in theory, at least–see more patients, thus making up the revenue that is lost through the reduced fees. PPOs enroll almost 50 percent of the American workers who are insured through their employers.

In addition to requiring a payment of a premium, as seen in Figure 4.6, a PPO often requires a copayment for visits. It does not require a primary care physician to oversee patients' care. Referrals to specialists are also not required. Premiums and copayments, however, are higher than in HMO or POS plans. Members choose from many in-network generalists and specialists. PPO members also can use out-of-network providers, usually for increased deductibles and coinsurance, higher copayments, or both.

EXAMPLE

A PPO member using an in-network provider pays a $20 copayment at the time of service, and the PPO pays the full balance of the charge for the visit. A member who sees an out-of-network provider pays a $40 copayment and is also responsible for coinsurance covering part of the visit charge.

As managed care organizations, PPOs also control the cost of health care by:

- *Directing patients' choices of providers:* PPO members have financial incentives to receive services from the PPO's network of providers.
- *Controlling the use of services:* PPOs have guidelines for appropriate and necessary medical care.
- *Requiring preauthorization for services:* PPOs may require preauthorization for nonemergency hospital admission and for some outpatient procedures.
- *Requiring cost-sharing:* PPO members are also required to pay copayments for general or specialist services.

Consumer-Driven Health Plans

Consumer-driven health plans (CDHPs) combine two elements. The first element is a health plan, usually a PPO, that has a high deductible (such as $2,000 for an individual) and low premiums. The second element is a special savings account that is used to pay medical bills before the deductible has been met. The savings account, which is similar to an individual retirement account (IRA), lets people put aside untaxed wages that they may use to cover their out-of-pocket medical expenses. Some employers contribute to employees' accounts as a benefit. Enrollment in CDHPs, as illustrated in Figure 4.6, has been increasing steadily in recent years.

Cost containment in consumer-driven health plans begins with consumerism–the idea that patients who themselves pay for health care services become more careful consumers. Both insurance companies and employers believe that asking patients to pay a larger portion of medical expenses reduces costs. To this are added the other controls typical of a PPO, such as in-network savings and higher costs for out-of-network visits.

THINKING IT THROUGH 4.5

If a patient has met the annual deductible for her health plan and the coinsurance rate is 35 percent, how much does she owe for a charge of $310? How much will the health plan pay?

TABLE 4.1 Health Plan Options

Plan Type	Provider Options	Cost-Containment Methods	Features
Indemnity plan	Any provider	• Few or none • Preauthorization required for some procedures	• Higher costs • Deductibles • Coinsurance • Preventive care usually not covered
Health maintenance organization (HMO)	HMO network providers only	• Primary care physician manages care; referral required • No payment for out-of-network nonemergency services • Preauthorization required	• Low copayment • Limited provider network • Covers preventive care
Point-of-service (POS)	Network or out-of-network providers	• Within network, primary care physician manages care	• Lower copayments for network providers • Higher costs for out-of-network providers • Covers preventive care
Preferred provider organization (PPO)	Network or out-of-network providers	• Referral not required for specialists • Discounted fees • Preauthorization for some procedures	• Higher cost for out-of-network providers • Preventive care coverage varies
Consumer-driven health plan (CDHP)	Usually network or out-of-network providers	• Increases patient awareness of health care costs • Patient pays directly until high deductible is met	• High deductible, low premium • Savings account

The most recent trend in health care plans is to replace copayments with coinsurance, thereby moving even more of the burden of health care onto the patient. The major types of plans are summarized in Table 4.1.

4.6 Eligibility and Benefits Verification

After scheduling an appointment, the front desk staff or the medical biller contacts the patient's health plan to verify the patient's eligibility for insurance benefits. Except in a medical emergency, where care is provided immediately and insurance is checked after the encounter, the following information should be obtained before a patient encounter:

- The patient's general eligibility for benefits
- The amount of the copayment for the visit, if one is required
- Whether the planned encounter is for a covered service that is medically necessary under the payer's rules

Factors Affecting General Eligibility

General eligibility for benefits depends on a number of factors. If premiums are required, patients must have paid them on time. For government-sponsored plans, like Medicaid, in which income is the criterion, eligibility can change monthly. For patients with employer-sponsored health plans, employment status can be the deciding factor:

- Coverage may end on the last day of the month in which the employee's active full-time service ends, such as for disability, layoff, or termination.
- The employee may no longer qualify as a member of the group. For example, many companies do not provide benefits for part-time employees. If a full-time employee changes to part-time employment, the coverage ends.
- An eligible dependent's coverage may end on the last day of the month in which the dependent status ends, such as for reaching the age limit stated in the policy.

If the patient's plan is an HMO that requires a primary care provider (PCP), the practice must verify that (1) the provider is a plan participant, (2) the patient is listed on the plan's enrollment master list, and (3) the patient is assigned to the PCP as of the date of service.

The office also checks with the payer to confirm whether the patient is currently covered. If online access is used, the office and the payer's provider representative exchange information over the Internet and via email messages. If the payer requires verification to be checked on the telephone, the provider representative is called. Based on the patient's plan, eligibility for these specific benefits may also need to be checked:

- Office visits
- Laboratory work
- Diagnostic X-rays
- Maternity services
- Pap smears
- Psychiatric visits
- Physical or occupational therapy
- Durable medical equipment (DME)
- Foot care

Checking Out-of-Network Benefits

If a patient has insurance coverage but the practice does not participate in the plan, the office staff checks whether the patient has out-of-network benefits. When the patient has out-of-network benefits, the payer's rules concerning copayments and coverage are followed. If a patient does not have out-of-network benefits, as is common when the health plan is an HMO, the patient is responsible for the entire bill, rather than simply a copayment. This must be communicated to the patient before the appointment.

Verifying the Amount of the Copayment and Coinsurance

The amount of the copayment, if required, must be checked. Sometimes the copay information on the insurance card is out of date, and the correct copay is different. If the plan requires coinsurance, the percentage of coinsurance the patient must pay also should be verified.

Determining Whether the Planned Encounter Is for a Covered Service

The office staff must also try to determine whether the planned encounter is for a covered service. If the service will not be covered, the patient can be made aware of the financial responsibility in advance.

The resources for determining what services are covered under a given plan include knowledge of the major plans held by the practice's patients, information from payer websites, and the electronic benefit inquiries described below. Most members of the medical administrative team are familiar with the services covered under typical plans. For example, most plans cover regular office visits, but they may not cover preventive services or some therapeutic services. For unusual or unfamiliar services, the office needs to query the payer.

Electronic Benefit Inquiries and Responses

Previously, to query a payer–to find out about coverage, about whether a patient was up to date on insurance premiums, or about what percentage the plan would pay for a given procedure–the staff member in charge of patient eligibility had to refer to the latest paperwork from the insurance company or phone a representative. This process has changed because of easy access to the Internet.

> **TIP**
>
> **X12 270/271 Eligibility for a Health Plan Inquiry and Response**
>
> The HIPAA Eligibility for a Health Plan transaction is also called the X12 270/271. The number 270 refers to the inquiry that is sent, and 271 to the answer returned by the payer.

Instead of making telephone calls or sending faxes, medical practices usually use electronic transactions to communicate with payers. Electronic transactions are the most efficient because they take only seconds. Most practice management programs have a feature that enables online inquiries to a payer to be sent from within the program. When an eligibility benefits transaction is sent, the computer program assigns a unique trace number to the inquiry. Often, eligibility transactions are sent the day before patients arrive for appointments.

The health plan responds to an inquiry with this information:

- Trace number, as a double-check on the inquiry
- Benefit information, such as whether the insurance coverage is active

- Covered period—the period of dates that the coverage is active
- Benefit units, such as the number of physical therapy visits
- Coverage level—who is covered, such as spouse and family or individual

The following information may also be transmitted:

- The copay amount
- The yearly deductible amount
- The coinsurance amount
- The out-of-pocket expenses
- The health plan's information on the insured's/patient's first and last names, dates of birth, and identification numbers
- The primary care provider

Online Eligibility Services

Some practice management programs also offer electronic eligibility checking through an online service. Rather than having the medical practice contact the payer directly, the online service acts as the relay, or go-between, for a practice and all the major payers. The online service provides a computer network for instant communication of clinical, financial, and administrative data with the major insurance payers. The responses retrieved via the service come directly from payers.

Procedures When the Patient Is Not Covered

If an insured patient's policy does not cover a planned service, the patient should be informed that the payer does not pay for the service and that he or she is responsible for the charges. For example, some plans do not pay for preventive services such as annual physical examinations. Many patients, however, consider preventive services a good idea and are willing to pay for them.

Some payers require the physician to use specific forms to tell the patient about noncovered services. These financial agreement forms, which patients must sign, prove that patients were told—before the services were given—about their obligation to pay the bill. Figure 4.10 is an example of a form used to tell patients in advance of the probable cost of procedures that are not going to be covered by their plan and to secure their agreement to pay.

Figure 4.10 Sample Financial Agreement for Patient Payment of Noncovered Services

Service to be performed: ____________________
Estimated charge: ____________________
Date of planned service: ____________________
Reason for exclusion: ____________________

I, ____________, a patient of ____________, understand the service described above is excluded from my health insurance. I am responsible for payment in full of the charges for this service.

THINKING IT THROUGH 4.6

Managed care organizations often require different payments for different services. The table below shows the copayments for an HMO health plan. Study the schedule, and answer these questions:

- How does the copayment amount for physical therapy compare with the copayment for seeing a specialist?
- What is the copayment amount for an emergency room visit? Is the copayment ever waived?
- Does this health plan cover chiropractic care? Contraceptives? Eye exams?
- How much does an insured have to pay on prescriptions each year before prescription benefits begin?

Example of Benefits Under an HMO

Service	Copayment
Primary Care Physician Visits During office hours After hours/home visits	 $25 copay $25 copay
Specialty Care During office hours For diagnostic outpatient testing Physical, occupational, speech therapy	 $35 copay $25 copay $25 copay
Surgery in Special-Purpose Unit	$250 copay
Hospitalization	$250 copay
Emergency Room (copay waived if admitted)	$50 copay
Maternity First OB visit Hospital	 $35 copay $250 copay
Mental Health Inpatient Outpatient	 $250 copay, 60 days 30% copay
Substance Abuse Detoxification Inpatient rehab (combined w/mental health amount) Outpatient rehabilitation	 $250 copay $250 copay 30% copay
Preventive Care Routine eye exam Routine gynecological exam Pediatric preventive dental exam	 Not covered $30 copay Not covered
Chiropractic Care (20 visits/condition)	$20 copay
Prescriptions Contraceptives Diabetic supplies 31–90 day supply	$15/$20/$20 copay; $150 deductible/calendar year Covered Covered $30/$40/$60 copay
Durable Medical Equipment	No copay

> **TIP**
>
> **HIPAA Referral Certification and Authorization**
>
> The electronic transaction that must be used for preauthorization or referral is the HIPAA Referral Certification and Authorization transaction, also called the X12 278.

4.7 Preauthorization, Referrals, and Outside Procedures

In addition to verifying a patient's eligibility for benefits, the medical administrative team needs to check for preauthorization or referral requirements that may be part of the patient's plan prior to the office visit. Preauthorization and referrals are required for many services in managed care plans, such as HMOs.

Preauthorization

A managed care payer often requires preauthorization before the patient sees a specialist, is admitted to the hospital, or has a particular procedure. The office's medical insurance specialist may request preauthorization over the phone, by email or fax, or in an electronic transaction. If the payer approves the service, it issues a preauthorization number that must be entered in the practice management program so it will be stored and appear later on the health care claim for the encounter. (This number may also be called a certification number.)

To help secure preauthorization, best practice is to:

- Be as specific as possible about the planned procedure when exchanging information with the payer.
- Collect and have available all diagnosis information related to the procedure, including any pertinent history.
- Query the provider about all procedures that may potentially be used to treat the patient, and then request preauthorization for all of them.

Referrals

Often, a physician needs to send a patient to another physician for evaluation and/or treatment. For example, an internist might send a patient to a gastroenterologist for a colonoscopy. In this case, the internist would be considered to be the **referring provider.** If a patient's plan requires it, the patient must obtain a **referral number** and a referral document for the specialist before the visit. Usually the office of the primary care physician contacts the payer to obtain the referral number and then prepares the referral document.

referring provider physician who refers the patient to another physician for treatment

referral number authorization number given by a referring physician to the referred physician

The referral document is either given to the patient to take to the visit or sent directly to the specialist on the patient's behalf. A paper referral document (see Figure 4.11) describes the services the patient is certified to receive. It is a specific set of instructions from the primary care physician that directs the patient to a specialist or facility for medically necessary care. This approval may instead be communicated electronically using the HIPAA referral transaction.

Referral Form

Label with Patient's Demographic & Insurance Information

Physician referred to: ______________________

Referred for:

- ❑ Consult only
- ❑ Follow-up
- ❑ Lab
- ❑ X-ray
- ❑ Procedure
- ❑ Other

Reason for visit: ______________________

Number of visits: __________

Appointment requested: Please contact patient; phone: __________

Primary care physician

Name: ______________________

Signature: ______________________

Phone: ______________________

Figure 4.11 Referral Document

The specialist's office handling a referred patient must:

- Check that the patient has a referral number
- Verify patient enrollment in the plan
- Understand restrictions to services, such as regulations that require the patient to visit a specialist in a specific amount of time after receiving the referral or that limit the number of times the patient can receive services from the specialist

Sometimes a managed care patient may "self-refer"—come for specialty care without a referral number when one is required. In such a case, the medical insurance specialist asks the patient to sign a form acknowledging responsibility for the services. A sample form is shown in Figure 4.12a.

In other cases, a patient who is required to have a referral document may not bring one. When this occurs, the medical insurance specialist asks the patient to sign a referral waiver document, such as that shown in Figure 4.12b, to ensure that the patient will pay for services if a referral is not documented in the time specified.

Outside Procedures

The medical administrative team is also responsible for scheduling patients for inpatient (defined as requiring an overnight stay) or outpatient admissions procedures. Most plans require preauthorization for such procedures if they are not emergencies.

After obtaining the preauthorization, the staff member in charge of scheduling outside appointments asks the doctor for an order that specifies all the

Member Self-Referral Acknowledgment

I, ____________________, understand that I am seeking the care of this specialty physician or health care provider, ____________________, without a referral from my primary care physician. I understand that the terms of my plan coverage required that I obtain that referral, and that if I fail to do so, my plan will not cover any part of the charges, costs, or expenses related to this specialist's services to me.

Signed,

____________________ ____________________

(member's name) (date)

****

Specialty physician or other health care provider:

Please keep a copy of this form in your patient's file

(a)

Referral Waiver

I did not bring a referral for the medical services I will receive today. If my primary care physician does not provide a referral within two days, I understand that I am responsible for paying for the services I am requesting.

Signature: ________________________________

Date: ____________________

(b)

Figure 4.12 (a) Self-Referral Document, (b) Referral Waiver

details related to the procedure, including when the results are required. The provider of the outside procedures requires such an order to do the medical work. The staff member then contacts the outside lab or hospital where the procedure will be performed to verify that the facility or referring physician accepts the patient's insurance. In preparation for the appointment, the staff member also:

- Finds out what days and times are available for scheduling the procedure
- Provides the facility with detailed information about the test or procedure
- Obtains instructions the patient needs in order to prepare for the procedure
- Contacts the operating room secretary about reserving a room and time, if required
- Provides the facility with the patient's demographics and insurance information for admission and billing purposes
- Obtains a telephone number and contact person for the patient to use when calling back to set up the appointment

After this information is obtained, the staff member can contact the patient with an idea of what times are available and provide the patient with

THINKING IT THROUGH 4.7

What is the difference between a preauthorization and a referral?

the phone number to use for making the appointment. The patient is also given instructions on how to prepare for the procedure. Patients generally feel less stressed about making an appointment for an inpatient or outpatient admissions procedure when given this information ahead of time.

chapter 4 summary

KEY TERMS

benefits	medical insurance	preexisting condition
chart number	new patient (NP)	premium
coinsurance	noncovered services	preregistration
copayment (copay)	nonparticipating (nonPAR) provider	preventive medical services
covered services	out-of-network	provider
deductible	out-of-pocket	referral number
demographics	participating (PAR) provider	referring provider
established patient (EP)	payer	schedule matrix
health plan	policyholder	schedule of benefits
indemnity plan	preauthorization	sponsor
managed care		

LEARNING OUTCOME	KEY CONCEPTS/EXAMPLES
4.1 Describe the primary methods used to schedule appointments.	In medical offices, most patient appointments are scheduled over the telephone, and some are scheduled online. If a patient requests an appointment via telephone (or in person after a visit), the offices' electronic scheduling program can be easily accessed to set up the appointment. If the medical office has a website, patients may have the option of scheduling appointments online through a patient portal. Patients can view an online calendar with available openings, select a time, and receive an email confirmation.
4.2 Differentiate between new and established patients.	A patient is classified as a new patient (NP) if he or she has not received any services from the provider (or another provider of the same specialty who is a member of the same practice) within the past three years. The patient is classified as an established patient (EP) if he or she has seen the provider (or another provider in the practice who has the same specialty) within the past three years.
4.3 List the three categories of information new patients provide during telephone preregistration and demonstrate use of the patient scheduler.	1. Patient demographics such as name, address, gender, date of birth, and telephone number 2. Basic information about insurance coverage 3. The reason for the visit

LEARNING OUTCOME	KEY CONCEPTS/EXAMPLES
4.4 Identify the information that needs to be verified for established patients when making an appointment.	When an established patient calls for an appointment, the front desk verifies that the demographic and insurance information on file for the patient is still up to date. The reason for the visit is determined so that the correct length of time can be scheduled. In addition, the patient's account is reviewed to check for any overdue amounts so that the patient can be asked to take care of them during the upcoming visit.
4.5 Describe covered and noncovered services under medical insurance policies.	Covered services are listed on each plan's schedule of benefits and usually include primary care, emergency care, medical specialists' services, and surgery. Managed care plans generally cover preventive medical services as well, including annual physical examinations, prenatal care, and screening procedures such as mammograms. The services for which the payer does not pay, called noncovered services, are listed separately in the medical insurance policy and may include dental services, eye examinations or eyeglasses, employment-related injuries, cosmetic procedures, infertility services, or experimental procedures. Many policies also do not offer prescription drug benefits.
4.6 List the three main points to verify with the payer regarding a patient's benefits prior to a visit.	The medical insurance specialist verifies: 1. The patient's general eligibility for benefits 2. The amount of the copayment for the visit (if one is required) 3. Whether the planned encounter is for a covered service that is medically necessary under the payer's rules
4.7 Explain when a preauthorization number or referral document is required for a patient's encounter.	Preauthorization from a payer is required to certify that the services the patient is scheduled to receive will be covered under the policy. A referral to another provider requires a similar certification, along with a referral letter from the referring physician with specific instructions regarding the medically necessary services that are being requested.

chapter 4 review

MATCHING QUESTIONS

Match the key terms with their definitions.

_____ 1. *[LO 4.5]* preexisting condition

_____ 2. *[LO 4.5]* indemnity plan

_____ 3. *[LO 4.5]* deductible

_____ 4. *[LO 4.5]* coinsurance

_____ 5. *[LO 4.5]* payer

_____ 6. *[LO 4.5]* benefits

_____ 7. *[LO 4.5]* provider

_____ 8. *[LO 4.5]* referral

_____ 9. *[LO 4.5]* premium

_____ 10. *[LO 4.5]* medical insurance

a. An amount that an insured person must pay, usually on an annual basis, for health care services before a health plan's payment begins.

b. Illness or disorder of a beneficiary that existed before the effective date of insurance coverage.

c. Health plan or program.

d. Person or entity that supplies medical or health services and bills for the services in the normal course of business.

e. The portion of charges that an insured person must pay for health care services after payment of the deductible amount.

f. Type of medical insurance that reimburses a policyholder for medical services under the terms of its schedule of benefits.

g. Money the insured pays to a health plan for a health care policy; usually paid monthly.

h. Financial plan that covers the cost of hospital and medical care.

i. Transfer of patient care from one physician to another.

j. The amount of money a health plan pays for services covered in an insurance policy.

MULTIPLE-CHOICE QUESTIONS

Select the letter that best completes the statement or answers the question.

1. *[LO 4.7]* The preauthorization number may also be called the _________ number.
   a. eligibility
   b. verification
   c. certification
   d. demographic

2. *[LO 4.1]* Websites that can be used by patients to make appointments or receive messages from their health care providers are known as _________.
   a. patient portals
   b. health care networks
   c. electronic health records
   d. medical alerts

3. *[LO 4.1]* Examples of different scheduling systems include open-hours scheduling, ________ scheduling, double-booking, and wave scheduling.
   a. rotating
   b. ripple
   c. stream
   d. flow

4. *[LO 4.3]* The process of gathering information about a new patient before an appointment is known as________.
   a. prerecording
   b. preregistration
   c. preauthorization
   d. predetermination

5. *[LO 4.5]* In most managed care insurance plans, patients must use network physicians to avoid paying higher charges. For this reason, patients check whether the provider is ________ in their plan.
   a. a practicing physician
   b. a participating provider
   c. an authorized provider
   d. a preferred provider

6. *[LO 4.5]* At the time an HMO member sees a provider, he or she pays a specified charge called the ________.
   a. copayment
   b. coinsurance
   c. premium
   d. deductible

7. *[LO 4.5]* The medical insurance policy for each health plan contains the ________ that summarizes the payments that may be made for medically necessary services received by policyholders.
   a. schedule of referrals
   b. diagnostic code list
   c. formulary of benefits
   d. schedule of benefits

8. *[LO 4.5]* Although there are many variations in the way health plans are structured, indemnity and ________ plans are the basis for all of them.
   a. workers' compensation
   b. individual
   c. managed care
   d. group

9. *[LO 4.5]* Medicaid is a government-sponsored health insurance program that covers ________.
   a. people who are 65 or older
   b. individuals who are disabled
   c. low-income individuals
   d. members of the uniformed services

10. *[LO 4.7]* A certification number for a procedure is the result of the ________ transaction and process.
    a. coordination of benefits
    b. referral and authorization
    c. claims status
    d. eligibility for a health plan

SHORT-ANSWER QUESTIONS

Define the following abbreviations.

1. *[LO 4.2]* EP ______________________
2. *[LO 4.5]* POS ______________________
3. *[LO 4.3]* nonPAR ______________________
4. *[LO 4.2]* NP ______________________
5. *[LO 4.3]* PAR ______________________
6. *[LO 4.5]* HMO ______________________
7. *[LO 4.5]* PPO ______________________
8. *[LO 4.5]* CDHP ______________________

APPLYING YOUR KNOWLEDGE

Sequencing Tasks

4.1 *[LO 4.1]* Assume that you are scheduling a follow-up appointment over the phone for a patient who was in the office several months ago for a heart condition. Number the steps below in the order that best accommodates the patient's needs while on the phone.
– Review the patient's account to see if there is an outstanding balance.
– Book the appointment.
– Ask the patient to verify the reason for the visit.
– Ask the patient to verify his or her name and date of birth.
– Ask the patient if he or she would like to set up a payment plan for an overdue balance of $250 from several earlier visits.
– Greet the patient while opening the scheduling program.
– Look for the first suitable day and time in the schedule.

Using Insurance Terms

4.2 *[LO 4.5]* The following passage describes a patient's insurance plan. Using the insurance terms provided after the passage, fill in the missing words.

If you have paid your ________ and your ________ policy is up to date, the ________ services, listed on your ________, will be paid by your insurance. However, you will still be responsible for the ________ for each visit.

medical insurance

copay

premium

covered

schedule of benefits

4.3 *[LO 4.5]* The following passage describes an insurance contract. Using the insurance terms provided after the passage, fill in the missing words.

________ is a written policy between an individual, called the ________, and a ________, an insurance company or government program that is the ________. The policyholder pays a specified amount of money called a ________. In exchange, the policyholder receives ________, defined by America's Health Insurance Plans (AHIP) as payments for covered medical services for a specific period of time.

policyholder

health plan

benefits

medical insurance

premium

payer

Calculating Amounts Due

Calculate the amounts billed in each of the following situations.

4.4 *[LO 4.5]* The patient is enrolled in a capitated HMO. Previously, the patient paid a $25 copay for mental health care services. Due to a change in policy, the patient is now required to pay 10 percent coinsurance. The provider charges $450 for a visit. What amount is the patient responsible for? How much will the health insurance plan pay for the visit? Which costs the patient more, the copay or the coinsurance?

____

____

4.5 *[LO 4.5]* A patient's total surgery charges are $4,300. The patient's health plan has a $100 annual deductible. The coinsurance percentage listed in the policy is 80-20. What does the patient owe? The plan?

____

____

4.6 *[LO 4.5]* A patient has a high-deductible consumer-driven health plan. The annual deductible is $3,000. Of that deductible, the patient has paid $400 this year. The patient now faces minor surgery, and the procedure will cost $2,200. What percentage of this cost will the insurance plan pay?

____

____

chapter 5

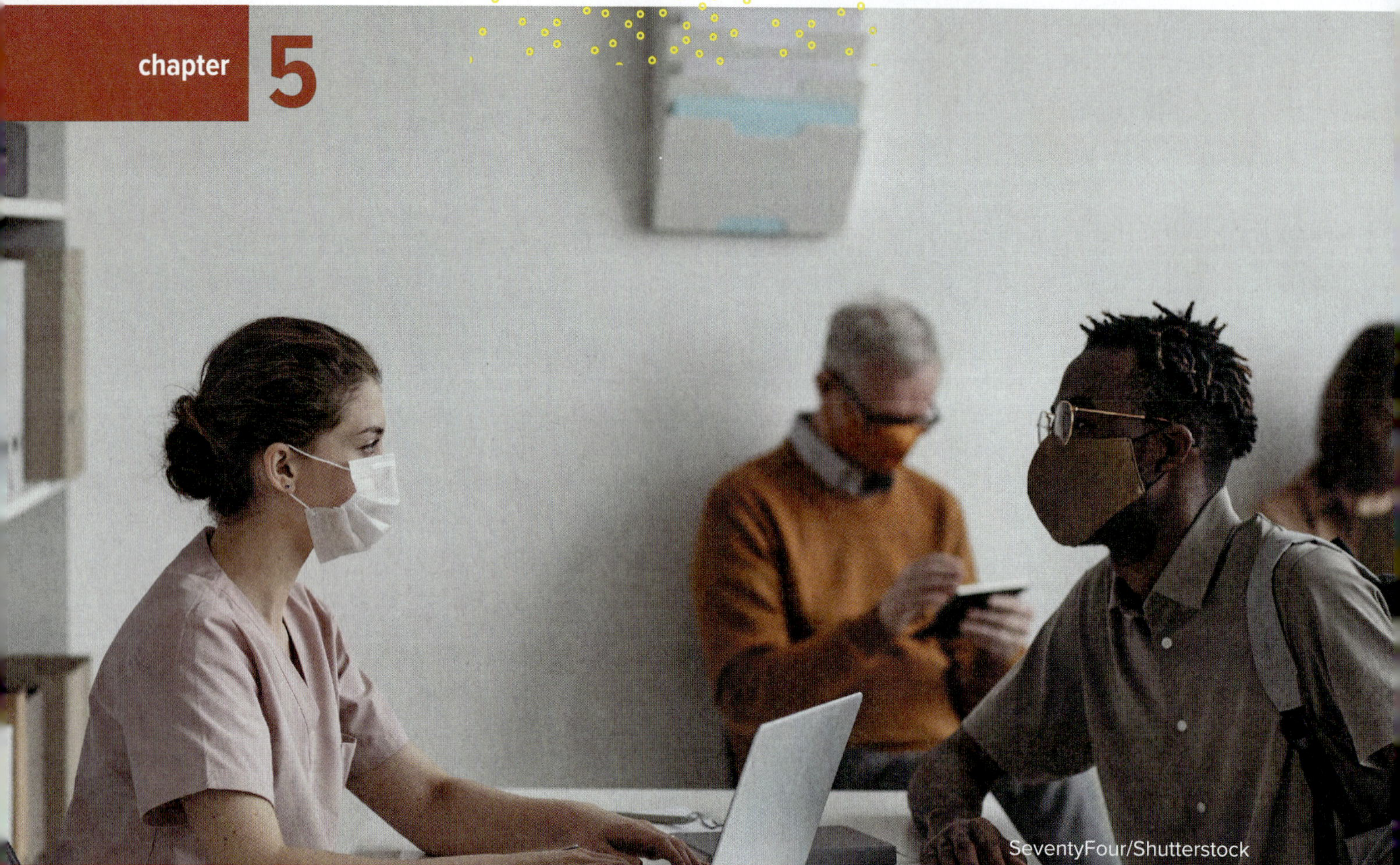

SeventyFour/Shutterstock

Office Visit: Check-In Procedures

LEARNING OUTCOMES

When you finish this chapter, you will be able to:

5.1 List the six types of information that are gathered as part of the registration process for new patients.

5.2 Determine which health plan is primary when there is more than one.

5.3 Describe the purpose of a practice's financial policy.

5.4 List the types of payments that may be collected from patients at check-in.

5.5 Discuss the advantages of tracking patients electronically during a visit.

An Ounce of Prevention

As a receptionist for a busy practice like the Trilogy Family Care Center, Laurie Harcourt is at her desk most of the day. Usually, she tries to go out for a short walk during her lunch break, but today she's decided to stay at her desk. Laurie came in this morning feeling a bit out of sorts—too bad, because the busy morning included two new patients, plus an emergency case she had to squeeze in! "I think I should double-check the two new patient records that I put into the system this morning."

She remembers the mistake she made when she chose the wrong insurance company from the pulldown menu. A simple slip of her cursor had caused a lot of trouble! Now Laurie makes a point of looking over her work.

The receptionist in the example has developed a number of habits that help her maintain her balance in the office. What self-awareness skills has she developed? Why are they important?

5.1 Patient Registration

Preregistration, as explained in Chapter 4, is the process of obtaining basic patient information and setting up an appointment time that suits the patient's needs. When patients arrive at the front desk for their appointments, registration staff follow the process of **registration** to obtain more detailed information about patients and their particular health plans before their encounters with providers.

registration process of gathering personal and insurance information about a patient before an encounter with a provider

Information for New Patients

If the patient is new to the practice, these six types of information are gathered:

1. Medical history
2. Detailed patient and insurance information
3. Identification verification
4. Financial agreement and authorization for treatment
5. Assignment of benefits statement
6. Acknowledgment of Receipt of Notice of Privacy Practices (NPP)

To communicate this information, a new patient fills out several forms and signs others.

Medical History Form

Each new patient is asked to complete a medical history form. This form asks for information about the patient's pertinent personal medical history, the family's medical history, and the patient's social history. Social history covers lifestyle factors such as smoking, exercise, and alcohol use. Some practices give printed forms to patients when they come in. Others make the form available for completion ahead of time by posting it online or mailing it to the patient. For patients with long medical histories, particularly elderly patients, the option to complete a medical history form ahead of time can be useful, as it can be difficult to recall this information prior to an appointment in a waiting room.

During the encounter, the physician reviews the information on the medical history form with the patient and documents the patient's answers and the physician's observations. The provider can enter this information into the EHR during the visit. EHRs offer providers a number of methods for documenting patients' histories and other clinical information during or after a visit. The methods range from traditional dictation to the use of medical history templates to voice-activated software. Chapters 6 and 7 discuss some of these methods.

Patient Information Form

patient information form form that includes a patient's personal, employment, and insurance data needed to complete a health care claim; also known as a registration form

New patients also complete a **patient information form.** Also referred to as a *patient registration form,* it is used to collect information about the patient, including employment and insurance data needed to complete an insurance claim. As with the medical history form, some practices provide patients with printed patient information forms to fill in when they arrive. Others make the form available for completion ahead of time by posting it online or mailing it to patients.

A patient information form, as illustrated in Figure 5.1, contains the following information:

- First name, middle initial, and last name
- Gender (typically assigned gender at birth or legal gender)
- Birth date, using four digits for the year
- Home address and telephone number (area code with seven-digit number)
- Marital status (*S* for single, *M* for married, *D* for divorced, *W* for widowed)
- Student status
- Social Security number
- E-mail address
- Allergies
- Employer's name, address, and telephone number
- For a patient who is a minor (under the age of majority according to state law) or has a medical power of attorney in place, meaning that another person is handling the patient's medical decisions, the responsible person's name, gender, birth date, address, Social Security number, telephone number, and employer information. In most cases, the responsible person is a parent, guardian, adult child, or other person acting with legal authority to make health care decisions on behalf of the patient. A minor's status as a full-time or part-time student is also recorded.
- The name of the patient's primary insurance carrier
- The insured's (policyholder's) name, the patient's relationship to the insured, and the insured's identification number and other details of the plan (group number, insurance address, telephone number, copay and deductible amounts)
- If the patient is covered by another insurance carrier, the name and policyholder information for that plan

FAMILY CARE CLINIC
285 Stephenson Boulevard
Stephenson, OH 60089-4000
614-555-0000

PATIENT INFORMATION FORM

Patient				
Last Name	First Name	MI	Sex __ M __ F	Date of Birth / /
Address	City	State	Zip	
Home Ph # ( )	Cell Ph # ( )	Marital Status	Student Status	
SS#	Email	Allergies		
Employment Status	Employer Name	Work Ph # ( )	Primary Insurance ID #	
Employer Address	City	State	Zip	
Referred By	Ph # of Referral ( )			

Responsible Party (Complete this section if the person responsible for the bill is not the patient)				
Last Name	First Name	MI	Sex __ M __ F	Date of Birth / /
Address	City	State	Zip	SS#
Relation to Patient __ Spouse __ Parent __ Other	Employer Name	Work Phone # ( )		
Spouse, or Parent (if minor):	Home Phone # ( )			

Insurance (If you have multiple coverage, supply information from both carriers)			
Primary Carrier Name		Secondary Carrier Name	
Name of the Insured (Name on ID Card)		Name of the Insured (Name on ID Card)	
Patient's relationship to the insured __ Self __ Spouse __ Child		Patient's relationship to the insured __ Self __ Spouse __ Child	
Insured ID #		Insured ID #	
Group # or Company Name		Group # or Company Name	
Insurance Address		Insurance Address	
Phone #	Copay $ Deductible $	Phone #	Copay $ Deductible $

Other Information

Is patient's condition related to: | Reason for visit:

__ Employment __ Auto Accident (if yes, state in which accident occurred: __) __Other Accident

Date of Accident: / / Date of First Symptom of Illness: / /

Financial Agreement and Authorization for Treatment

I authorize treatment and agree to pay all fees and charges for the person named above. I agree to pay all charges shown by statements, promptly upon their presentation, unless credit arrangements are agreed upon in writing.

Signed: ______________________________

I authorize payment directly to FAMILY CARE CLINIC of insurance benefits otherwise payable to me. I hereby authorize the release of any medical information necessary in order to process a claim for payment in my behalf.

Date: ______________________________

Figure 5.1 Patient Information (Registration) Form

It is important to understand the difference between the insured and the patient. The insured is the holder of the insurance policy that covers the patient. When patients have their own insurance policy, the patient and the insured are the same person. However, if a patient is covered by someone else's policy, such as a spouse's, that person is the insured. As mentioned in Chapter 4, when the patient is not the insured, the insured is usually a spouse, divorced spouse, guardian, or other relation. Other terms for insured are **guarantor,** *policyholder,* and *subscriber.* In a PM/EHR system, the guarantor is the individual who agrees to take financial responsibility for the patient.

guarantor person who is the insurance policyholder for a patient of the practice; agrees to financial responsibility for a patient

Identification Verification

For an insured new patient, the front and the back of the insurance card are scanned or photocopied and added to the patient's chart at registration. All data from the card that the patient has written on the patient information form are double-checked against the insurance card for accuracy before being entered into the practice's patient database.

Most insurance cards have the following information (see Figure 5.2):

- Group identification number
- Date on which the member's coverage became effective
- Member name
- Member identification number
- The health plan's name, type of coverage, copayment requirements, and frequency limits or annual maximums for services; sometimes the annual deductible
- Claim submission procedure and contact information
- Preauthorization/preadmission requirements
- Optional items, such as prescription drugs that are covered, with the copayment requirements

A common error message on returned or rejected insurance claims relates to the misspelling of the patient's name. Payers want the name of the patient on a claim to be exactly as it is shown on the insurance card. It is important, therefore, to check the patient information form to make sure the patient has not used a nickname, skipped a middle initial, or otherwise changed the name from the way it appears on the insurance card and thus in the health plan's records.

TIP

Spelling Counts!

Never assume spelling of a patient's name. When registering new patients and recalling established patient records, it is important to verify the correct spelling of their names.

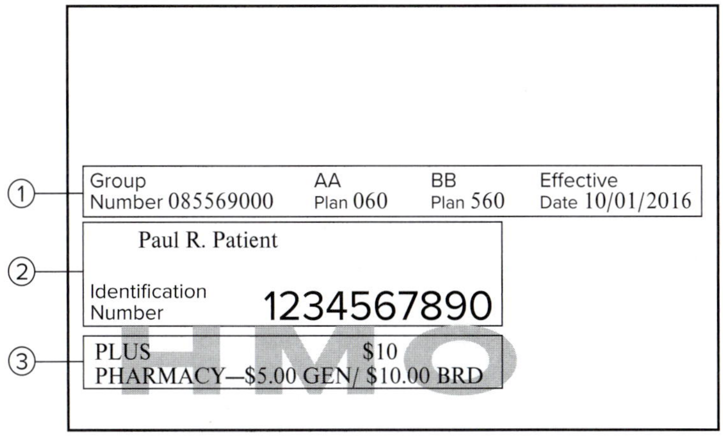

1. ***Group identification number***
   The 9-digit number used to identify the member's employer.

   Plan codes
   The numbers used to identify the codes assigned to each plan: used for claims submissions when medical services are rendered out-of-state.

   Effective date
   The date on which the member's coverage became effective.

2. ***Member name***
   The full name of the cardholder.

   Identification number
   The 10-digit number used to identify each plan member.

3. ***Health plan***
   The name of the health plan and the type of coverage; usually lists any copayment amounts, frequency limits or annual maximums for home and office visits; may also list the member's annual deductible amount.

   Riders
   The type(s) of riders that are included in the member's benefits (DME, Visions).

   Pharmacy
   The type of prescription drug coverage; lists copayment amounts.

Figure 5.2 An Example of an Insurance Card

EXERCISE 5.1

Add a New Patient to the EHR

EHRclinic

A new patient walked into Trilogy Family Medical Care Center for urgent care. After he completes his new patient paperwork, you must create a patient account and register him as a new patient.

Your instructor may assign this exercise to you in Connect. Exercise steps and EHRclinic Help Guides can be downloaded at http://www.mhhe.com/pmehr2.

Patient Identification Many practices also require the patient to present a photo ID card, such as a driver's license. The practice scans the photo ID and stores it in the EHR, where it can be called up for billing purposes or to verify the patient's identity when the patient arrives for a visit. Trilogy Family Care Center uses the new hand scanner technology for patient identification. Patients place a hand in the holder each time they check in for an appointment.

Assignment of Benefits

Physicians usually submit claims for patients and receive payments directly from the payers. This saves patients paperwork and expedites payments to providers. The policyholder must authorize this procedure by signing and dating an **assignment of benefits** statement. This statement authorizes the provider to **accept assignment** for the patient—that is, to submit claims for the patient and receive payments directly from the payer. The assignment of benefits may be a separate form, as in Figure 5.3, or an entry on the patient information form. In Figure 5.1, an assignment of benefits statement is displayed at the bottom of the form: "I authorize payment directly to Trilogy Family Care Center of insurance benefits otherwise payable to me."

assignment of benefits authorization by a policyholder that allows a health plan to pay benefits directly to a provider

accept assignment participating physician's agreement to accept the allowed charge as full payment

Financial Agreement and Authorization for Treatment

"I authorize treatment and agree to pay all fees and charges for the person named above. I agree to pay all charges shown by statements, promptly upon their presentation, unless credit arrangements are agreed upon in writing." This is a typical financial agreement and authorization for treatment statement. Like the assignment of benefits, this information may be provided on a separate form or as an entry on the patient information form, as in the example in Figure 5.1.

> **TIP**
>
> **Who Is Requesting PHI?**
>
> Although the HIPAA Privacy Rule permits sharing PHI for treatment, payment, and operations (TPO) purposes without authorization, it also requires verification of the identity of the person who is asking for the information. The person's authority to access PHI must also be verified. If the requestor's right to the information is not certain, the best practice is to have the patient authorize the release of PHI.

Acknowledgment of Receipt of Notice of Privacy Practices

HIPAA (see Chapter 3) requires medical practices to give each patient a copy of their Notice of Privacy Practices (NPP) document at the time of the patient's first encounter and at least once every three years thereafter, and

Figure 5.3 Assignment of Benefits Form

Assignment of Benefits

I hereby assign to Family Care Clinic, any insurance or other third-party benefits available for health care services provided to me. I understand that Family Care Clinic has the right to refuse or accept assignment of such benefits. If these benefits are not assigned to Family Care Clinic, I agree to forward to Family Care Clinic all health insurance and other third-party payments that I receive for services rendered to me immediately upon receipt.

Signature of Patient/Legal Guardian: ____________________

Date: ____________

then to have the patient sign a separate form called an Acknowledgment of Receipt of Notice of Privacy Practices. This form indicates that the patient has received the document that states how the provider intends to protect the patient's rights to privacy under HIPAA.

The patient's acknowledgment is scanned and stored along with the patient's chart in the EHR. If the EHR program uses an electronic format for the Notice of Privacy Practices and acknowledgment, the documents may be read and signed online.

Other Forms and Documents

In addition to the six types of information just discussed, depending on the office's policies, several other forms and documents may be exchanged as part of the registration process.

Release Authorization

While the HIPAA Privacy Rule does not require an authorization to release patients' PHI for treatment, payment, and operations (TPO) purposes, state law may be more stringent and may require a release authorization. For this reason, many practices routinely have patients sign release of information statements at the time of registration. Release statements are either separate documents or part of the patient information form. On the patient information form in Figure 5.1, the release of information statement–"I hereby authorize the release of any medical information necessary in order to process a claim for payment in my behalf"–is included with the other authorizations at the bottom of the form. Trilogy Family Care Center patients also sign a form that includes the names of other individuals who are authorized to receive information about the patient, such as a sister, parents, or a spouse.

Forms Required by Particular Health Plans

At times, patients' health plans require the practice to inform beneficiaries in writing about the patients' likely financial responsibility. One of the most typical examples of such plan requirements is in the Medicare program. By statute, Medicare does not provide coverage for all services and procedures. Claims are denied for services that are excluded by Medicare and for services not considered reasonable and necessary for the patient.

Physicians who participate in the Medicare program agree to not bill patients for services that Medicare declares are not reasonable and necessary unless the patients were informed ahead of time in writing and agreed to pay for the services. Local coverage determinations (LCDs) and national coverage determinations (NCDs) issued by Medicare help sort out medical necessity issues. LCDs and NCDs contain detailed and updated information about the coding and medical necessity of specific services.

If a provider thinks that a procedure will not be covered by Medicare because it is not reasonable and necessary, the patient is notified of this before the treatment by means of a standard **advance beneficiary notice of noncoverage (ABN)** from CMS (see Figure 5.4). A filled-in form is given to the patient for signature. The ABN form is designed to:

- Identify the service or item that Medicare is unlikely to pay for
- State the reason Medicare is unlikely to pay
- Estimate how much the service or item will cost the beneficiary if Medicare does not pay

advance beneficiary notice of noncoverage (ABN) Medicare form used to inform a patient that a service to be provided is not likely to be reimbursed by Medicare

(A) **Notifier(s):**
(B) **Patient Name:** *(C)* **Identification Number:**

ADVANCE BENEFICIARY NOTICE OF NONCOVERAGE (ABN)

NOTE: If Medicare doesn't pay for ***(D)***_____________ below, you may have to pay.

Medicare does not pay for everything, even some care that you or your health care provider have good reason to think you need. We expect Medicare may not pay for the ***(D)***_____________ below.

*(D)*_______________	*(E)* **Reason Medicare May Not Pay:**	*(F)* **Estimated Cost:**

WHAT YOU NEED TO DO NOW:

- Read this notice, so you can make an informed decision about your care.
- Ask us any questions that you may have after you finish reading.
- Choose an option below about whether to receive the ***(D)***____________ listed above.

  Note: If you choose Option 1 or 2, we may help you to use any other insurance that you might have, but Medicare cannot require us to do this.

(G) **OPTIONS:** **Check only one box. We cannot choose a box for you.**

☐ **OPTION 1.** I want the ***(D)***_________ listed above. You may ask to be paid now, but I also want Medicare billed for an official decision on payment, which is sent to me on a Medicare Summary Notice (MSN). I understand that if Medicare doesn't pay, I am responsible for payment, but **I can appeal to Medicare** by following the directions on the MSN. If Medicare does pay, you will refund any payments I made to you, less co-pays or deductibles.

☐ **OPTION 2.** I want the ***(D)***_________ listed above, but do not bill Medicare. You may ask to be paid now as I am responsible for payment. **I cannot appeal if Medicare is not billed.**

☐ **OPTION 3.** I don't want the ***(D)***_________ listed above. I understand with this choice I am **not** responsible for payment, and **I cannot appeal to see if Medicare would pay.**

(H) **Additional Information:**

This notice gives our opinion, not an official Medicare decision. If you have other questions on this notice or Medicare billing, call **1-800-MEDICARE** (1-800-633-4227/**TTY**: 1-877-486-2048).

Signing below means that you have received and understand this notice. You also receive a copy.

(I) **Signature:**	*(J)* **Date:**

According to the Paperwork Reduction Act of 1995, no persons are required to respond to a collection of information unless it displays a valid OMB control number. The valid OMB control number for this information collection is 0938-0566. The time required to complete this information collection is estimated to average 7 minutes per response, including the time to review instructions, search existing data resources, gather the data needed, and complete and review the information collection. If you have comments concerning the accuracy of the time estimate or suggestions for improving this form, please write to: CMS, 7500 Security Boulevard, Attn: PRA Reports Clearance Officer, Baltimore, Maryland 21244-1850.

Form CMS-R-131 (03/08) Form Approved OMB No. 0938-0566

Figure 5.4 Advance Beneficiary Notice of Noncoverage (ABN)

The purpose of the ABN is to help the beneficiary make an informed decision about services that might have to be paid out-of-pocket. Medicare expects providers to know that certain services will not be covered. If a provider performs such a service without informing the patient in advance, the provider will not be allowed to bill the patient and thus will not be paid for the service.

When provided, the ABN must be verbally reviewed with beneficiaries or with their representatives, and questions posed during that discussion must be answered before the form is signed. The form must be provided in advance to allow the beneficiary or representative time to consider options and make an informed choice. Either the physician or another member of the practice's health care team presents the ABN. After the form has been completely filled in and signed, a copy is given to the beneficiary or representative. In all cases, the provider must retain the original notice on file.

EXERCISE 5.2

Record Receipt of Required Documents EHRclinic

You have created a new patient registration for a walk-in patient. He has signed his Acknowledgment of Receipt of Notice of Privacy Practices and an authorization for his visit records to be sent to his primary care physician. Record receipt of these documents in the patient's EHR.

Your instructor may assign this exercise to you in Connect. Exercise steps and EHRclinic Help Guides can be downloaded at http://www.mhhe.com/pmehr2.

Information for Established Patients

When established patients appear for appointments, their patient and insurance information is already stored in the practice management program. Registration staff, though, must ask returning patients whether any pertinent personal or insurance information has changed. This update process is important because different employment, marital status, dependent status, or plans may affect patients' coverage. Patients sometimes alert the practice about changes, such as new addresses or employers, in advance of an appointment.

To make sure information is current, most practices periodically ask established patients to review and sign off on their patient information forms when they come in. This review should be done at least once a year. A good time is an established patient's first appointment in a new year. The file is also checked to be sure that the patient has been given a current Notice of Privacy Practices.

THINKING IT THROUGH 5.1

The registration process requires the patient to fill out many forms and to sign papers that may be difficult to understand. In addition, the patient may be under time constraints or may not be feeling well. In what ways can the medical administrative team show empathy to the patient? What advantages can be gained by establishing a clear line of communication with the patient during the registration process?

If the insurance coverage of an established patient has changed, both sides of the new card are copied, and all data are checked. Many practices routinely scan or copy the card at each visit as a safeguard.

EXERCISE 5.3

Edit Patient Demographics

EHRclinic

An established patient arrives for her appointment. Upon registration, she indicates that she has a new address and insurance. Update the patient's demographics and insurance information in her EHR.

Your instructor may assign this exercise to you in Connect. Exercise steps and EHRclinic Help Guides can be downloaded at http://www.mhhe.com/pmehr2.

EHRclinic TIP

EHRclinic

Patient Demographics

In EHRclinic, patient demographics can be accessed and edited in the Patient info tab when scheduling an appointment, within the patient's face sheet, or in the Patient information box in the patient database.

5.2 Other Insurance Plans: Coordination of Benefits

primary insurance plan health plan that pays benefits first when a patient is covered by more than one plan

secondary insurance plan health plan that pays benefits after the primary plan pays when a patient is covered by more than one plan

The registration staff also examines the patient information form and insurance card to see if other coverage is in effect. A patient may have more than one insurance carrier. The staff member, using the coordination of benefits guidelines described below, must then determine which carrier is the **primary insurance plan**—the plan that pays first when more than one plan is in effect—and which is the **secondary insurance plan**—an additional policy that provides benefits. Tertiary insurance, a third payer, is possible. Some patients have supplemental insurance, a "fill-the-gap" insurance plan that covers parts of expenses, such as coinsurance, that they must otherwise pay out-of-pocket under the primary plan.

Determining the primary insurance is important because this payer is sent the first claim for the encounter. A second claim is sent to the secondary payer after the payment is received for the primary claim. After both plans have made payments, any unpaid bills are submitted to the patient.

The HIPAA Coordination of Benefits transaction is used to send the necessary data to payers. This transaction is also called the ASC X12N 837—the same transaction used to send electronic claims—because it goes along with the claim.

EXERCISE 5.4

Add a Patient's Primary Insurance Information

EHRclinic

You registered a new patient who walked into Family Care Medical Center for urgent care, and you documented receipt of his required documents. Now you will need to add the patient's primary insurance to his EHR.

Your instructor may assign this exercise to you in Connect. Exercise steps and EHRclinic Help Guides can be downloaded at http://www.mhhe.com/pmehr2.

Coordination of Benefits

Deciding which payer is primary is also important because insurance policies contain a provision called **coordination of benefits (COB).** The coordination of benefits guidelines ensure that when a patient has more than one policy, maximum appropriate benefits are paid, but without duplication. Under the law, to protect the insurance companies, if the patient has signed an assignment of benefits statement, the provider is responsible for reporting any additional insurance coverage to the primary payer.

coordination of benefits (COB) clause in an insurance policy that explains how the policy will pay if more than one insurance policy applies to the claim

Coordination of benefits in government-sponsored programs such as Medicare and Medicaid follow specific guidelines. Medicaid, for example, always pays last. If the patient has coverage through any other insurance plan or if the claim is covered by another program, such as Medicare or workers' compensation, the other plan is billed first, and information from that payer is forwarded to Medicaid. For this reason, Medicaid is known as the payer of last resort, since it is always billed after another plan has been billed when other coverage exists.

Guidelines for Determining the Primary Plan

How do patients come to have more than one plan in effect? Possible answers are that a patient may have coverage under more than one group plan, such as a person who has both employer-sponsored insurance and a policy from union membership. A person may have primary insurance coverage from an employer but also be covered as a dependent under a spouse's insurance, making the spouse's plan the person's additional insurance. General guidelines for determining the primary insurance are shown in Table 5.1.

TABLE 5.1 Determining Primary Coverage
• If the patient has only one policy, it is primary.
• If the patient has coverage under two plans, the plan that has been in effect for the patient for the longest period of time is primary. (However, if an active employee has a plan with the present employer and is still covered by a former employer's plan as a retiree or a laid-off employee, the current employer's plan is primary.)
• If the patient is also covered as a dependent under another insurance policy, the patient's plan is primary.
• If an employed patient has coverage under the employer's plan and additional coverage under a government-sponsored plan, the employer's plan is primary. For example, if a patient is enrolled in a PPO through employment and is also on Medicare, the PPO is primary.
• If a retired patient is covered by a spouse's employer's plan and the spouse is still employed, the spouse's plan is primary, even if the retired person has Medicare.
• If the patient is a dependent child covered by both parents' plans and the parents are not separated or divorced (or if the parents have joint custody of the child), the primary plan is determined by the birthday rule.
• If two or more plans cover a dependent child of separated or divorced parents who do not have joint custody of their child, the child's primary plan is determined in this order (or by court order): • The plan of the custodial parent • The plan of the spouse of the custodial parent if remarried • The plan of the parent without custody

birthday rule guideline that determines which of two parents with medical coverage has the primary insurance for a child; the parent whose day of birth is earlier in the calendar year is considered primary

financial policy practice's rules governing payment for medical services from patients

A common issue involves determining which of two parents' plans is primary for a child. If both parents cover dependents on their plans, the child's primary insurance is usually determined by the **birthday rule.** This rule states that the parent whose day of birth is earlier in the calendar year is primary. For example, Rachel Foster's mother and father both work and have employer-sponsored insurance policies. Her father, George Foster, was born on October 7, 1971, and her mother, Myrna, was born on May 15, 1972. Since the mother's date of birth is earlier in the calendar year (although the father is older), her plan is Rachel's primary insurance. The father's plan is secondary for Rachel. If both parents have the same birthdate (day and month), then the plan that has been in effect the longest is considered to be the primary insurance.

THINKING IT THROUGH 5.2

When a patient has secondary insurance, the claim for the secondary payer is sent after the claim to the primary payer is paid. Why is that the case? What information do you think the medical biller provides to the secondary payer?

Note that if a dependent child's primary insurance does not provide for the complete reimbursement of a bill, the balance may usually be submitted to the other parent's plan for consideration.

EXERCISE 5.5

Add a Patient's Secondary Insurance Plan EHRclinic

A patient arrives for her appointment at Family Care Medical Center. Upon registration, she informs you that she has a secondary insurance plan through her husband. Update the patient's secondary insurance information in the EHR.

Your instructor may assign this exercise to you in Connect. Exercise steps and EHRclinic Help Guides can be downloaded at http://www.mhhe.com/pmehr2.

5.3 Financial Policy of the Practice

As part of the check-in procedures, patients should always be reminded of their financial obligations according to practice procedures. New patients are given information about the practice's financial policy so they understand that they are responsible for payment of charges that are not paid by their health plans. The practice's **financial policy** on payment for services is usually either displayed at the reception desk or included in a new patient information packet. An example of a financial policy is shown in Figure 5.5.

THINKING IT THROUGH 5.3

Who is ultimately responsible for payment of charges incurred for medical services?

Figure 5.5 Example of a Financial Policy

We sincerely wish to provide the best possible medical care. This involves mutual understanding between the patients, doctors, and staff. We encourage you, our patient, to discuss any questions you may have regarding this payment policy.

Payment is expected at the time of your visit for services not covered by your insurance plan. We accept cash, check, MasterCard, and Visa.

Credit will be extended as necessary.

Credit Policy
Requirements for maintaining your account in good standing are as follows:

1. All charges are due and payable within 30 days of the first billing.
2. For services not covered by your health plan, payment at the time of service is necessary.
3. If other circumstances warrant an extended payment plan, our credit counselor will assist you in these special circumstances at your request.

We welcome early discussion of financial problems. A credit counselor will assist you.

An itemized statement of all medical services will be mailed to you every 30 days. We will prepare and file your claim forms to the health plan. If further information is needed, we will provide an additional report.

Insurance
Unless we have a contract directly with your health plan, we cannot accept the responsibility of negotiating claims. You, the patient, are responsible for payment of medical care regardless of the status of the medical claim. In situations where a claim is pending or when treatment will be over an extended period of time, we will recommend that a payment plan be initiated. Your health plan is a contract between you and your insurance company. We cannot guarantee the payment of your claim. If your insurance company pays only a portion of the bill or denies the claim, any contact or explanation should be made to you, the policyholder. Reduction or rejection of your claim by your insurance company does not relieve the financial obligation you have incurred.

The policy should explain what is required of the patient and when payment is due. For example, the policy may state the following:

Assigned claims	After your insurance claim is processed by your insurance company, you will be billed for any amount you owe. You are responsible for any charges that are denied or are not paid by the carrier. All patient accounts are due within thirty days of the date of the invoice.
Unassigned claims	Payment for the physician's services is expected at the end of your appointment unless you have made other arrangements with our practice manager.
Copayments	Copayments must be paid before patients leave the office.

If patients have large bills that they are unable to pay immediately, financial arrangements for series of payments may be made (see Figure 5.6). The patient may begin with a prepayment followed by monthly amounts. Such arrangements are governed by federal and state laws.

5.4 Estimating and Collecting Payment

Another aspect of check-in procedures is estimating and collecting payments from patients. Chapter 10 explains how most time-of-service payments are collected at checkout after the encounter. However, depending on

Figure 5.6 Financial Arrangement for Services Form

Patient Name and Account Number

Total of All Payments Due

FEE	$________	
PARTIAL PAYMENT	$________	
UNPAID BALANCE	$________	
AMOUNT FINANCED	$________	(amount of credit we have provided to you)
FINANCE CHARGE	$________	(dollar amount the interest on credit will cost)
ANNUAL PERCENTAGE RATE	$________	(cost of your credit as a yearly rate)
TOTAL OF PAYMENTS DUE	$________	(amount paid after all payments are made)

Rights and Duties

I (we) have reviewed the above fees. I agree to make ________ payments in monthly installments of $________, due on the ________ day of each month payable to ________, until the total amount is paid in full. The first payment is due on ________. I may request an itemization of the amount financed.

Delinquent Accounts

I (we) understand that I am financially responsible for all fees as stated. My account will be overdue if my scheduled payment is more than 7 days late. There will be a late payment charge of $________ or ________% of the payment, whichever is less. I understand that I will be legally responsible for all costs involved with the collection of this account including all court costs, reasonable attorney fees, and all other expenses incurred with collection if I default on this agreement.

Prepayment Penalty

There is no penalty if the total amount due is paid before the last scheduled payment.

I (we) agree to the terms of the above financial contract.

________________________ ________

Signature of Patient, Parent, or Legal Representative Date

________________________ ________

Witness Date

________________________ ________

Authorizing Signature Date

office policy, some payments, including copayments, outstanding balances, and partial payments, may be collected from patients at check-in.

Copayments

Copayments are routinely collected during check-in. Payments may be made by cash, check, or credit or debit card. When a payment is made, a receipt is given to the patient. The copayment amount depends on the type of service and on whether the provider is in the patient's network. Copays for out-of-network providers are usually higher than for in-network providers. Different copay amounts may be required for office visits to primary care physicians (PCPs), for visits to specialists, and for lab work, radiology services such as X-rays, and surgery.

Established patients' copayment requirements are stored in the practice management program along with their insurance data. When the patient's appointment is selected in the practice management program at check-in, the scheduling screen displays the copayment amount due for the visit. If the plan's copayment requirements change, the patient informs the practice, and the amounts are easily updated in the program.

EXERCISE 5.6

Collect a Patient's Copayment

EHRclinic

A walk-in patient was seen by a provider at Trilogy Family Care Center. Before leaving, he is required to pay his copayment. Record the copayment and provide the patient with a receipt.

Your instructor may assign this exercise to you in Connect. Exercise steps and EHRclinic Help Guides can be downloaded at http://www.mhhe.com/pmehr2.

Outstanding Balances

In many practices, if a patient owes a balance to the practice, this amount is also collected at check-in, or arrangements for payment are made. Practice management programs usually have shortcut keys or quick check buttons for determining whether the patient has an overdue amount. Usually, the appointment scheduler that comes with the practice management program will also display this information. If the patient's account is overdue, the receptionist can talk with the patient about the possibility of making a payment while the patient is at the desk.

EXERCISE 5.7

Collect Payment Toward an Outstanding Balance

EHRclinic

Upon a patient's check-in, you identify that there is an outstanding balance owed. After discussing this, the patient agrees to make a payment toward the balance. Post the payment and provide the patient with a receipt.

Your instructor may assign this exercise to you in Connect. Exercise steps and EHRclinic Help Guides can be downloaded at http://www.mhhe.com/pmehr2.

Partial Payment

While insurance companies require physician practices to collect copayments from patients when they come in for care, some medical offices are now asking patients for partial payment of the office visit charges during check-in to increase cash flow. The amount of the partial payment is usually a percentage of the estimated patient responsibility for the procedure. For example, if the patient is expected to owe $200 for a procedure and practice policy is to collect 50 percent, the patient is asked to pay $100 on the day of the encounter and to expect to be billed $100 after the claim is processed. Since it is not always possible to estimate a patient's financial obligation accurately at check-in, offices usually base the patient's share on the average charge for the scheduled service. The prepayments are low enough that few patients overpay.

5.5 Patient Tracking

Patient tracking features are used during patient encounters to track the status of each appointment (this includes whether the appointment was kept, canceled, or rescheduled) as well as to track where patients are during the different steps of the encounter (this includes whether a patient has checked in, is in the exam room, is with a provider, or has checked out). In most PM and EHR

patient tracking features
function attached to the electronic scheduler that is used during a patient encounter to track where the patient is during the different steps of the encounter

programs, the patient tracking features are attached to the electronic scheduler. Tracking where patients are during a visit is especially helpful in large practices that see many patients at a time and may be double-booking them. Any member of the medical administrative team can see a patient's whereabouts at a glance.

Depending on the reporting capacity of the program, various reports can be created using the patient tracking information. For example, a report can be created that lists canceled appointments for all providers during the last week. If the scheduling program has a timing feature that keeps track of the amount of time patients spend for each part of a visit, more-detailed reports can be generated that list the average amount of time patients are being seen by physicians or the average time patients spend in the waiting room. The office manager can study the results of the tracking reports to help improve the day-to-day functions of the office.

EHRclinic tracks patients' activity throughout the encounter. As patients complete the stages of the encounter, the system updates the tracking status, as shown in Figure 5.7. Filters can also be used to identify which patients are in each stage of the tracking system, including:

- Checked-in waiting
- Patient intake
- Specific provider
- Ready for provider
- Ready for treatment
- In treatment
- Ready for checkout
- Checked out

EXERCISE 5.8

Utilize the Patient Tracker

EHRclinic

A patient has arrived for his appointment. Check him into the system, and use the EHRclinic Patient Tracker to review his status.

Your instructor may assign this exercise to you in Connect. Exercise steps and EHRclinic Help Guides can be downloaded at http://www.mhhe.com/pmehr2.

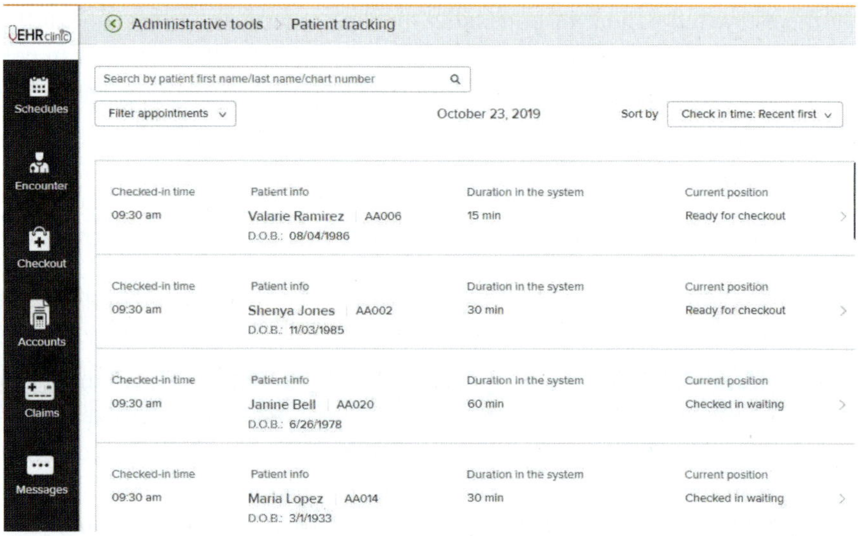

Figure 5.7 EHRclinic Patient Tracker

chapter 5 summary

KEY TERMS

accept assignment
advance beneficiary notice of noncoverage (ABN)
assignment of benefits
birthday rule
coordination of benefits (COB)
financial policy
guarantor
patient information form
patient tracking features
primary insurance plan
registration
secondary insurance plan

LEARNING OUTCOME	KEY CONCEPTS/EXAMPLES
5.1 List the six types of information that are gathered as part of the registration process for new patients.	The six types of information are: 1. Medical history form 2. Patient information form 3. Insurance card 4. Assignment of benefits 5. Financial agreement and authorization for treatment 6. Acknowledgment of Receipt of Notice of Privacy Practices (NPP)
5.2 Determine which health plan is primary when there is more than one.	The primary health plan is determined by following the coordination of benefits rules: - The plan that has been in effect for the patient for the longest period of time is primary. - If the patient is also covered as a dependent under another insurance policy, the patient's plan is primary. - If an employed patient has coverage under the employer's plan and additional coverage under a government-sponsored plan, the employer's plan is primary. - If the patient is a dependent child covered by both parents' plans and the parents are not separated or divorced or if the parents have joint custody of the child, the primary plan is determined by the birthday rule. - If two or more plans cover a dependent child of separated or divorced parents who do not have joint custody of their child, the child's primary plan is determined in this order (or by court order): (1) the plan of the custodial parent; (2) the plan of the spouse of the custodial parent if remarried; (3) the plan of the parent without custody.
5.3 Describe the purpose of a practice's financial policy.	The financial policy explains what is required of the patient and when payment is due.

LEARNING OUTCOME	KEY CONCEPTS/EXAMPLES
5.4 List the types of payments that may be collected from patients at check-in.	These payments may be collected at check-in or at the time of service: - Copayments - Balances - Partial payments
5.5 Discuss the advantages of tracking patients electronically during a visit.	Tracking allows the staff to know patients' whereabouts. Tracking reports can be used to improve day-to-day functions of the office. Tracking information also creates a record of a patient's appointment history.

chapter 5 review

MATCHING QUESTIONS

Match the key terms with their definitions.

_____ 1. *[LO 5.2]* coordination of benefits

_____ 2. *[LO 5.3]* financial policy

_____ 3. *[LO 5.2]* birthday rule

_____ 4. *[LO 5.1]* guarantor

_____ 5. *[LO 5.1]* assignment of benefits

_____ 6. *[LO 5.2]* secondary insurance

_____ 7. *[LO 5.1]* accept assignment

_____ 8. *[LO 5.2]* primary insurance plan

_____ 9. *[LO 5.1]* patient information form

_____ 10. *[LO 5.1]* registration

a. Health plan that pays when a patient is covered by more than one plan.

b. Guidelines that ensure that when a patient has more than one policy, maximum appropriate benefits are paid, but without duplication.

c. Patient registration form.

d. Explains who is responsible for charges not paid by the carrier.

e. Subscriber.

f. Participating physician's agreement to consider the allowed charge as full payment.

g. Authorization to allow benefits to be paid directly to a provider.

h. Process of gathering personal and insurance information about a patient at check-in.

i. First plan to be billed.

j. The parent whose day of birth is earlier in the calendar year holds the primary plan.

MULTIPLE-CHOICE QUESTIONS

Select the letter that best completes the statement or answers the question.

1. *[LO 5.5]* _____ are used during patient encounters to track where patients are during the different steps of the encounter.
   a. Patient information forms
   b. Records of treatment and progress
   c. Patient tracking features
   d. Capitated plans

2. *[LO 5.1]* The medical history form contains all of the following EXCEPT _____.
   a. lifestyle factors, such as exercise and alcohol use
   b. medical conditions of family members
   c. details of prior surgeries, if any
   d. previous occupations held

3. *[LO 5.1]* The ______ form is used to collect basic demographic information about the patient.
   a. encounter
   b. patient information
   c. authorization
   d. coordination of benefits
4. *[LO 5.1]* Each of the terms below refers to the insured EXCEPT ______.
   a. guarantor
   b. policyholder
   c. subscriber
   d. preferred provider
5. *[LO 5.1]* The policyholder authorizes the physician to submit insurance claims for patients and receive payments directly by signing the ______ statement.
   a. assignment of benefits
   b. release authorization
   c. participating provider
   d. indemnity plan
6. *[LO 5.1]* If a provider thinks that a procedure will not be covered by Medicare, the patient is notified of this before the treatment by means of the ______ form.
   a. assignment of benefits
   b. advance beneficiary notice of noncoverage
   c. release authorization
   d. nonparticipating provider
7. *[LO 5.2]* ______ ensure that when patients have more than one policy, maximum appropriate benefits are paid.
   a. Prior authorization numbers
   b. Guarantors
   c. Coordination of benefits guidelines
   d. Walkout receipts
8. *[LO 5.2]* The process used to determine the primary insurance carrier if both parents cover dependents on their health insurance plans is called the ______.
   a. schedule of referrals
   b. birthday rule
   c. gender rule
   d. schedule of benefits
9. *[LO 5.3]* The financial policy of the practice addresses all of the following topics EXCEPT ______.
   a. assigned claims
   b. unassigned claims
   c. copayments
   d. referred claims
10. *[LO 5.2]* What health plan is considered the payer of last resort and is never primary in the event that there is another plan?
    a. Medicare
    b. Medicare
    c. TRICARE
    d. CHAMPVA

SHORT-ANSWER QUESTIONS

Define the following abbreviations.

1. *[LO 5.1]* ABN ______________________

2. *[LO 5.2]* COB ______________________

3. *[LO 5.1]* LCD ______________________

APPLYING YOUR KNOWLEDGE

Gathering Information

5.1 *[LO 5.1]* In the following list, put a *Y* (for *Yes*) before an item if it is routinely collected at registration and an *N* (for *No*) if it is not.

a. _____ Notice of Privacy Practices
b. _____ medical history
c. _____ insurance information
d. _____ copy of last bank statement
e. _____ copy of insurance card
f. _____ copy of living will
g. _____ advance beneficiary notice
h. _____ financial agreement and authorization for treatment
i. _____ assignment of benefits statement
j. _____ National Provider Identifier (NPI)
k. _____ Acknowledgment of Receipt of Notice of Privacy Practices
l. _____ HIPAA X12 837 transaction
m. _____ assignment of health care proxy

5.2 *[LO 5.1]* Refer to Tom Bridgewater's insurance card, and answer the following questions.

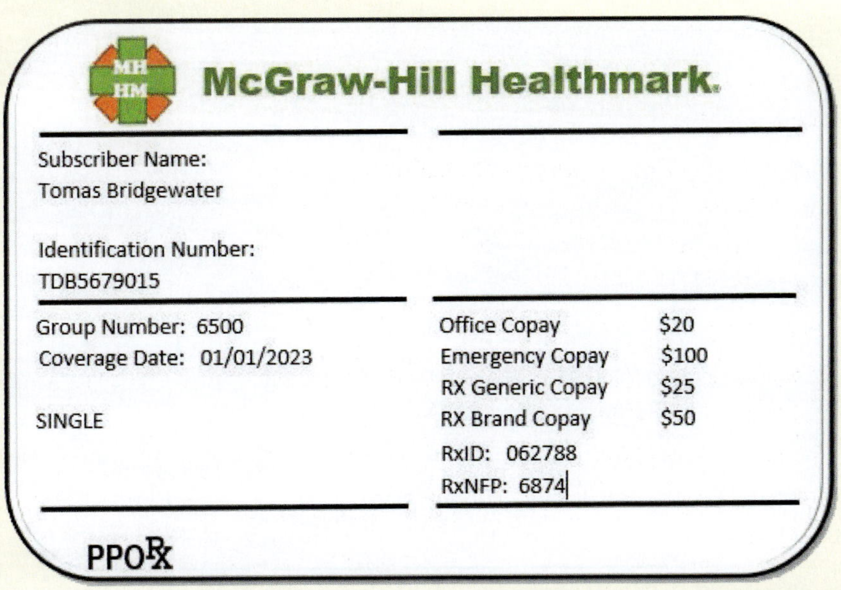
McGraw-Hill Healthmark.

Subscriber Name:
Tomas Bridgewater

Identification Number:
TDB5679015

Group Number: 6500
Coverage Date: 01/01/2023

SINGLE

Office Copay	$20
Emergency Copay	$100
RX Generic Copay	$25
RX Brand Copay	$50

RxID: 062788
RxNFP: 6874

PPORx

a. What is the member's name? ______
b. What is the member's ID number? ______
c. What is the amount of the copayment due when the patient goes to the emergency room? ______
d. What is the date on which the coverage became effective? ______
e. What is the copayment for generic prescriptions? ______
f. What type of insurance plan does the patient have? ______

Evaluating Information

Consider the following situations.

5.3 *[LO 5.2]* Maria is twelve years old and is an established patient. She has flu symptoms and is checking in for an appointment. Her family has gone through a number of changes since Maria's last visit. Her parents are divorced, and her mother has recently remarried. Maria now lives full time with her mother and stepfather. Her mother is no longer working and does not have an independent health plan. However, her father and stepfather both have health insurance plans that include her. Which plan is Maria's primary health plan? Why?

____

____

5.4 *[LO 5.3]* Le'Andre's medical bills are quite large. He would like to make a financial arrangement that would allow him to make monthly payments. What steps do you need to take to facilitate this?

____

____

5.5 *[LO 5.2]* Tasha Maritski is enrolled in an indemnity plan through her employment. She is also a Medicare beneficiary. Who is her primary payer, the indemnity plan or Medicare, and why?

____

____

chapter 6

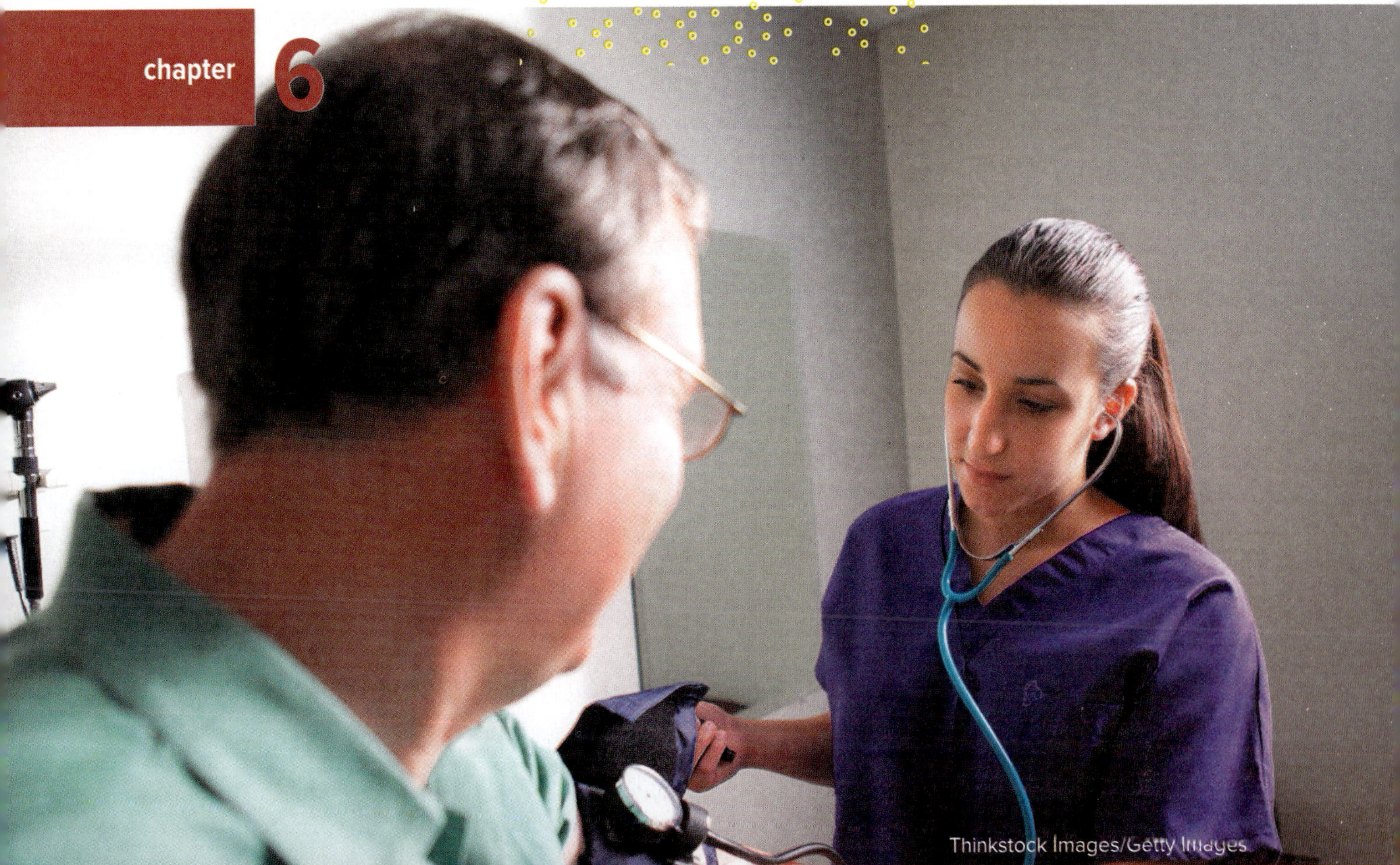
Thinkstock Images/Getty Images

Office Visit: Patient Intake

LEARNING OUTCOMES

When you finish this chapter, you will be able to:

6.1 Identify the four stages of patient flow.

6.2 Discuss the main sections of the patient chart.

6.3 Describe the elements of a patient's past medical, family, and social history.

6.4 Explain how allergies and intolerances are entered in the patient chart.

6.5 Describe the procedure used to enter patient medications and immunizations.

6.6 Explain how the chief complaint and history of present illness are obtained.

6.7 Explain how a patient's vital signs are recorded in the patient chart.

The Trade-Off. . .

Trilogy Family Care Center has had their new PM/EHR program for a little over a month.

Tiffany Patel, the consultant helping with the implementation, has come by to see how things are going. She finds out that Alex Horowitz, the medical assistant, has been writing down some of the patient information on paper during patient intake and entering it in the EHR later in the day. She catches up with Alex on his afternoon break and asks him about it.

"It's fine if they have one or two medications, but some of these patients have eight or ten," Alex responded. "How am I supposed to enter all those while in the exam room with the patient? I like to try and make the patient comfortable, especially when they are new to the practice. It's pretty hard to do that if you have your nose in the computer," said Alex.

As you read this chapter, think about the problem that Alex is experiencing. Is he doing the right thing by making notes on paper and entering them later? Do you see any possible consequences of not entering medications while in the exam room with the patient? Can you think of a solution to this problem?

6.1 Patient Flow in the Physician Office

patient flow the progression of patients from the time they enter the office for a visit until they exit the system by leaving the office after a visit

Where does the information in a patient chart come from? Much of it comes from activities that occur during the stages of patient flow. The term **patient flow** refers to the progression of patients from the time they enter the office for a visit until they exit the system by leaving the office after a visit. A typical patient flow consists of four stages (see Figure 6.1).

Note: The term *medical assistant* is used often throughout this book to refer to the person performing clinical tasks. In actual practice, the person performing the task may also be a nurse or other health care professional.

Check-in

During check-in, the patient arrives at the office and proceeds to the front desk. The front desk staff member checks the patient in, recording the time he or she arrived. This places the patient in the queue of patients waiting to see the provider. The staff member confers with the patient to determine whether any information, such as a change in insurance or employment, needs to be updated in the patient record. The patient may be asked for payment at the time of check-in. Once check-in is complete, the patient takes a seat in the waiting room.

Figure 6.1 The Stages of Patient Flow

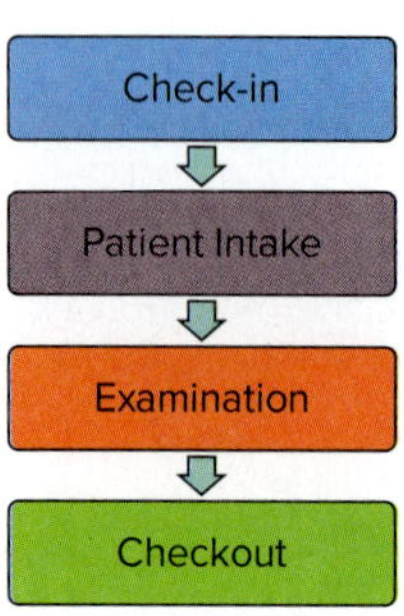

Patient Intake

The patient is escorted to the exam room, where the medical assistant conducts an interview to obtain detailed information. The interview varies depending on the nature of the visit and whether the patient is new or established. Generally, the purpose of the interview is to:

- Obtain past medical, family, and social history
- Review allergies and medications
- Determine the chief complaint

Once the interview is complete, the medical assistant measures the patient's vital signs and prepares the patient for the examination. After the medical assistant has completed these tasks, the provider is notified that the patient is ready to be seen.

Examination

The provider reviews the patient's previous records, and then enters the room and examines the patient. During the encounter, the provider may order lab work or diagnostic tests. Medications may be prescribed. The provider develops a treatment plan and completes the examination. The details of the encounter must be documented. Some providers document the patient encounter during the visit, while others prefer to document the encounter later that same day.

Checkout

The patient leaves the exam room and proceeds to the checkout desk. During checkout, the office staff gives the patient any additional information required, such as patient education materials or lab work instructions. If necessary, a follow-up appointment is scheduled. Before the patient leaves, the staff member collects any payment that is due, if it was not collected during check-in.

This chapter provides detailed instructions on how to perform the steps that are completed by a medical assistant, nurse, or another member of the clinical staff. The steps completed by the physician or other health care provider are covered in Chapter 7.

Table 6.1 lists the steps of patient flow for a typical office visit. It shows both the tasks performed in a paper office and those performed in an office with an integrated practice management/electronic health record (PM/EHR) system.

Information Collected During Patient Flow

The clinical information collected during patient flow and recorded in the patient's chart includes the following:

- **Vital signs and other measurements** **Vital signs** are measurements of a patient's temperature, respiratory rate, pulse, and blood pressure. Although height, weight, and head circumference (for children) are measurements, they are often grouped with vital signs during patient intake.
- **Chief complaint** The **chief complaint (CC)** is a brief description of the patient's current problem in his or her own words.
- **Progress notes** **Progress notes** are notes documenting the care delivered to a patient, and the medical facts and clinical thinking relevant to diagnosis and treatment.
- **Past, family, and social history (PFSH)** **Past, family, and social history (PFSH)** is a commonly used abbreviation for past medical, family, and social history.
- **Past medical history** The **past medical history (PMH)** is the patient's history of medical problems, including chronic conditions, surgeries, and hospitalizations. This includes any illness (past or present) for which the patient has received treatment.

vital signs measurements of a patient's temperature, respiratory rate, pulse, and blood pressure

chief complaint (CC) patient's description of the symptoms or reasons for seeking medical care

progress note note documenting the care delivered to a patient, and the medical facts and clinical thinking relevant to diagnosis and treatment

past, family, and social history (PFSH) patients' answers to physicians' questions about their personal medical histories, medical events in their families, and factors relating to their social environments

past medical history (PMH) the patient's history of medical problems, including chronic conditions, surgeries, and hospitalizations

TABLE 6.1 Patient Flow in a Paper Office and an Office with a PM/EHR

Step	Paper Office	PM/EHR Office
Pre-visit	Charts pulled for patients with appointments.	Daily schedule viewed in EHR.
Check-in	Patient completes or updates patient information form and HIPAA forms.	Patient completes or updates patient information form and HIPAA forms, which are scanned and stored in EHR.
	Insurance card and driver's license are photocopied.	Insurance card and driver's license are scanned and stored in EHR.
	Front desk looks in patient chart to see notes about overdue balance.	System alerts front desk if patient has overdue balance.
	Encounter form is placed in patient chart.	No paper encounter form is needed (now electronic).
	Chart is placed in bin for medical assistant (MA) or nurse; light turned on to notify MA or nurse that patient is checked in and ready for exam.	Message is sent in EHR to notify MA or nurse that patient has checked in and is ready for exam.
	Patient is escorted to exam room.	Patient is escorted to exam room.
Patient Intake	If new patient, MA or nurse interviews patient and writes past medical, family, and social history in patient chart.	If new patient, MA or nurse interviews patient and records past medical, family, and social history in EHR.
	MA or nurse reviews and updates medications and allergies in paper chart.	MA or nurse reviews and updates medications and allergies in EHR.
	MA or nurse records chief complaint in paper chart.	MA or nurse records chief complaint in EHR.
	MA or nurse takes vital signs and records them on paper form.	MA or nurse takes vital signs and enters them directly into patient chart in EHR.
	MA or nurse uses flag or light to notify physician that patient is ready; patient chart is placed in bin for physician.	MA or nurse sends electronic message in EHR to notify physician that patient is ready.
Examination	Physician picks up chart from bin, enters exam room, and reviews information in the chart.	Physician reviews patient chart in EHR, including today's vital signs and chief complaint.
	Physician examines patient.	Physician examines patient.
	Physician documents exam in paper chart during visit or later in the day. May use dictation.	Physician documents exam in EHR. May use templates.
	If prescription is required, physician writes it and gives it to patient.	If prescription is required, physician enters electronic prescription and transmits it to patient's pharmacy.
	If follow-up, referral, or tests are required, physician writes information on encounter form.	If follow-up, referral, or tests are required, physician enters orders in EHR.
	If patient education materials are required, physician notes that on encounter form, and checkout staff member locates paper materials to give to patient.	If patient education materials are required, physician prints them directly from EHR and hands them to patient.
	If additional procedures are required, physician uses flag or light system to alert medical assistant or nurse.	If additional procedures are required, physician sends electronic message to medical assistant or nurse.
	Medical assistant or nurse performs procedures.	Medical assistant or nurse performs procedures.
	If labs are required, MA or nurse locates paper form to write lab orders.	If labs are required, MA or nurse enters lab orders in EHR; order is transmitted electronically to lab.
	MA or nurse records additional procedures on encounter form.	MA or nurse records additional procedures in EHR.
	Patient leaves exam room and proceeds to checkout desk.	Patient leaves exam room and proceeds to checkout desk.

(continued)

TABLE 6.1 (continued)		
Step	**Paper Office**	**PM/EHR Office**
Checkout	Coder reviews documentation in paper chart, assigns codes, and records them on encounter form. Patient chart with instructions for follow-up, referral, tests, and so on and encounter form arrive at checkout desk. Checkout staff member writes instructions for referral, tests, and so on; schedules follow-up appointment; and completes appointment card for patient. Checkout staff reviews encounter form to see whether payment is due. Payment is collected and recorded on encounter form; patient is given handwritten receipt. Billing staff member reviews charges and payments on encounter form. Billing staff member enters charges and payments in PM.	Coder reviews documentation in EHR and assigns codes on electronic encounter form in EHR. Electronic message is sent to checkout desk with instructions for follow-up, referral, tests, and so on and link to electronic encounter form. Checkout staff member prints instructions for referral, tests, and so on from EHR; schedules follow-up appointment; and prints appointment reminder for patient. Encounter information is transmitted electronically from EHR to PM. Billing staff member reviews charges and payments in PM and clicks button to electronically post charges in PM. Checkout staff member views patient account in PM to see whether payment is due. Payment is collected and entered in PM; receipt is printed.

- **Family history** The **family history (FH)** details medical events among members of the patient's family, including the ages, living status, and diseases of siblings, children, parents, and grandparents. This includes diseases related to the chief complaint as well as any hereditary diseases.
- **Social history** The **social history (SH)** is information about the patient's tobacco use, alcohol and drug use, sexual history, relationship status, and other significant social facts that may contribute to the care of the patient.
- **Allergies** A list of the patient's known allergies, including reactions to each one.
- **Medication list** Includes all currently prescribed medications as well as over-the-counter medications and nontraditional therapies. Dosage and frequency should be noted.
- **History of present illness (HPI)** The **history of present illness (HPI)** is a description of the course of the present illness, including how and when the problem began, up to the present time. The HPI includes everything related to the illness or condition, including aggravating and alleviating factors, associated symptoms, previous treatment and diagnostic tests, related illnesses, and risk factors.

The following parts of patient flow will be discussed in greater detail in Chapter 7.

- **Review of systems (ROS)** The **review of systems (ROS)** is an inventory of body systems in which the patient reports signs or symptoms he or she is currently having or has had in the past.

family history (FH) a detailed record of medical events among members of the patient's family, including the ages, living status, and diseases of siblings, children, parents, and grandparents

social history (SH) information about the patient's tobacco use, alcohol and drug use, sexual history, relationship status, and other significant social facts that may contribute to the care of the patient

history of present illness (HPI) a description of the course of the present illness, including how and when the problem began, up to the present time

review of systems (ROS) an inventory of body systems in which the patient reports signs or symptoms he or she is currently having or has had in the past

THINKING IT THROUGH 6.1

Table 6.1 compares the patient flow performed in an office using paper records with an office using computerized records. Explain why an office with computerized records is likely to have fewer medical errors.

- **Diagnosis and assessment** The physician's thinking about the cause of the patient's problem as well as any tests performed to come to this determination.
- **Plan and treatment** The physician's thinking about the intervention that will be necessary to cure or manage the patient's condition, including medications, procedures, and lifestyle changes.

6.2 The Patient Chart

Most of the information in an electronic health record program such as EHRclinic is stored in the electronic version of the patient chart. The first step in creating a patient chart in EHRclinic is to select "Manage practice data" in the Tools menu and then clicking on "Patient information." New patient charts can be initiated, and established patients can be selected by name or chart number from this screen (see Figure 6.2).

Patient Information

The "Patient information" screen is used to document patient demographics and insurance carriers. When a new patient chart is created or an established patient is selected, the "Patient information" dialog box opens (see Figure 6.3). When established patient information is updated during the check-in process, this dialog box will be used. This is also the area where new patient chart numbers are generated by the EHRclinic system.

> **TIP**
>
> **Accuracy Is Everything!**
>
> When working in patient charts, it is critical that patient information is entered accurately. Take care to ensure that numbers are correct, and that names, addresses, and emails are spelled correctly. If you are unsure, ask the patient for clarification.

Figure 6.2 The Patient Information Screen

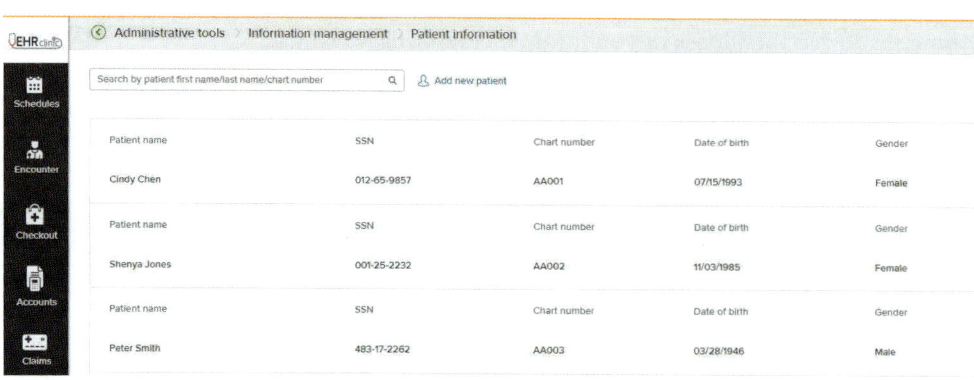

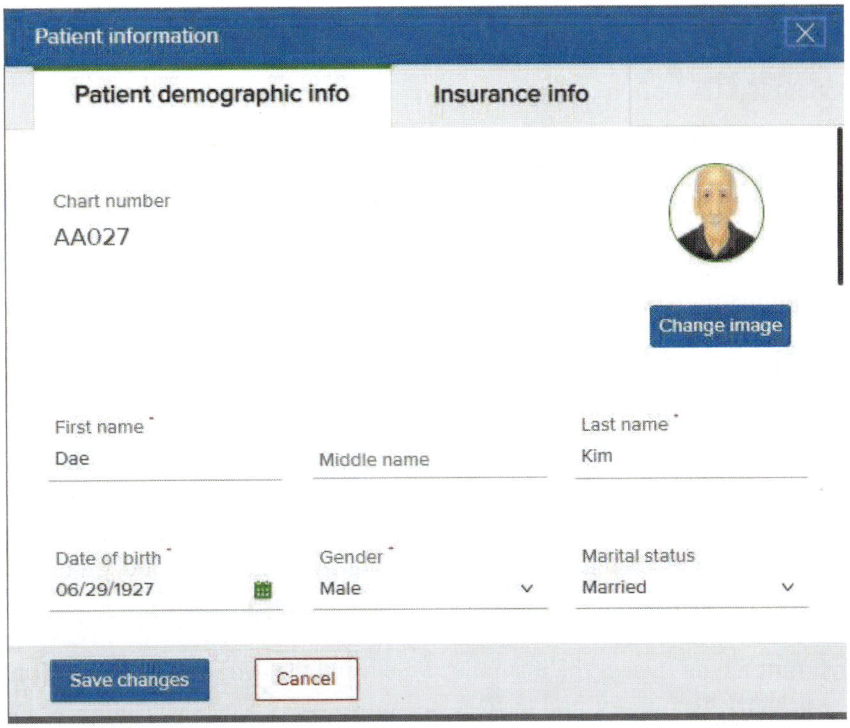

Figure 6.3 Patient Demographics and Insurance Dialog Box

The Patient Demographic Tab

In the "Patient demographic info" tab (shown in Figure 6.3), identifying information about a patient is documented. This information often comes from a patient registration form, and it includes:

Change image Upload the patient's image (typically taken from the driver's license or state identification card) and select it to save it to the patient's chart.

Patient name Enter the patient's first, middle, and last names, taking care to ensure that the names are spelled correctly and are input in the right fields.

Patient ID The patient's chart number is generated upon initiating a new patient chart.

Gender Enter the patient's gender. In EHRclinic, this refers to the gender assigned at birth and the legal gender on the patient's birth certificate.

Marital status Select marital status from the drop-down.

Address Enter the patient's address, including street, city, state, and zip code.

Phone numbers Enter the patient's home, work, and cell phone numbers, including area codes.

Student status Select student status from the drop-down.

Employment status Select employment status from the drop-down.

Email Enter the patient's e-mail, taking care to ensure that it is accurately recorded.

SSN Enter the patient's Social Security number.

Other identifiers Using information identified in the patient registration form, enter the patient's preferred language, race, ethnicity, and religion. The patient has the option to decline answering these questions.

Insurance carrier Select the patient's insurance carrier from the drop-down. If the insurance carrier is not listed, it will need to be added to the insurance database.

Patient insurance ID Enter the patient's insurance identification (ID) number, as listed on the insurance card.

The Insurance Information Tab

While basic information, such as the insurance carrier name and patient ID number, is listed in the "Patient demographic" tab, the patient's detailed insurance information is entered in the "Insurance info" tab (shown in Figure 6.4). This dialog box is used to record primary, secondary, and tertiary insurance information and to edit existing data, including:

Insurance type Select the insurance type using the drop-down. The options are primary, secondary, and tertiary insurance types. This determines which insurance carrier is billed first, second, or third. A new entry should be created for each insurance type the patient carries.

Insurance carrier Select the patient's insurance carrier from the drop-down. If the insurance carrier is not listed, it will need to be added to the insurance database.

Patient insurance ID Enter the patient's insurance identification (ID) number, as listed on the insurance card.

Figure 6.4 Insurance Information Dialog Box

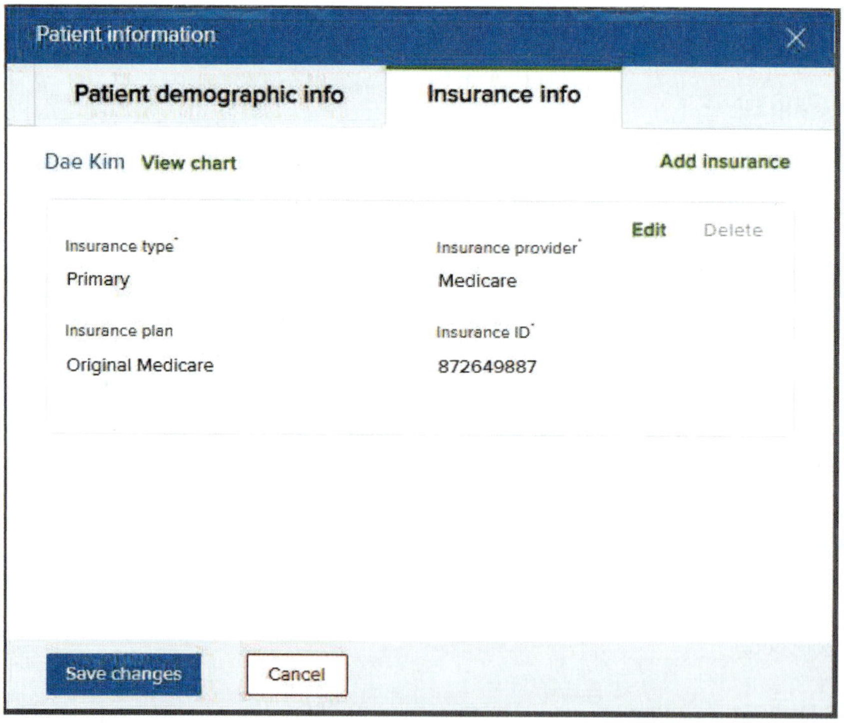

Verify active After verifying the patient's insurance, record Yes if the plan is active and No if it is not active.

Patient responsibility Select whether the patient has a copayment or a coinsurance responsibility.

Deductible Record the patient's deductible amount. If the patient does not have a deductible, record 0.

Dates of coverage Enter the patient's effective start and end dates of coverage.

Guarantor If the patient acts as his or her own guarantor, select Yes. If another person is the patient's guarantor, select No. If No is selected, a guarantor must be added by clicking on "Add guarantor."

Group insurance ID Enter the patient's group ID number, listed on the insurance card.

EXERCISE 6.1

Create a New Patient Chart

EHRclinic

A new patient arrives for her appointment at Trilogy Family Care Center. She has completed her new patient paperwork and hands you her patient registration form, state-issued driver's license, and insurance card. Create a new patient chart and record the information provided.

Your instructor may assign this exercise to you in Connect. Exercise steps and EHRclinic Help Guides can be downloaded at http://www.mhhe.com/pmehr2.

TIP

Source Documents

Documents provided by another entity (the patient, insurance company, etc) with the intention of sharing information are called *source documents.* Source documents provided by patients include patient registration paperwork, identification such as a driver's license, and insurance cards. Special care should be taken to ensure that information obtained from source documents should be accurately entered into the PM or EHR system.

Not all sections of the Patient Chart screen are discussed in this chapter. The focus is on providing an overall understanding of the features of an EHR system, and a closer look at the tasks often performed by allied health professionals. Chapter 7 discusses the sections of the chart used by physicians and other health care providers. The chart folders discussed in this chapter include:

- Past Medical History
- Social History
- Family History
- Allergies

- Medications/Immunizations
- Chief Complaints
- Vital Signs

6.3 Medical History

The medical history section of the patient chart in EHRclinic includes five sections:

- **Patient (past) medical history** Chronic illnesses, injuries, medical diagnoses, and other health information
- **Problem list** An extension of the past medical history that lists current, ongoing problems
- **Surgical history** List of the patient's historical surgical procedures and their approximate dates
- **Social history** Medically relevant information about the patient's life, such as marital status, tobacco and alcohol use, habits, and work
- **Family history** Medically relevant information about the patient's family, including major diseases and chronic conditions

The Face Sheet

Each section of the patient's medical history is recorded with other information in the patient's face sheet. As shown in Figure 6.5, the face sheet is an at-a-glance snapshot of the patient's medical status. An EHRclinic's face sheet is initially shown with each section collapsed (closed). They can be expanded (opened) individually by clicking the title bar, or they can all be opened by clicking "Expand all." When each section is expanded, the patient's details can be seen.

The EHRclinic face sheet sections include:

- Patient information
- Patient (past) medical history
- Problem list
- Surgical history
- Family medical history

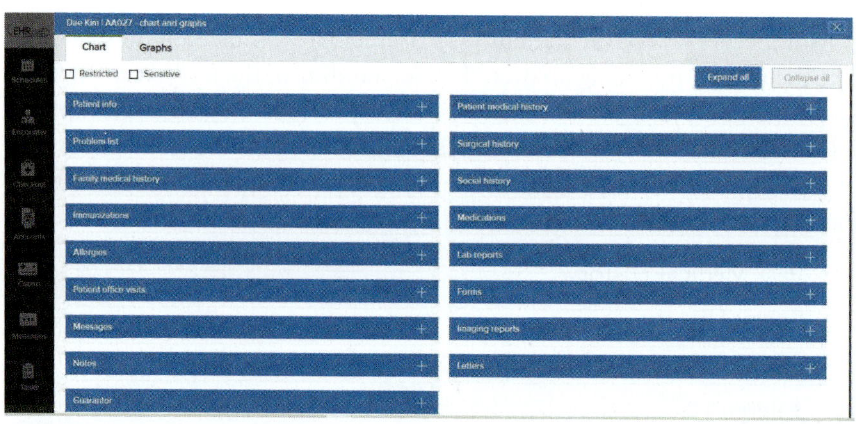

Figure 6.5 The Patient Face Sheet

- Social history
- Immunizations
- Medications
- Allergies
- Lab reports
- Patient office visits
- Forms
- Messages
- Imaging reports
- Notes
- Letters
- Guarantor information

EXERCISE 6.2

Build a New Patient's Face Sheet

After the new patient's chart is created, you will begin creating the face sheet. Complete the patient history sections of the face sheet, including the patient medical history, problem list, surgical history, family medical history, and social history.

Your instructor may assign this exercise to you in Connect. Exercise steps and EHRclinic Help Guides can be downloaded at http://www.mhhe.com/pmehr2.

EHRclinic TIP

Past History Dates

When recording elements of a patient's past medical history, it is ideal to add dates of occurrence, if known. Approximate dates, such as the month and year, can be added if the patient is unsure.

6.4 Allergies

When a new medication is prescribed for a patient, EHRclinic checks whether the patient has any allergies or intolerances. While an allergy is a relative rare condition in which the immune system responds to a medication and causes adverse effects, an intolerance or sensitivity is generally a milder reaction and does not involve the immune system. For example, an antibiotic may cause stomach upset, which is considered an intolerance and not an allergy. Intolerance can sometimes be eliminated by taking medication with food or by lowering the dosage.

Patient allergies are recorded and stored in the Allergies section of the patient's face sheet. When this section is expanded, the allergy box is displayed. Information about all allergies and intolerances is listed here (see Figure 6.6).

In addition to adding, editing, or deleting allergy data, the program also records relevant information to give the provider a better understanding of the circumstances surrounding the allergies or intolerances.

Figure 6.6 Allergies Section of the Face Sheet

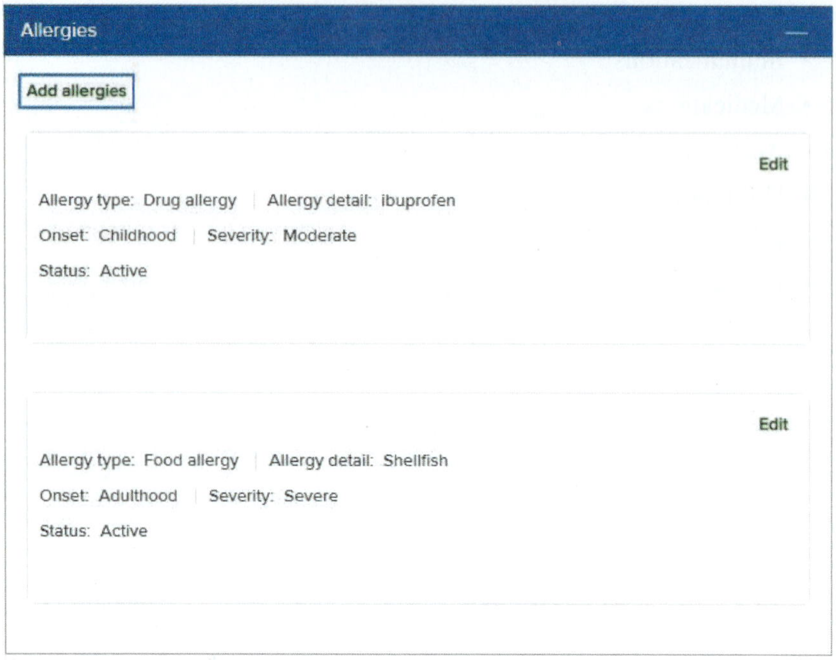

If a patient reports that there are no known allergies (drugs, food, environmental), this information should also be recorded. Failure to document this results in the provider not knowing if there are no allergies or if a member of the health care team simply forgot to record them. Additionally, allergies should be reviewed and updated with every patient encounter to ensure that the most accurate and current information is documented.

The Allergies Dialog Box

To add a patient's allergies and intolerances, click the "Add allergies" button in the Allergies section of the face sheet. When the button is clicked, the Allergies dialog box is displayed (see Figure 6.7). When an allergy or intolerance is added, it becomes viewable in the patient's face sheet.

The fields in the Allergies dialog box include:

Allergy type Identifies if the allergy or intolerance is related to a drug, food, or environmental factor. If a patient reports that there are no known allergies, this information would be reported here, and the dialog box would be closed.

Allergy details Enter the name of the drug, food, or environmental allergy. A new allergy list should be created for each allergy.

Onset Select the allergy or intolerance onset–Childhood, Adulthood, or Unknown–from the drop-down list.

Date/time identified Enter the date and time (if known) the patient's first allergic reaction occurred.

Severity Select the severity of the allergy–Very mild, Mild, Moderate, or Severe–from the drop-down list.

Status Select the allergy or intolerance status–Active or Inactive–from the drop-down list.

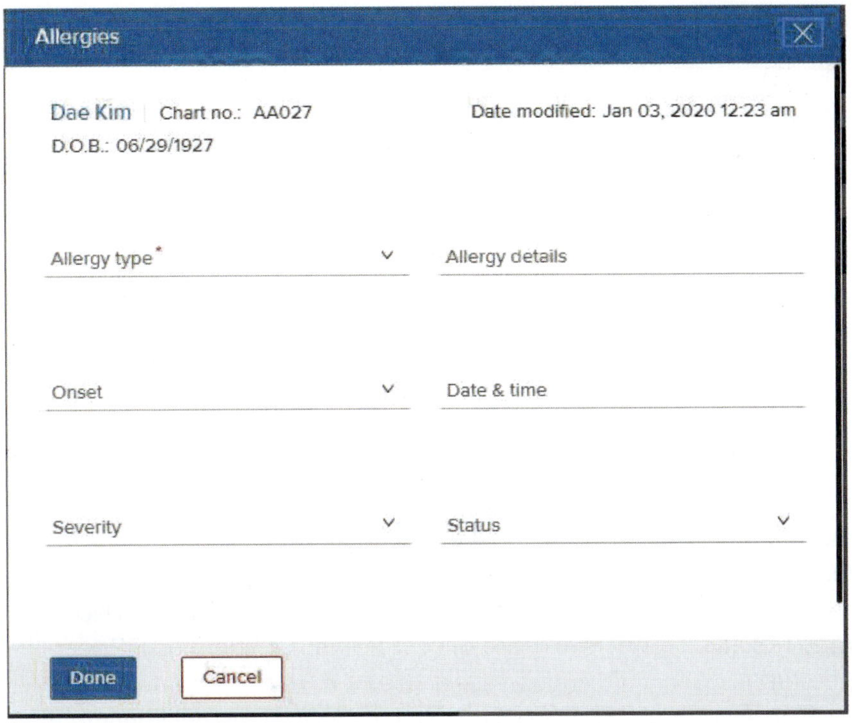

Figure 6.7 The Allergies Dialog Box

Adverse reaction Enter a brief description of the patient's reaction.

Other sensitivities Enter a brief description of other sensitivities related to the allergy or intolerance record.

After each field in the dialog box is complete for an allergy entry, select Done. *Note:* If the medical assistant does not have enough information to complete any of the fields, those fields should remain blank.

EXERCISE 6.3

Add Allergies to a New Patient's Face Sheet

EHRclinic

As you are completing the new patient's face sheet, add the drug, food, and environmental allergies that she listed on her patient information form.

Your instructor may assign this exercise to you in Connect. Exercise steps and EHRclinic Help Guides can be downloaded at http://www.mhhe.com/pmehr2.

6.5 Medications

In many medical offices, a medical assistant is responsible for reviewing medication lists with patients when they come in for an office visit. The patient or a family member is asked to look at the list of current medications and indicate whether anything has changed. Medications that have been added, discontinued, or changed are noted in the patient chart. This process is called *medication reconciliation,* and it is an important part of the patient intake process so the provider can identify if there are any issues with a patient's medications and how they are being taken.

Another important aspect of a patient's chart is maintenance of the immunization record. When a new patient's face sheet is created, historic immunizations should be documented based on the patient's immunization

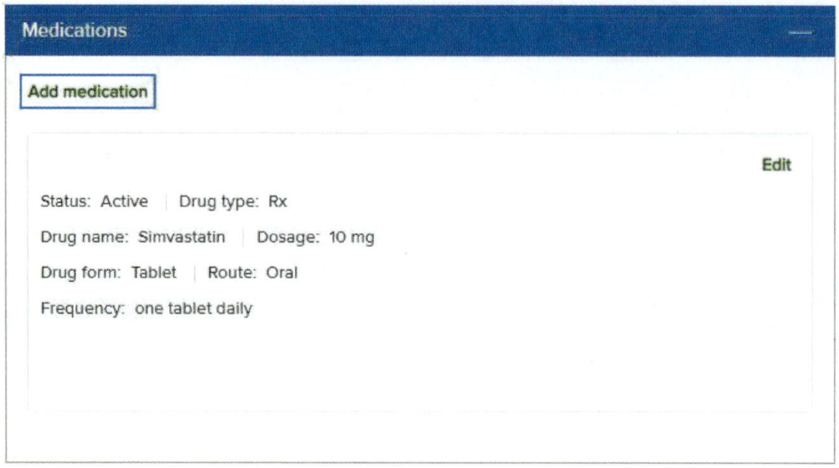

Figure 6.8 Medications Section of the Face Sheet

record. For an established patient, new immunizations are also recorded in the Immunizations section of the face sheet.

Figure 6.8 shows the expanded Medications section of a patient's face sheet. In EHRclinic, providers also use the Medications section for E-Prescribing (creating electronic prescriptions).

This section covers how to record patient medications and immunizations in the patient chart. Creating and refilling prescriptions are covered in Chapter 8.

The Medication Dialog Box

All prescription and over-the-counter drugs are recorded in the Medication dialog box (see Figure 6.9).

The Medications section of the face sheet lists a patient's current medications, including information about the dose and frequency. The process of recording a patient's current medications begins with clicking the "Add

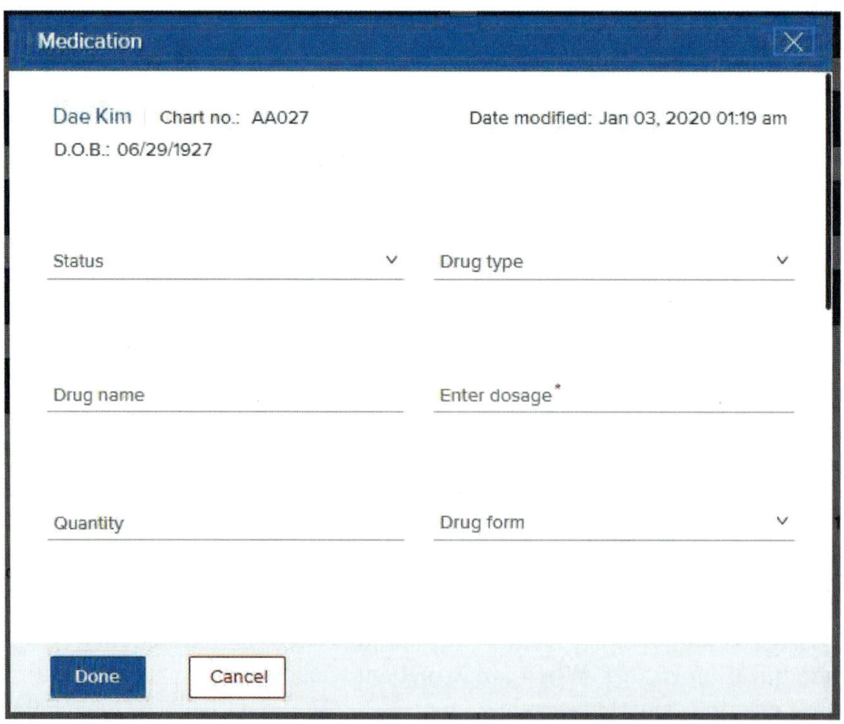

Figure 6.9 The Medication Dialog Box

medication" button in the Medications section of the face sheet. When this button is clicked, the Medication dialog box appears (see Figure 6.9). This is the same dialog box that is used by a physician to manage medication refills and prescribe new medications. In this chapter, the dialog box is used to record the patient's current medications, not to create a new prescription. As a result, only the fields used to record a patient's current medications are discussed in this section. The remaining fields are covered in Chapter 8.

The fields in the Medication dialog box include:

Status Using the drop-down list, identify if the medication is active or inactive. Active drugs can be edited to inactive status when they are discontinued, either because the drug therapy has concluded or because the medication was not effective.

Drug type Identify if the drug is a prescription or over-the-counter medication. Over-the-counter drugs do not require a prescription from a provider; however, it is important that they are recorded in the patient's chart to prevent drug interactions.

Drug name Enter the medication name. Be sure that the drug name is entered accurately (look the drug name up in a drug dictionary if you are not sure).

Enter dosage Enter the drug's dosage. Don't forget to add units of measurement. For example, record 20 mg to indicate that the patient takes 20 milligrams of a particular drug.

Drug form Select the drug form—Oral Solution, Injectable Solution, Tablet—from the drop-down list. If the drug form is other than listed in the drop-down list, do not select any option (the other routes will be covered in the Route drop-down list).

Route Select the route of administration from the drop-down list.

Dose timing Enter the time the drug should be taken—for instance, in the evening, before bed, with meals, and so on.

Frequency Enter how often the medication is taken. For example, 1 tab twice a day.

Quantity This field is optional and is used to enter the quantity of a medication that a patient would use for the duration of treatment or one month. For example, if a patient takes a drug twice a day, then the quantity will be 60 tablets for one month.

Duration Specify how long the patient is taking the medication. Either type the number in days or leave blank if the medication is taken continuously, such as for a chronic condition.

Diagnosis Enter the diagnosis for which the medication was prescribed.

Default provider If the prescription has been written by a provider in the current practice, enter the prescribing physician's name. If the medication was prescribed by a provider outside of the practice, enter "outside provider" in the provider field.

EXERCISE 6.4

Add Medications to a New Patient's Face Sheet

As you are interviewing the new patient during the intake process, she brings out a bag of her medication bottles. Record her prescription and over-the-counter medications in the Medications section of the face sheet.

Your instructor may assign this exercise to you in Connect. Exercise steps and EHRclinic Help Guides can be downloaded at http://www.mhhe.com/pmehr2.

The Immunization Dialog Box

Immunizations are recorded in the Immunizations section of the face sheet. To add a historic or new immunization, click the "Add immunization" button, which will open the Immunization dialog box (see Figure 6.10).

The fields in the Immunization dialog box include:

Immunization type Select the immunization type from the drop-down list.

Ordering physician Enter the name of the ordering provider.

Follow up directions Enter follow-up directions, if given.

Dosage Enter the dosage, including units of measurement. If the immunization is a one-dose unit, enter the total volume of medication. For example, 0.5 mL.

Manufacturer Enter the manufacturer of the immunization.

Lot number Enter the lot number listed on the immunization packaging. This is important in case there is a recall.

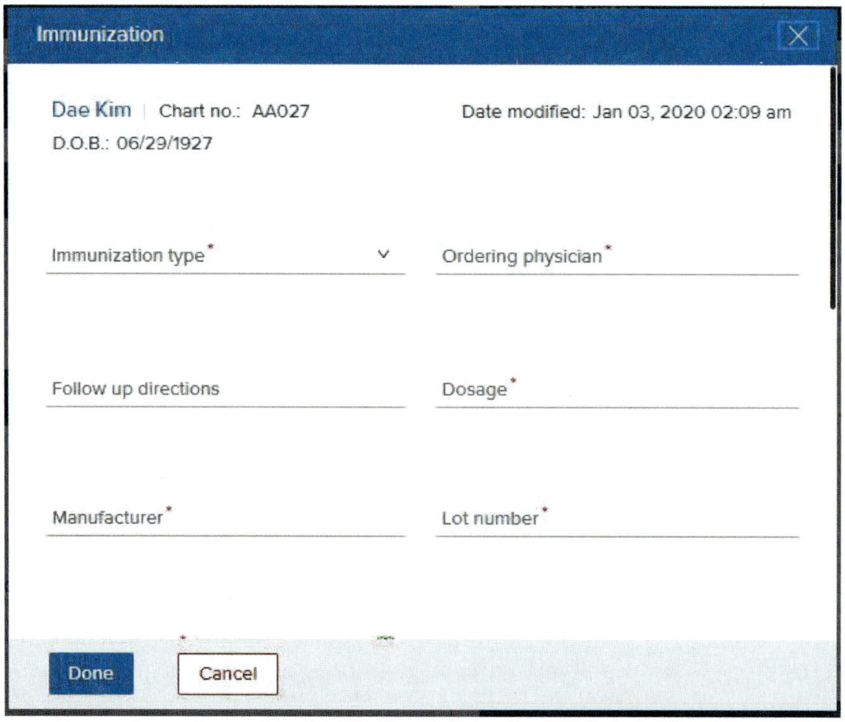

Figure 6.10 The Immunization Dialog Box

Expiration date Enter the expiration date listed on the packaging. Always check the expiration date before administering a drug or immunization. If it is expired, discard the medication according to the practice's protocol.

Site of administration If the immunization is injected, select the side of administration, such as left or right.

Site If the immunization is injected, select the location from the drop-down menu.

Adverse effects Note any adverse effects that the patient experienced after administration of the immunization. If no adverse effects were observed or reported, enter None.

VIS given Select whether a Vaccine Information Statement (VIS) was given. In real-world EHR software, the version of the VIS used would also be recorded.

Follow up directions provided Enter any follow-up directions, such as "Return in 48 to 72 hours to have PPD skin test read."

Patient instructed to return on Select the date the patient should return if a follow-up visit to the provider is needed.

Immunization start date Select the date of the first immunization in a series or the date of administration for a single-dose immunization.

Next dose due date Select the approximate date of return, indicated by when the next immunization is due. For example, a hepatitis B vaccine is given in a series of three immunizations over six months, or a tetanus booster is due after 10 years.

EXERCISE 6.5

Maintain an Immunization Record EHRclinic

During the patient interview, the new patient provides you with her vaccine record sheet. Record her past immunizations in the Immunizations section of the face sheet.

Your instructor may assign this exercise to you in Connect. Exercise steps and EHRclinic Help Guides can be downloaded at http://www.mhhe.com/pmehr2.

6.6 The Chief Complaint and HPI

In most practices, the chief complaint (CC) and history of present illness (HPI) are entered into the progress note for the patient's visit during the patient interview that occurs during intake. Progress notes are also referred to as *office visits* in EHRclinic.

In EHRclinic, the chief complaint and HPI are listed in the office visit or progress note in the *subjective* section. This area of the note is reserved for documenting information that is provided by the patient to describe the reason for the visit, the symptoms, and supporting detail as experienced by the patient. A template box to the right of the office visit notes can be used to efficiently enter information into these fields.

Chief Complaint

The chief complaint is typically the reason for the patient's visit. While patients may have more than one issue to discuss, the chief complaint narrows it down to a concise description. Chief complaints are subjective, meaning that they are personal to the patient. For example, a patient may have a chief complaint of "stomach pain," which describes how he or she is interpreting the problem. It is important to capture patients' chief complaint as they describe it. In other words, avoid revising the description; you may be changing what the patient is trying to describe.

EXAMPLES

During the patient interview, the medical assistant will obtain a chief complaint. This question is usually framed as, "What brings you in to see the provider today?" or something similar. The patient will then respond with a reason for the visit, such as an injury, illness, physical exam, and so on.

If the visit is routine with no problems, this should be noted, such as:

Complete physical exam

Follow-up blood pressure

School physical

If a problem is identified, then it should be recorded as "complaining of (C/O). . ." and described concisely in the patient's own words. The duration is often included in the chief complaint. For example:

C/O sore throat x 2 days

C/O fatigue

C/O "stomach pain" x 1 week

Note that "stomach pain" is recorded with quotation marks to indicate that this is the patient's description. It may be tempting to record this using medical terminology, such as C/O abdominal pain; however that isn't how the patient described the pain.

History of Present Illness

The history of present illness (HPI) expands on the information provided in the chief complaint. Obtaining an accurate and detailed HPI is the first step in determining the cause of a patient's problem. During the patient interview, the HPI is obtained by asking the patient questions about various aspects of their chief complaint. Like the chief complaint, the HPI is recorded in the subjective area of the office visit or progress note because these questions are answered from the patient's personal experience.

While the creation of progress notes is introduced in this section, Chapter 7 covers progress notes in detail.

6.7 Vital Signs

Patients' vital sign measurements are entered in the Patient Intake tab of a patient encounter. The dialog box displayed in Figure 6.11 lists a patient's vital signs and measurements, including height, weight, BMI (which is auto-calculated), systolic and diastolic blood pressure, pulse, respirations, pain scale, temperature, head circumference (for children), and SpO2 (pulse oximetry). Vital signs taken over a period of time can be viewed in a table or a graph.

The Vital Signs Dialog Box

Once a patient has checked in, EHRclinic will move the electronic chart to Encounters. The three tabs in Encounters–Patient Intake, Provider Encounter, and Plan Review–relate to the office visit. Upon selecting the patient's name in the Patient Intake tab, the Vital Signs dialog box will be displayed.

The fields in the Vital Signs (New) dialog box include:

Date and time The current date and time are automatically displayed.

Height Enter the patient's height. To change the height values to inches or centimeters, go to Settings and revise these preferences.

Weight Enter the patient's weight. To change the weight values to pounds or kilograms, go to Settings and revise these preferences.

BMI When the height and the weight are both recorded, the BMI will automatically be recorded.

Systolic (S) Enter the patient's systolic blood pressure.

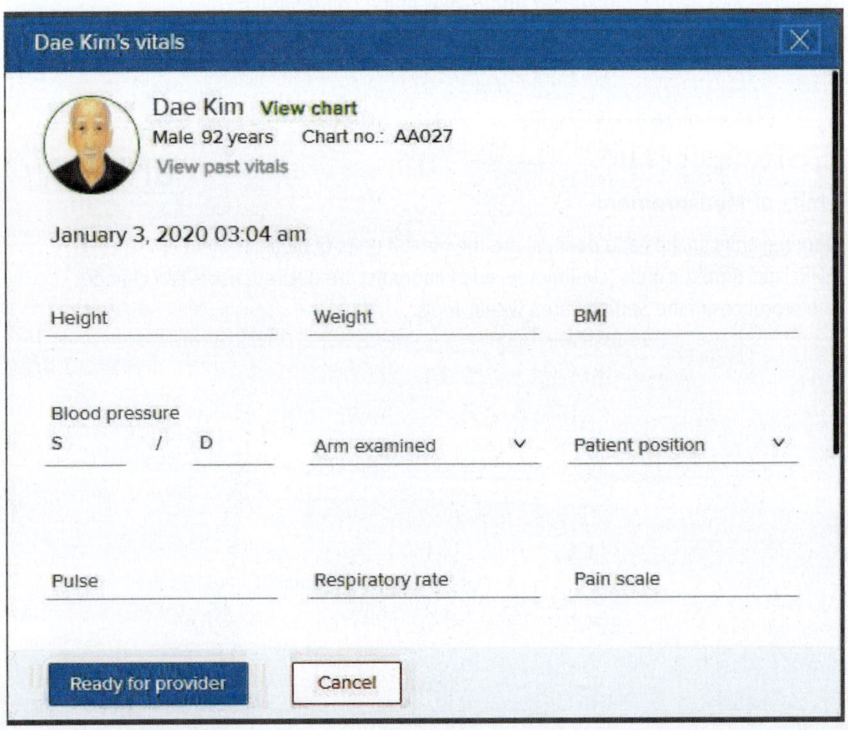

Figure 6.11 The Vital Signs Dialog Box

Diastolic (D) Enter the patient's diastolic blood pressure.

Arm examined Select the arm used for the blood pressure reading–right or left–from the drop-down list.

Patient position Select the patient's position–sitting, standing, or lying–from the drop-down list.

Pulse Enter the patient's pulse (heart rate per minute). It will be recorded as BPM for beats per minute.

Respiratory rate Enter the number of respirations per minute.

Pain scale If the patient reports pain, record the pain on a scale of 1 to 10.

Temperature Enter the patient's temperature. To change the temperature values to Fahrenheit (F) or Celsius (C), go to Settings and revise these preferences.

Temperature type Select the route the temperature was measured from the drop-down list.

Head circumference Enter the patient's head circumference in inches or centimeters. (This is used to monitor growth in children.)

EXERCISE 6.6 Record a Patient's Vitals

EHRclinic

You have obtained the height and weight and vital signs of the new patient. Record the measurements in the Vital Signs dialog box in EHRclinic.

Your instructor may assign this exercise to you in Connect. Exercise steps and EHRclinic Help Guides can be downloaded at http://www.mhhe.com/pmehr2.

EHRclinic TIP

EHRclinic

Units of Measurement

Imperial units (inches and pounds) are the default units of measurement in EHRclinic. If metric units (centimeters and kilograms) are desired, users can change the prerences in the Settings area within Tools.

chapter 6 summary

KEY TERMS

chief complaint (CC)
family history (FH)
history of present illness (HPI)
past, family, and social history (PFSH)
past medical history (PMH)
patient flow
progress notes
review of systems (ROS)
social history (SH)
vital signs

LEARNING OUTCOME	KEY CONCEPTS/EXAMPLES
6.1 Identify the four stages of patient flow.	The four stages of patient flow are check-in, patient intake, examination, and checkout. 1. During check-in, the front desk staff member checks the patient in, recording the time he or she arrived; confers with the patient to determine whether any information, such as a change of insurance or employment, needs to be updated in the patient record; and may ask the patient for payment. 2. In the patient intake stage, the patient is escorted to the exam room, and the medical assistant obtains detailed information from the patient, including past medical, family, and social history; allergies and medications; and the chief complaint. The medical assistant measures the patient's vital signs and prepares the patient for the examination. 3. During the examination stage, the provider examines the patient. The provider may order lab work or diagnostic tests and may prescribe medications. The provider develops a treatment plan and completes the examination. 4. The patient leaves the exam room and proceeds to the checkout desk. During checkout, the office staff member gives the patient any additional information required, such as patient education materials or lab work instructions. If necessary, a follow-up appointment is scheduled. Before the patient leaves, the staff member collects any payment that is due if it was not collected during check-in.
6.2 Discuss the main sections of the patient chart.	There are two main sections used to generate a new patient chart and to edit established patient chart data. 1. Patient Demographic tab–used to document identifying information about a patient (demographics). Data is typically obtained from the patient registration form. 2. Insurance Information tab–used to detail the patient's insurance information. Data is obtained from the patient's insurance card.

LEARNING OUTCOME	KEY CONCEPTS/EXAMPLES
6.3 Describe the elements of a patient's past medical, family, and social history.	Five sections are included in the medical history section of the patient chart in EHRclinic. These are documented in the patient's face sheet in an electronic health record. 1. Patient (Past) Medical History 2. Problem List 3. Surgical History 4. Social History 5. Family History
6.4 Explain how allergies and intolerances are entered in the patient chart.	Patient allergies and intolerances are recorded and stored in the Allergies section of the patient's face sheet. 1. Click the Allergies section in the face sheet. 2. Click the "Add allergies" button to open the Allergies dialog box. 3. Enter the allergy details (type, name, onset, date/time identified if known, severity, status, and a description). 4. Click Done to add the allergy/intolerance. 5. Complete these steps for each allergy.
6.5 Describe the procedure used to enter patient medications and immunizations.	Prescription and over-the-counter medications are recorded and stored in the Medications section of the patient's face sheet. 1. Click the Medications section in the face sheet. 2. Click the "Add medication" button to open the Medication dialog box. 3. Enter the medication details (status, type, drug name, dosage, drug form, route, timing, frequency, quantity, duration, diagnosis, and provider). 4. Click Done to add the medication. 5. Complete these steps for each drug.
6.6 Explain how the chief complaint and history of present illness are obtained.	Enter the chief complaint as the title of a new progress note: 1. Click the Chart button on the toolbar. 2. When the Patient Lookup dialog box appears, enter letters in the Last Name field and press Enter. 3. Select the patient from the list, and click the OK button to open the chart. 4. Click the Note button on the toolbar. 5. Click just to the right of the -* symbol, and enter the chief complaint. 6. To sign the note, enter ^*Shared_Note_Signature*.

LEARNING OUTCOME	KEY CONCEPTS/EXAMPLES
	7. Click the OK button to save the note. A dialog box appears asking whether you are permanently done with the note. Click the No button. The Enter Signature dialog box appears. 8. Enter the signature PIN in the Signature field. 9. Press the OK button. The Progress Notes dialog box closes.
6.7 Explain how a patient's vital signs are recorded in the patient chart.	1. Click the Vital Signs folder. The Vital Signs dialog box appears. 2. Click the New button. The Vital Signs (New) dialog box opens. 3. Enter the patient's vital signs in the appropriate fields– Weight, Height, Temperature, OFC, Pulse, Systolic, Diastolic, Posturals, BP Location, Respirations, and Oximetry. For example, to enter a patient's height, click in the first Height field and enter the patient's height in feet. Then click in the second Height box to enter the inches measurement. 4. When finished, click the OK button to save your entries. 5. Click the Close button to close the Vital Signs (New) dialog box.

chapter 6 review

MATCHING QUESTIONS

Match the key terms with their definitions.

_____ 1. *[LO 6.1]* past medical history (PMH)

_____ 2. *[LO 6.1]* progress note

_____ 3. *[LO 6.1]* patient flow

_____ 4. *[LO 6.1]* family history

_____ 5. *[LO 6.1]* social history

_____ 6. *[LO 6.1]* history of present illness

_____ 7. *[LO 6.1]* review of systems

_____ 8. *[LO 6.1]* past, family, and social history (PFSH)

a. Information about the patient's tobacco use, alcohol and drug use, sexual history, relationship status, and other significant social facts that may contribute to the care of the patient.

b. Note documenting the care delivered to a patient, and the medical facts and clinical thinking relevant to diagnosis and treatment.

c. Progression of patients from the time they enter the office for a visit until they exit the system by leaving the office after a visit.

d. Patient's history of medical problems, including chronic conditions, surgeries, and hospitalizations.

e. Detailed record of medical events among the patient's relatives, including the ages, living status, and diseases of siblings, children, parents, and grandparents.

f. A commonly used abbreviation for past medical, family, and social history.

g. An inventory of body systems in which the patient reports signs or symptoms he or she is currently having or has had in the past.

h. A description of the course of the present illness, including how and when the problem began, up to the present time.

MULTIPLE CHOICE QUESTIONS

Select the letter that best completes the statement or answers the question.

1. *[LO 6.1]* The _________ is the patient's history of medical problems, including chronic conditions, surgeries, and hospitalizations.
   a. past medical history
   b. progress note
   c. family history
   d. social history

2. *[LO 6.1]* The ________ is information about the patient's tobacco use, alcohol and drug use, sexual history, relationship status, and other significant social facts that may contribute to the care of the patient.
   a. past medical history
   b. progress note
   c. family history
   d. social history

3. *[LO 6.1]* The ________ details medical events among members of the patient's family, including the ages, living status, and diseases of siblings, children, parents, and grandparents.
   a. past medical history
   b. progress note
   c. family history
   d. social history

4. *[LO 6.1]* The ________ documents the care delivered to a patient and the medical facts and clinical thinking relevant to diagnosis and treatment.
   a. past medical history
   b. progress note
   c. family history
   d. social history

5. *[LO 6.3]* An at-a-glance snapshot of a patient's medical status in an EHR is called a ________.
   a. progress note
   b. face sheet
   c. problem list
   d. history report

6. *[LO 6.5]* The Rx/Medications dialog box lists ________ medications.
   a. current
   b. ineffective
   c. historical
   d. newly prescribed

7. *[LO 6.6]* The subjective main reason for the patient's visit is known as the ________.
   a. history of present illness
   b. chronic illness
   c. chief complaint
   d. past medical history

8. *[LO 6.4]* A(n) ________ is a mild reaction to a medication and does not involve an immune system response.
   a. intolerance
   b. anaphylactic reaction
   c. skin rash
   d. allergy

9. *[LO 6.7]* What is automatically calculated when a patient's height and weight are recorded in the Vital Signs dialog box?
   a. Temperature
   b. Systole
   c. BMI
   d. Head circumference

10. *[LO 6.2]* Patient registration forms, insurance cards, and other type types of information provided for entry into an EHR are known as ________.
   a. information pages
   b. data elements
   c. source documents
   d. electronic activities

SHORT ANSWER QUESTIONS

Define the following abbreviations.

1. *[LO 6.1]* SH ____________________
2. *[LO 6.1]* PMH ____________________
3. *[LO 6.1]* FH ____________________
4. *[LO 6.1]* HPI ____________________
5. *[LO 6.1]* ROS ____________________
6. *[LO 6.1]* PFSH ____________________
7. *[LO 6.1]* CC ____________________

APPLYING YOUR KNOWLEDGE

Answer the questions below in the space provided.

6.1 *[LO 6.1]* Why is it important for medical practices to collect information about a patient's family history and social history?

____

____

6.2 *[LO 6.5]* Describe the medication reconciliation process. Why is it important to perform medication reconciliation with every patient encounter?

____

____

6.3 *[LO 6.4]* Why are patients' allergies and/or intolerances recorded in the EHR?

____

____

chapter 7

Office Visit: The Progress Note

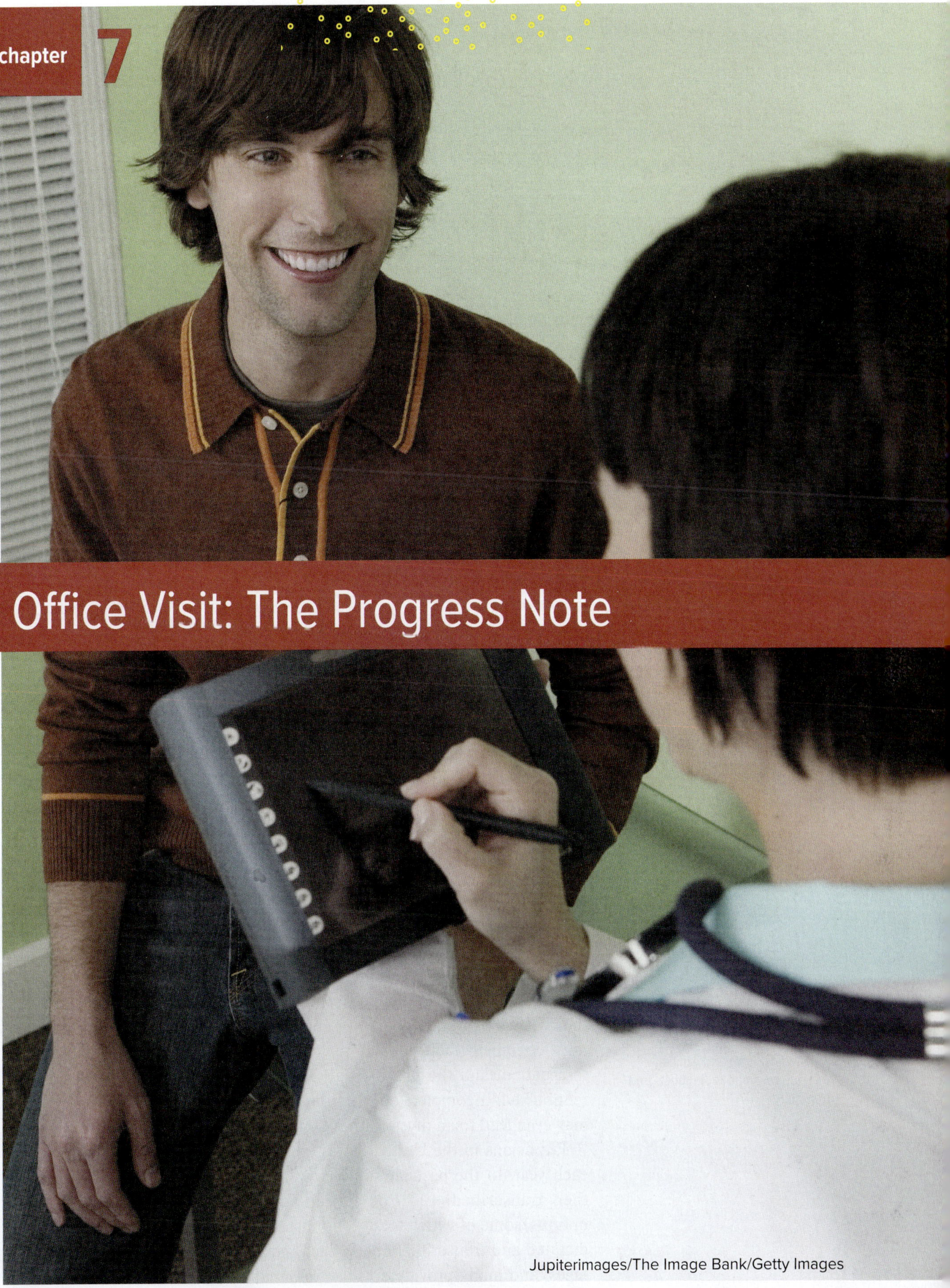

Jupiterimages/The Image Bank/Getty Images

LEARNING OUTCOMES

When you finish this chapter, you will be able to:

7.1 Discuss the methods of entering documentation in an EHR.

7.2 Explain the SOAP method of documenting encounters.

7.3 Build a patient encounter in EHRclinic, including the chief complaint, review of systems, physical exam, diagnosis, and treatment.

Adjusting to Change

Remember Alex Horowitz, the medical assistant who was wondering how to enter long lists of patient medications in the EHR? He is not the only one having difficulty adjusting to the new workflow.Dr. Katherine Yan uses the EHR to order medications and lab work, but she still dictates her progress notes and has Alex type them in the EHR.

Dr. Patricia McGrath, on the other hand, finds that using the EHR's templates makes her more efficient. "I spend less time documenting visits," she said. "I had to spend time learning how to use the templates, but now I wouldn't go back to dictation."

Alex feels overwhelmed. In addition to learning how to use the EHR for recording medications and vital signs, he stays late each day to enter Dr. Yan's progress notes, something he never had to do before. He finds that since the EHR was installed, he has to spend more time on tasks, not less.

In this chapter, you will learn about the different methods of entering progress notes in an EHR. As you read the chapter and complete the exercises, think about how Dr. Yan and Dr. McGrath enter progress notes.

7.1 Methods of Entering Physician Documentation in an EHR

progress note note documenting the care delivered to a patient, and the medical facts and clinical thinking relevant to diagnosis and treatment

Every service submitted for payment, including medical care, diagnostic tests, consultations, surgeries, and other services eligible for payment, must be documented in the patient's medical record. Documentation is directly linked to the financial health of the practice and is typically done through the creation of **progress notes** for encounters. To be reimbursed, the provider must document each service provided to the patient. If a treatment is given to a patient and the provider fails to document it, the service will not be reimbursed. Incomplete or inaccurate records may result in claim denials or may even lead to an investigation of possible fraudulent and abusive actions.

Physicians in the United States create more than a billion clinical notes each year. In the past, these notes were handwritten or were dictated and then transcribed. Electronic health records offer providers additional options, some of which totally eliminate the need for both written notes and dictated and transcribed notes. Each method has advantages and disadvantages, and many providers use a combination of methods. In this chapter, you will learn about the different documentation methods, and you will practice entering patient progress notes in an EHR.

Dictation and Transcription

Dictation is the process of recording spoken words that will later be transcribed into written form. Dictation and transcription have been the traditional method of documenting patient encounters. The flow of dictation is illustrated in Figure 7.1. A medical provider dictates the medical note into a telephone or a recording device. A medical transcriptionist receives the dictation and transcribes it on a computer. After review, the final computerized word processing file is emailed to the health care provider, or the file is transferred to a website and is later downloaded by the provider. It is then reviewed and added to the patient's electronic record.

In **digital dictation,** physicians dictate using a microphone and/or a headset connected to a computer. Dictation can also be spoken into a smartphone or a personal digital assistant (PDA). The spoken words are saved as a digital audio file, which can be transferred to a transcriptionist via a secure website.

Dictation corresponds intuitively to the physician's usual way of working. It allows the physician to describe a patient's condition in his or her

dictation the process of recording spoken words that will later be transcribed into written form

digital dictation the process of dictating using a microphone, a headset connected to a computer, a smartphone, or a PDA

Figure 7.1 Flowchart of Traditional Dictation and Transcription

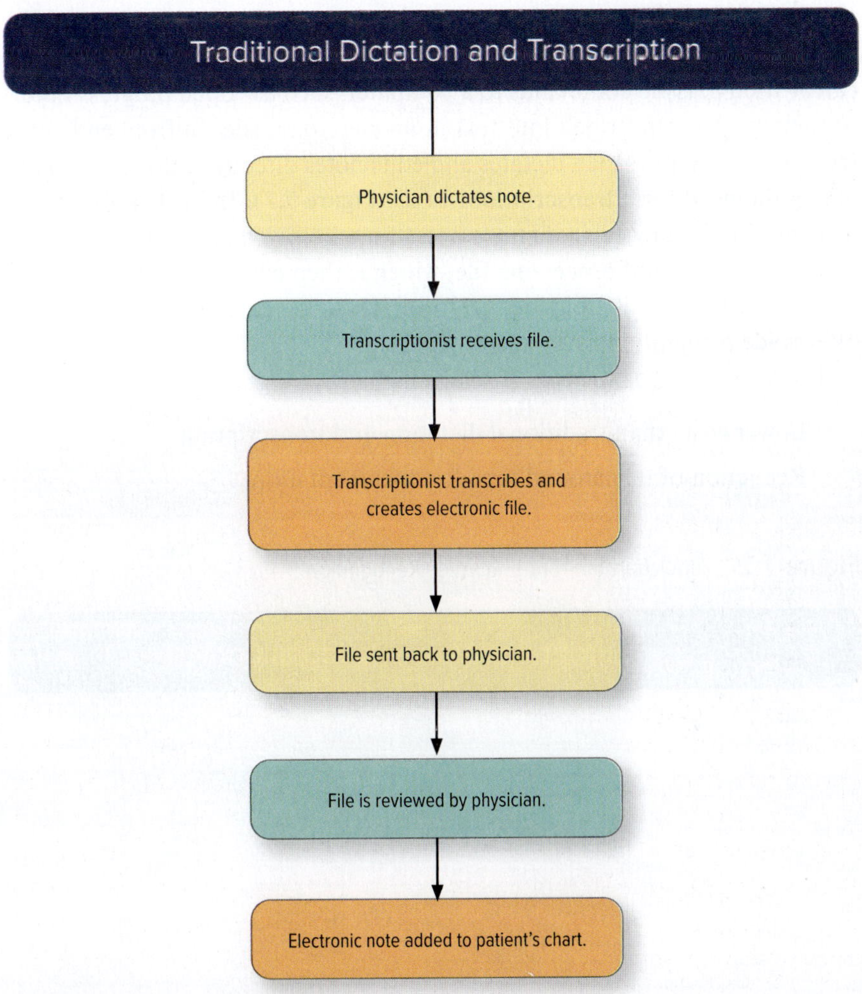

own words, reflecting both content and context. Physicians can dictate anytime, anywhere, using a telephone, a computer, or another recording device. By using this traditional method of documenting patient care, providers need not change the way they practice to accommodate an EHR system.

The benefits of dictation and transcription are as follows:

- Physicians who are uncomfortable with computers in the examination room can still use an EHR.
- Dictation retains the narrative form of documentation that promotes detail, context, and comprehensiveness.
- The method does not require additional training for physicians.

The drawbacks of dictation include these:

- Dictated reports are not immediately accessible.
- Dictation incurs transcription costs.
- The physician or an assistant must review and edit files.
- Detail is more likely to be omitted or forgotten if data are not captured at the point of care.

Voice Recognition Software

voice recognition software software that recognizes spoken words

Even after a successful transition to an EHR, some physicians prefer to continue using dictation as a means of entering information. Voice recognition programs make this a viable, cost-effective solution for some offices. **Voice recognition software** is software that recognizes spoken words. The words can be used to issue commands to a computer, such as "open progress note," or they can be transcribed into text in an electronic file. In front-end voice recognition, the physician dictates and edits notes directly in the EHR, eliminating the need for a transcriptionist (see Figure 7.2). In background voice recognition, the physician dictates notes that are saved as an electronic text file, similar to a word processing file, which is then edited by a transcriptionist. After editing, it is uploaded to the EHR (see Figure 7.3). Most EHRs offer voice recognition as an add-on module.

The advantages of voice recognition include:

- Lower costs than traditional dictation and transcription
- Reduction of turnaround time for documentation

Figure 7.2 Flowchart of Front-End Voice Recognition

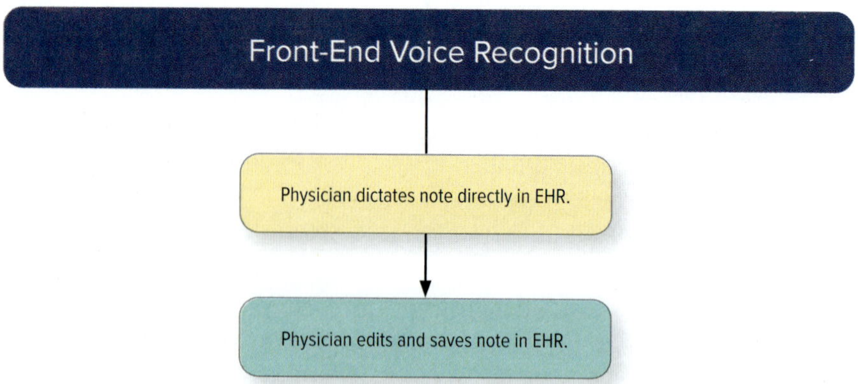

Figure 7.3 Flowchart of Background Voice Recognition

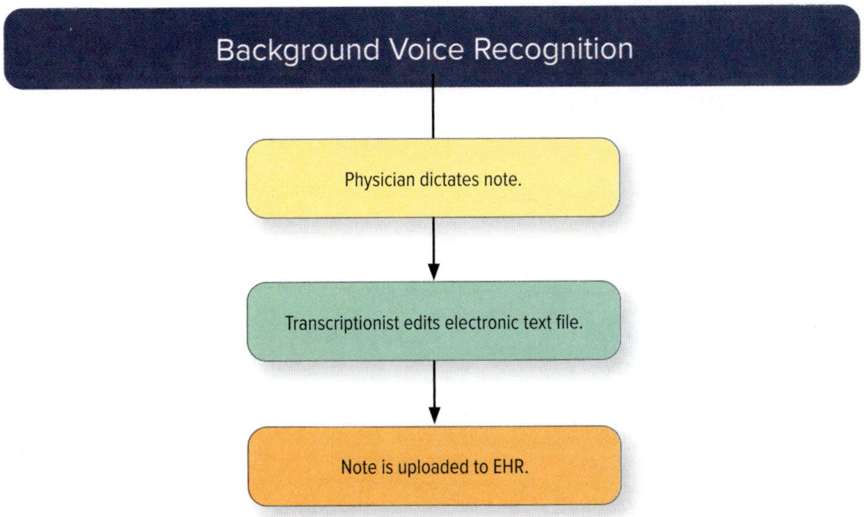

The disadvantages of voice recognition include:

- The possibility of an unacceptable accuracy rate if interference such as background noise is present
- The costs associated with purchasing voice recognition equipment and software

Templates

Another method of entering documentation in an EHR is through the use of templates. A **template** is a preformatted file that serves as a starting point for a new document. When a template is used, only patient-specific information must be typed into the note. The rest of the information is entered by clicking on labels in the templates and making selections from a list of choices.

template preformatted note that contains selections appropriate to the medical condition or type of visit

Templates in an EHR are similar to macros in a word processing program. Macros automate repetitive tasks, such as inserting the current date at the beginning of every letter. In an EHR, a template presents the physician with the most common entries for a specific type of office visit. For example, a template for a fifty- to sixty-four-year-old well-woman examination would contain a list of common menopausal symptoms. Rather than typing in the entry "hot flashes" or "night sweats," the physician clicks Yes or No next to the entry for the condition. If more information is required, clicking a special label in the template causes a list of additional information to be displayed.

Offices commonly use a number of different templates, depending on patients' ages and illnesses and the purposes of the visits. For example, an office might use one template for a middle-aged well-woman checkup, another for a routine checkup of a two-year-old female, and another for a diabetes follow-up visit. Specialists commonly have a set of templates unique to their specialty. Most EHRs provide templates for text-heavy parts of the patient's chart, such as medical history, family history, social history, and progress notes.

Figures 7.4 illustrates sections of three different progress note templates: middle-aged well-woman exam, two-year-old female well-child exam, and type II diabetic follow-up examination.

Figure 7.4
Sample Templates from an EHR

Well-woman template (excerpt)

GYN History: No concerns DELETE
Gravida 0 Past Pregnancies Post-Menopausal
Average interval between menses: DEL 28-31 days MenstrInt irregular P1
Length of menses: DEL DurDay P1
Flow: DEL MenstrFlo normal heavy light P1
Dysmenorrhea: DEL yes no controlled with NSAIDs controlled with OCPs H8
Post-coital bleeding: DEL yes no R7
Intermenstrual bleeding: DEL yes no R7
Pelvic pain: DEL yes no R7
Dyspareunia: DEL yes no R7
Vaginal discharge: DEL yes no VAG D/C DETAILS R7
GYN surgery: DEL GYNSURG none P1
Contraception: DEL Contracep P3 |

Menopausal Symptoms: none N/A DELETE
Hot flashes: DEL yes no tolerable intolerable R1
Night sweats: DEL yes no R1
Sleep disturbances: DEL yes no R11
Vaginal dryness: DEL yes no R7
Mood/cognitive disturbances: DEL yes no R11

Well-child template, female (excerpt)

Nutrition:
Milk: DEL Milktype MilkDrink
Table food: DEL TableFood varied diet

Developmental Milestones:
Knows 3-5 body parts: DEL yes no
Climbs stairs: DEL yes no
Scribbles spontaneously: DEL yes no
2 word sentences: DEL yes no
Points to named body parts: DEL yes no |
Removes clothing: DEL yes no
50 word vocabulary: DEL yes no

Objective:
Height Percentile DEL
Weight Percentile DEL
Complete Exam Girl 2-10 YO

Type 2 diabetic template (excerpt)

Glucose Monitoring: none DELETE
Accucheck frequency: DEL Not Checking QDay BID TID frequency
Fasting glucose: DEL blood sugars
Post prandial: DEL blood sugars

Most Recent HbA1C: DEL D1
Blood Pressure Range: DEL Not Checking Systolic / Diastolic * H3
Most Recent Lipid Panel:
DEL D1
Most Recent BMP:
DEL D1
Urine Microalbumin: DEL D1
Retinal Examination: DEL No Retinal Exam recorded in health maintenance unknown P1
Foot Exam: DEL No Foot Exam recorded in health maintenance unknown P1
Pneumovax Vaccine: DEL No Pneumovax vaccine recorded in health maintenance section UTD Not UTD Declines Pneumovax Postpones Pneumovax P1
Influenza Vaccine: DEL No Influenza vaccine recorded in health maintenance section UTD Not UTD Declines Influenza Postpones Influenza P1

Past Medical History/Complications of Diabetes: DELETE

The advantages of templates are as follows:

- Once learned, templates can be more efficient.
- Data can be searched and analyzed electronically.
- The physician is less likely to omit information.

The disadvantages of templates include these:

- It takes time to learn how to use them effectively.
- Standardized content may not apply to all patients.
- Entries may not capture the uniqueness of each patient.

THINKING IT THROUGH 7.1

Most EHRs offer providers the option of using templates to enter progress notes, which can reduce the time it takes to enter notes. However, not all providers use templates. Given that over a billion notes are created each year, why do you think some providers have not switched to this method of documenting patient visits?

7.2 Progress Notes

In EHR software, progress notes can be entered using a variety of methods, including the methods described earlier—dictation and transcription, voice recognition software, and templates. A combination of techniques can also be used in some EHR systems. EHRclinic utilizes point-of-care entry with templates—meaning that the providers enter the notes during the patient encounter.

SOAP Format

In this chapter, progress notes are entered in the SOAP format. **SOAP** is a widely used format for documenting patient encounters. It stands for *subjective, objective, assessment,* and *plan.* A sample SOAP note is illustrated in Figure 7.5.

SOAP format used to enter progress notes; it stands for *subjective, objective, assessment,* and *plan*

symptoms subjective indication of a disease or conditon as experienced by an individual

Subjective

The subjective section describes the patient's condition is his or her own words, including the degree of pain or discomfort, the presence of nausea or dizziness, when the problem first started, and any additional description that the patient provides.

In a SOAP note, the chief complaint (CC), history of present illness (HPI), and review of systems (ROS) are reported as subjective information because these elements of the medical record refer to a patient's **symptoms** as they are experienced by the patient.

EXAMPLES

CC: C/O sore throat x 3 days

HPI: Patient states he developed a sore throat 3 days ago. He has taken ibuprofen, which has alleviated some of the discomfort. Associated symptoms include chills, fatigue, and headaches.

(Continued)

(*Continued*)

The chief complaint of a sore throat and HPI describing chills, fatigue, and headaches are subjective symptoms because the patient is experiencing them. The ROS will also be documented to provide any other information or symptoms related to the patient's body systems.

signs objective evidence of a disease or condition

physical exam (PE) examination of the bodily functions and condition of an individual; typically reported as a body system assessment

Objective

The objective section of a note includes **signs** that can be measured, seen, heard, touched, felt, or smelled, including such vital signs as temperature, pulse, respiration, skin color, and swelling, measurements, and the results of diagnostic tests. The results of the **physical exam (PE)** are also reported as objective findings.

HSU, EDWIN
#HSUEDWI
11/12/2016

SUBJECTIVE
Edwin says he recently had a cold, which seemed to resolve. He rolled over during the night and experienced acute facial pain and was aware that he had what he calls a "killer headache." He characterizes the pain as an 8 out of 10. Blowing his nose produces a thick, greenish-yellow mucous and bending over at all makes the pain intensify.

OBJECTIVE
Patient is a well-developed, well-nourished Asian male who is holding his head during the examination.
Vitals: 101.6° F P: 88 (reg) R: 14 BP: 124/84 WT: 208 lbs
HEENT: There is copious greenish-yellow drainage from the nose. Exquisite tenderness over the frontal sinuses, more marked on the right than on the left.
Chest: Clear to auscultation and percussion without wheezing, rales, or rhonchi.
Heart: Normal rate and rhythm without murmurs, gallops, or thrills.
Allergies: None.

ASSESSMENT
Acute sinusitis.

PLAN
He was given a prescription for erythromycin, 500 mg b.i.d. × 10 days (#20) and told he will need to take the medication until it is all gone, even if he begins to feel better. Also advised that he may use certrizine, 5 mg daily for decongestant relief, which is available over the counter, until the nasal congestion clears. To stay off work until his temperature returns to normal. Reminded to stay well hydrated. To call the office if his temperature is not down within 24 hours.

Patricia McGrath, MD

Figure 7.5 Sample SOAP Note

EXAMPLES

Wt: 163 pounds
BP: 118/74 mm/Hg left arm, sitting
P: 88 bpm
R: 16 rpm
T: 101.4°F oral
SPo2: 98% room air, at rest

Physical exam (PE) indicates pharyngeal erythema (redness of the throat) tonsillary hypertrophy with exudate (enlarged tonsils with pus formation), and swollen lymph nodes.

Rapid strep test - positive for strep A

The vital signs, PE, and diagnostic test are considered to be objective findings because they can be seen (redness of the throat and swelling of the tonsils), felt (swollen lymph nodes), and measured (fever and positive strep test).

Assessment

The assessment section of a note contains the physician's diagnosis of the patient's condition. Typically, the subjective information provided by the patient and the objective findings are reviewed to determine the diagnosis.

EXAMPLES

Dr. McGrath reviews the patient's subjective and objective findings to positively diagnose the patient with strep throat. Some indications that support this diagnosis are:

Patient reports symptoms of a sore throat, chills, fatigue, and headaches.

Objective signs include fever, observations of a red and inflamed throat, and a positive strep test.

Plan

The plan section of a note contains the provider's plan for treatment of the patient, such as laboratory, imaging, or radiological tests; medications; and procedures. The plan section may also include a referral to a specialist, patient directions, and follow-up care instructions.

EXAMPLES

Once a positive diagnosis of strep throat has been made, Dr. McGrath determines the following treatment plan:

- Prescribe amoxicillin 500 mg, one tablet twice a day for 10 days
- Take over-the-counter ibuprofen for pain relief and fever reduction
- Increase fluids
- Rest
- Practice infection control at home to avoid spreading to others
- Call the clinic if symptoms worsen or do not improve within 7 days

7.3 Building an OV in EHRclinic

office visit (OV) an encounter between a patient and provider in which new or existing health issues, concerns, or symptoms can be discussed

As described earlier in this chapter, the review of systems (ROS) and physical exam (PE) are essential components of documenting a patient's **office visit (OV)** encounter. These provide valuable insight for determining a patient's diagnosis and developing a treatment plan.

Flow of an OV in EHRclinic

In EHRclinic, an office visit begins with the patient's appointment. An appointment must first be added to the schedule to access a new OV in the patient's chart. Once the patient arrives for the appointment, he or she is checked into the system, which is described in greater detail in Chapter 5.

After the patient has checked in, the OV is moved to Encounters, where the following takes place:

- **Patient intake** The patient's measurements (height and weight) and vital signs are recorded.
- **Provider encounter** The patient is ready for office visit documentation. This is where the medical assistant records the chief complaint and present illness. The provider then records the review of systems and physical examination. The diagnosis, patient procedures, treatment, referrals, and follow-up are also recorded here. When the OV is complete, it is marked "Ready for treatment," at which time the provider must provide an electronic signature. In EHRclinic, a user's electronic signature is his or her password. In the office visit screen, three tabs are shown, and users can toggle back and forth between the patient chart, the patient vitals, and the provider notes (OV), as shown in Figure 7.6.
- **Plan review** When the OV has been signed and marked "Ready for treatment," it is moved to the plan review area. In this area, any treatment provided will be marked as not started, in progress, or complete. When all treatments and procedures have been marked complete, the encounter can be designated as "Ready for checkout," where the billing and coding process begins.

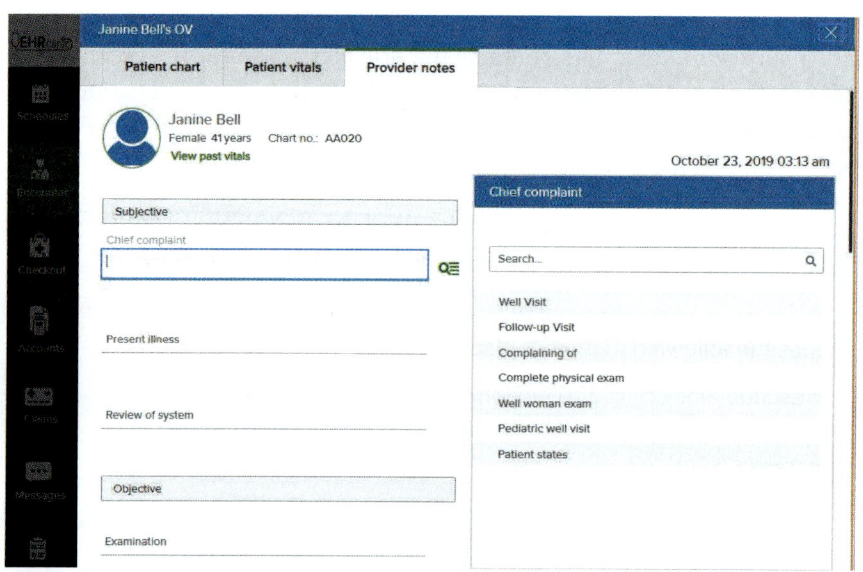

Figure 7.6 Office Visit Screen

Documenting the Provider Encounter

EHRclinic OV notes are set up in SOAP format. Initially, the MA will perform a patient interview to gather the reason for the patient's visit. Then, the provider completes the remainder of the visit or has an MA working as a scribe to document the details of the visit. The following are elements of an OV in EHRclinic.

Chief Complaint

The chief complaint (CC) is the reason for the patient's visit. This is documented concisely and using the patient's own words or description and the duration of the symptoms, if applicable.

Present Illness

The present illness (PI or HPI) expands on the chief complaint by providing clarification through better descriptions and details.

Review of Systems

Information provided in the review of systems (ROS) is typically obtained by having the patient complete a form. The form inventories each body system and allows patients to check off symptoms or write in their own. For example, the gastrointestinal section of the form might include symptoms such as diarrhea, constipation, blood in the stool, nausea, vomiting, and heartburn. The items checked by the patient are recorded in the ROS section of the encounter.

Physical Examination

The physical exam information (PE) is recorded by the provider. These are objective findings based on a physical review of body systems. Providers use methods such as auscultation (listening), palpation (feeling), percussion (listening), inspection (seeing), and mensuration (measurement) to perform the PE.

Diagnosis

The diagnosis or suspected diagnosis is recorded as part of the *assessment* in a SOAP note. In an EHRclinic encounter, the diagnosis is recorded by performing a search within the office visit template. The search is conducted through the ICD database maintained by practice administrators. ICD codes will be discussed in greater detail in Chapter 9.

Plan

The Plan section of an EHRclinic OV includes treatment ordered by the provider. This is set up in such a way that procedure (CPT) codes are selected as treatment is ordered, which helps to build the encounter form for billing and coding (covered in Chapter 9 and Chapter 11). The CPT code database is also maintained by practice administrators, and new codes can be added as needed.

The Plan section includes search databases for the following:

- Prescriptions
- Labs
- E/M coding (encounters)
- Procedures
- Imaging
- Immunization
- Medications
- Follow-up
- Other treatment (patient education and referrals)

This information is then pulled to the Plan Review to be marked off as it is completed. Later, it will be used to build the encounter form and will be linked to the diagnosis code(s) selected for claim submission.

Correcting Errors in an EHR

Every effort should be made to ensure accurate documentation of patient information and encounters. Health care practices should therefore develop procedures that facilitate the entry of correct information because this improves the billing and coding process and contributes to patient safety in their continuity of care. Consider what might happen if a patient's medications were incorrectly documented or if a provider added an inaccurate entry to the patient's EHR. There are also legal considerations because any documented information is defended as being the true account of a patient's care.

Despite the precautions to ensure accurate documentation, mistakes do occur occasionally. It is important that errors are corrected immediately upon discovery, but certain principles must be applied to making the corrections. Medical records can be amended as long as the relevant information can be recovered to correct improper alterations of the historical record. For example, the original entry must not be permanently deleted from the EHR if an error is corrected.

addendum information provided in an EHR that is not available in the original entry; adding to an original entry or correcting an erroneous entry

In many EHR systems, errors are corrected by entering an **addendum.** An addendum is an entry that is added after an original entry. It can be used to add information to the original entry or to correct an error. In the event of an error or addition, the addendum should be timely, should include the reason for the new entry, and should be signed by the person adding it.

EXERCISE 7.1 Maintain SOAP Templates

EHRclinic

Dr. McGrath has provided some new SOAP templates that she would like to have added to EHRclinic. Using the practice database for templates, add the new templates to the system.

Your instructor may assign this exercise to you in Connect. Exercise steps and EHRclinic Help Guides can be downloaded at http://www.mhhe.com/pmehr2.

EXERCISE 7.2 Build an Office Visit Note

EHRclinic

You have recorded the vital signs for the patient you were working with in Chapter 6. Acting as a medical assistant, you will record the patient's chief complaint and present illness. Then, you'll act as the provider and finish building the rest of the patient's office visit. Mark the OV as complete in the plan review.

Your instructor may assign this exercise to you in Connect. Exercise steps and EHRclinic Help Guides can be downloaded at http://www.mhhe.com/pmehr2.

EHRclinic TIP

EHRclinic

Completing an Office Visit

In EHRclinic, the chief complaint, present illness, review of systems, and examination can be completed by entering free text or by selecting preformatted text.

chapter 7 summary

KEY TERMS

addendum
dictation
digital dictation
office visit (OV)
physical exam (PE)
progress note
signs
SOAP
symptoms
template
voice recognition software

LEARNING OUTCOME	KEY CONCEPTS/EXAMPLES
7.1 Discuss the methods of entering documentation in an EHR.	Progress notes may be entered by the following methods: • Dictation and transcription, in which a provider dictates the medical note into a telephone or a recording device and a medical transcriptionist transcribes it on a computer. After review, the final computerized word processing file is emailed to the health care provider, or the file is transferred to a website and is later downloaded by the provider. It is then reviewed and added to the patient's electronic record. • Digital dictation, in which the physician dictates using a microphone and/or a headset connected to a computer, a smartphone, or a PDA. The spoken words are saved as a digital audio file, which can be transferred to a transcriptionist via a secure website. • Voice recognition software, which transcribes spoken words into text in an electronic file. In front-end voice recognition, the physician dictates and edits notes directly in the EHR, eliminating the need for a transcriptionist. In background voice recognition, the physician dictates notes that are saved as an electronic text file, which is then edited by a transcriptionist. After editing, it is uploaded to the EHR. • Templates, which are preformatted notes that contain selections appropriate to the medical condition or type of visit. When a template is used, only patient-specific information must be typed into the note. The rest of the information is entered by clicking on labels in the templates and making selections from a list of choices. • Directly typing into the EHR (point-of-care documentation).

LEARNING OUTCOME	KEY CONCEPTS/EXAMPLES
7.2 Explain the SOAP method of documenting encounters.	SOAP notes refer to organizing documentation by *subjective, objective, assessment,* and *plan* information. • Subjective information is provided by the patient. This includes the chief complaint, history of present illness, and the review of systems, in which patients describe symptoms or experiences for each of their body systems. • Objective information includes signs that can be measured, seen, heard, touched, felt, or smelled by others. Vital signs, measurements, physical exam findings, and the results of diagnostic tests are also reported in the objective section of a patient's encounter. • Assessment refers to the provider's determination of a diagnosis. The subjective and objective findings are reviewed to form a diagnosis or suspected diagnosis. • Plans refer to the treatment of the suspected diagnosis. The plan can include medications prescribed, laboratory or imaging tests, procedures, referrals, directions, and follow-up instructions.
7.3 Build a patient encounter in EHRclinic, including the chief complaint, review of systems, physical exam, diagnosis, and treatment.	• The chief complaint and present illess record details about the reason for the patient's visit. • A review of systems (ROS) details the symptoms the patient is experiencing, as catalogued by each body system. This is recorded as subjective information in the office visit. • The physical exam records the provider's physical assessment of each body system, especially as it relates to the ROS. This is recorded as objective information in the office visit. • The provider determines a diagnosis based on the subjective and objective information provided. • The Plan section of an office visit encounter includes prescriptions, labs, E/M coding, procedures, imaging, immunizations, medications, follow-up, and referrals.

chapter 7 review

MATCHING QUESTIONS

Match the key terms with their definitions.

_____ 1. *[LO 7.2]* review of systems

_____ 2. *[LO 7.2]* signs

_____ 3. *[LO 7.2]* symptoms

_____ 4. *[LO 7.1]* digital dictation

_____ 5. *[LO 7.2]* SOAP

_____ 6. *[LO 7.1]* dictation

_____ 7. *[LO 7.1]* progress note

_____ 8. *[LO 7.2]* physical exam

_____ 9. *[LO 7.1]* voice recognition software

_____ 10. *[LO 7.1]* template

a. Using a microphone or headset connected to a computer to record the findings of an encounter.

b. A computer program that can recognize spoken words.

c. The process of recording spoken words that will later be transcribed into written form.

d. Examination of the bodily functions of an individual.

e. A preformatted file that serves as a starting point for a new document.

f. Objective evidence of a disease or condition

g. Format used to enter progress notes.

h. Inventory of body systems in which the patient reports symptoms

i. Subjective indication of a disease or condition as experienced by the individual

j. Documentation of the care delivered to the patient.

MULTIPLE-CHOICE QUESTIONS

Select the letter that best completes the statement or answers the question.

1. *[LO 7.1]* During _____, a provider voice-records the details of a patient encounter so that it will be transcribed into written form for entry in the EHR.
   a. superscription
   b. transcription
   c. subscription
   d. dictation

2. *[LO 7.2]* An elevated temperature, cyanotic skin color, malodorous wound, and swelling of the extremities are examples of _____.
   a. diseases
   b. symptoms
   c. signs
   d. assessments

3. *[LO 7.2]* Point-of-care entry refers to the provider entering notes ______.
   a. prior to the patient encounter
   b. during the patient encounter
   c. after the patient encounter
   d. using dictation

4. *[LO 7.1]* ______ transcribes spoken words into text in an electronic file.
   a. digital dictation
   b. dictation
   c. voice recognition software
   d. all of the these

5. *[LO 7.3]* A patient's vital signs are recorded during the ______.
   a. provider encounter
   b. check-in process
   c. plan review
   d. patient intake

6. *[LO 7.2]* In a *SOAP* note, the chief complaint, HPI, and ROS are reported as ______ information.
   a. subjective
   b. objective
   c. assessment
   d. plan

7. *[LO 7.2]* Subjective information reported in the CC, HPI, and ROS are also known as ______ because they are experienced by the patient.
   a. signs
   b. qualifiers
   c. assessments
   d. symptoms

8. *[LO 7.1]* Which of the following is an advantage of using voice recognition software?
   a. Data can be searched and analyzed electronically
   b. The provider is less likely to omit information
   c. The provider does not need to review or edit files
   d. Reduction of turnaround time for documentation

9. *[LO 7.2]* Which of the following is reported as objective findings?
   a. Chief complaint
   b. Review of systems
   c. History of present illness
   d. Physical exam

10. *[LO 7.2]* A provider diagnoses a patient with hypertension. In which element of the *SOAP* note would this be reported?
    a. Subjective
    b. Objective
    c. Assessment
    d. Plan

SHORT-ANSWER QUESTIONS

Define the following abbreviations.

1. *[LO 7.2]* PE ____________________
2. *[LO 7.2]* ROS ____________________
3. *[LO 7.2]* S (in SOAP) ____________________
4. *[LO 7.2]* O (in SOAP) ____________________
5. *[LO 7.2]* A (in SOAP) ____________________
6. *[LO 7.2]* P (in SOAP) ____________________
7. *[LO 7.3]* OV ____________________

APPLYING YOUR KNOWLEDGE

Answer the questions below in the space provided.

7.1 *[LO 7.1]* In your own words, explain the advantages that voice recognition software can offer a provider.

____

____

7.2 *[LO 7.3]* Explain the advantages offered by electronic prescribing.

____

____

7.3 *[LO 7.2]* Match each item with its SOAP description (S = subjective; O = objective; A = assessment; and P = plan).

a. Rash ____________________

b. T: 98.2°F ____________________

c. Referral to physical therapy ____________________

d. Coughing ____________________

e. Headache ____________________

f. Bleeding ____________________

g. Hypothyroidism ____________________

h. Follow up in 7 days ____________________

i. Conjunctivitis ____________________

j. Loss of smell ____________________

chapter 8

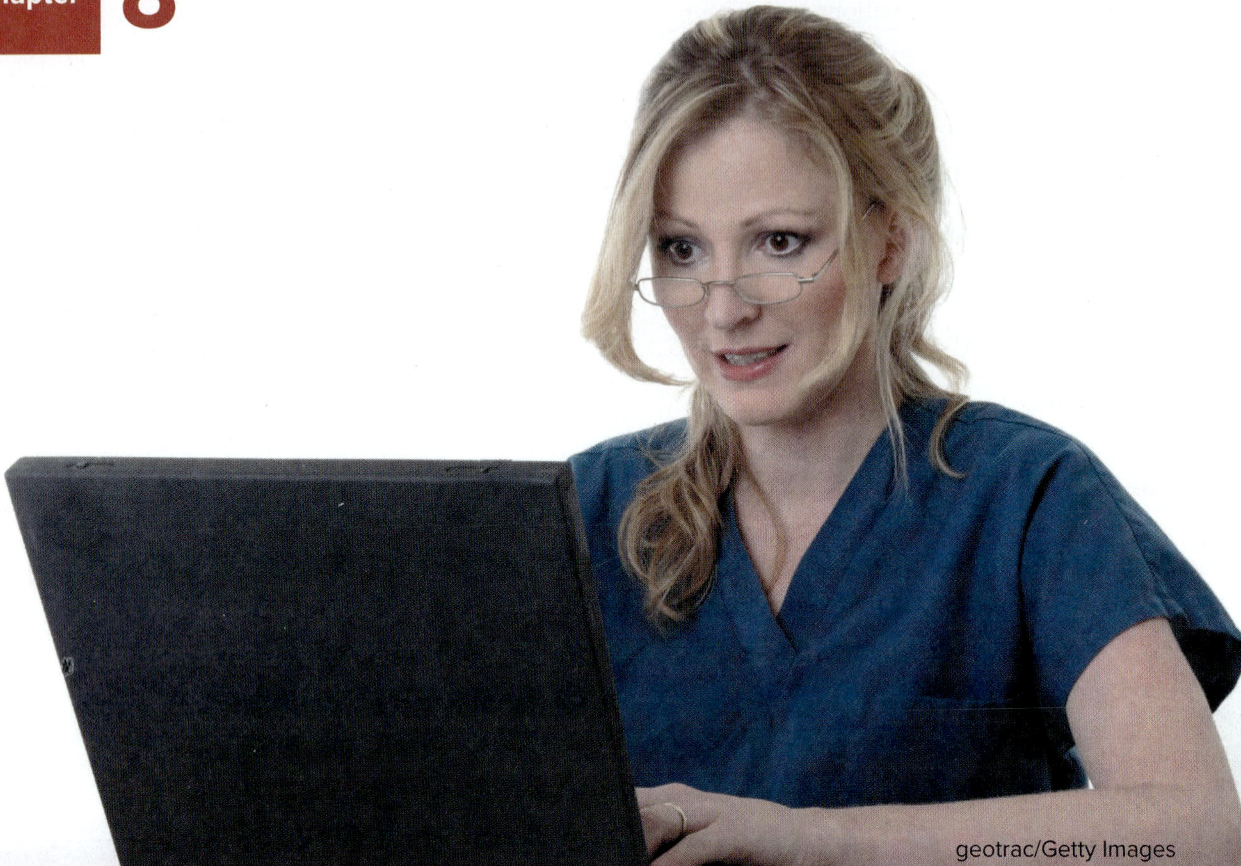
geotrac/Getty Images

Office Visit: Electronic Orders

LEARNING OUTCOMES

When you finish this chapter, you will be able to:

8.1 Explain why E-Prescribing reduces some medical errors.

8.2 Explain why ordering and receiving test results electronically is more efficient than paper methods.

8.3 Explain how orders are processed in an EHR.

Beneficial Questions

"Good morning, Trilogy Family Care Center. This is Laurie, how may I help you?" Leila Patterson is calling and says that she thinks she lost her order for her annual mammogram. She would like to stop in at the office and pick up a new order. She is also asking to pick up a prescription for a refill of her blood pressure medication. Laurie explains that the practice's new EHR system sends electronic orders to the radiology department and also has an E-Prescribing feature that can send prescription refills to the pharmacy electronically. Leila is thrilled that she doesn't need to come to the office to pick up her mammogram order and prescription.

Reflect on the ability of electronic health record systems to send orders and prescriptions electronically. What are the advantages of doing this? Can you think of any disadvantages? How do electronic orders and prescriptions promote patient safety?

8.1 E-Prescribing and Electronic Health Records

Once a provider has finished examining a patient, he or she may decide to order a medication. In an electronic health record, this is known as E-Prescribing. By writing prescriptions electronically, providers can avoid many of the mistakes that occur with handwritten prescriptions.

The benefits of E-Prescribing include:

- Prevents drug errors by providing access to a patient's prescription history to reduce the chance of the wrong drug being dispensed.
- Automated clinical decision support is provided by the use of databases to provide the most common prescribing information, such as dosage, strength, and frequency.
- Provides clinical alert notifications of allergies, drug interactions, and duplicate therapies.
- Promotes efficiency in the **medication reconciliation** process by the availability of electronic drug lists and **drug interaction checkers.**
- Tracks whether prescriptions have been filled to monitor patient compliance with drug therapy.
- Reduces the number of lost prescriptions because E-Prescribed prescriptions are transmitted directly to the pharmacy.
- Allows providers to prescribe and monitor **controlled substances** electronically and in the same manner as other prescriptions.

medicaton reconciliation the process of identifying the most accurate and current list of all medications taken by a patient; includes name, dosage, frequency, and route, and compares medical records to external lists of medications (such as from the patient or the pharmacy)

drug interaction checker tool to identify potentially harmful and unsafe combinations of prescription medications

controlled substance drug whose use and possession are regulated by law

drug-drug interactions reaction between two or more drugs in which the efficacy and/or side effects of at least one of the drugs is increased or decreased

drug-diagnosis warning a warning given by an E-Prescribing system when a patient's reported diagnosis does not support the drug being prescribed

Safety Checks

E-Prescribing (ERX) also provides a number of built-in safety checks. For example, when a provider selects a drug for a patient, the EHR checks for drug allergies, **drug-drug interactions,** and other potential conflicts using information in the patient's medical record, including past history, allergies, and a complete medication list. Figure 8.1 shows a **drug-diagnosis warning** that appeared when lisinopril, a popular drug for high blood pressure, was prescribed for a woman with type II diabetes.

Figure 8.1 A Drug–Diagnosis Warning in an EHR

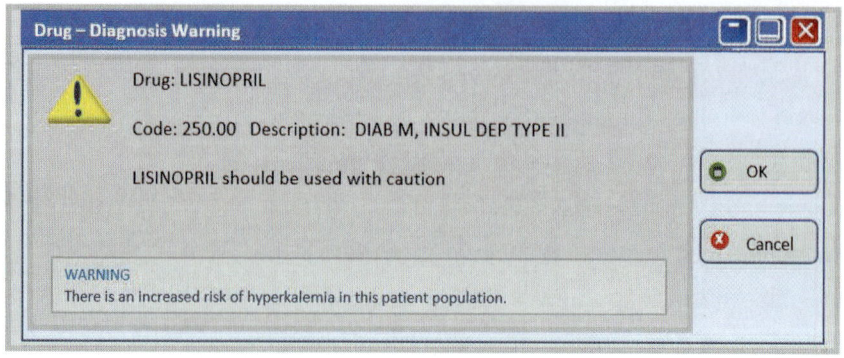

Formulary Check

formulary list of a plan's selected drugs and their proper dosages

The EHR also checks that the medication is in the formulary of the patient's health plan. A **formulary** is a list of pharmaceutical products and dosages deemed by a health care organization to be the best, most economical treatments for a condition or disease. Many health plans reimburse patients for drugs listed in the formulary only, so it is essential for the provider to have this information before the patient leaves the office. If a medication is not in the formulary, the EHR can suggest an alternative drug. Since the medications in formularies change from time to time, the formulary data in the EHRs are updated regularly.

Some EHRs even check whether the medication is in stock at the patient's preferred pharmacy. It is much better to know that a drug is in stock before the patient goes to pick it up at the pharmacy. E-Prescribing also gives the pharmacy time to prepare the prescription so the patient will not have to wait once he or she arrives.

The steps required to refill a patient prescription in a paper-based office and in an electronic office illustrate the advantages of E-Prescribing (see Figures 8.2 and 8.3).

THINKING IT THROUGH 8.1

E-Prescribing eliminates errors that arise from illegible handwriting, and it also provides a number of safety checks. How does it also play a role in increasing the likelihood that a patient will actually take the medication prescribed?

E-Prescribing in EHRclinic

In EHRclinic, the Medications section of the patient's face sheet is used to order new medications and monitor current, historical, or ineffective medications. Figure 8.4 shows a patient's Medications box listing current medications.

Prescribing medications The Medications box is used to enter new prescriptions or refill current prescriptions. The fields in the Medication dialog box were discussed in Chapter 6, including Date, Status, Medication, Dosage, Quantity, Drug Form, Route, Frequency, Duration, and refill information. To prevent errors in prescribing, it is critical that these fields be completed accurately.

Figure 8.2 Prescription Refill in a Paper-Based Office

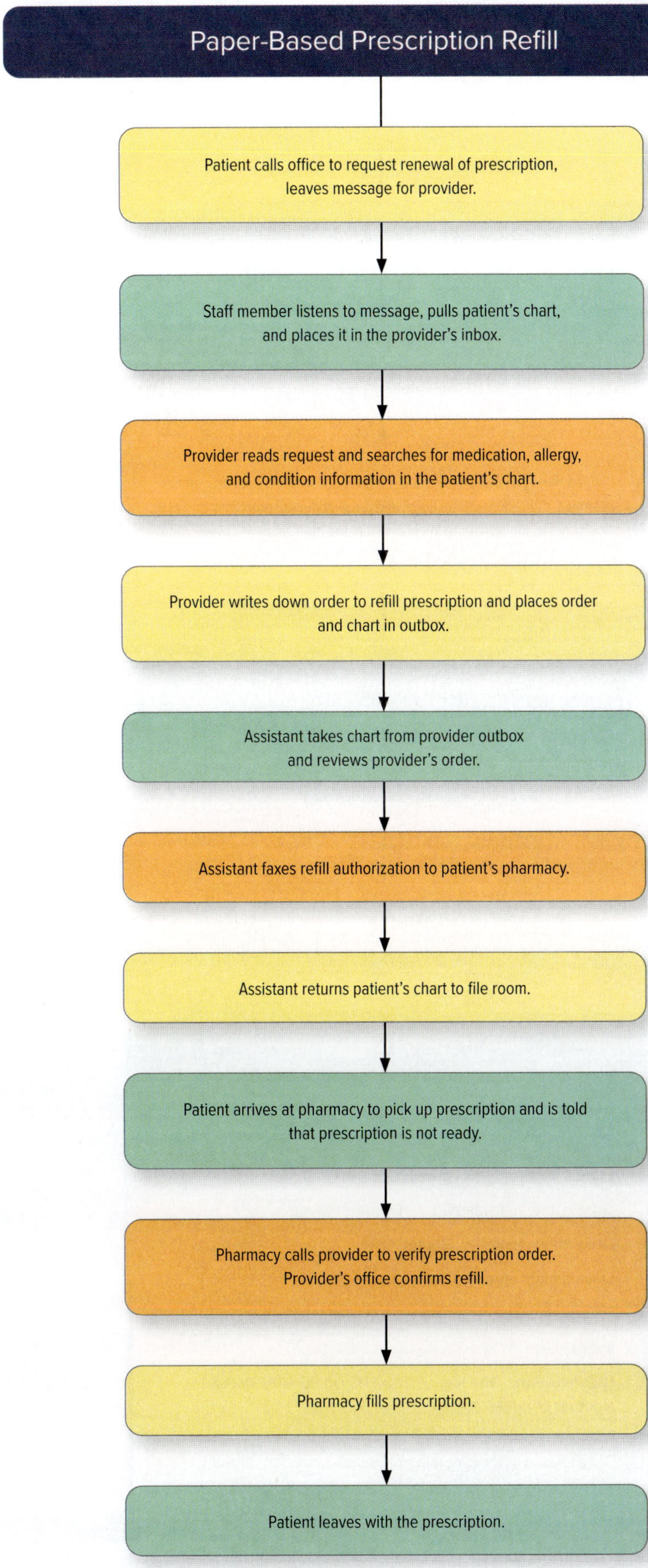

Figure 8.3 Prescription Refill in an Electronic Office

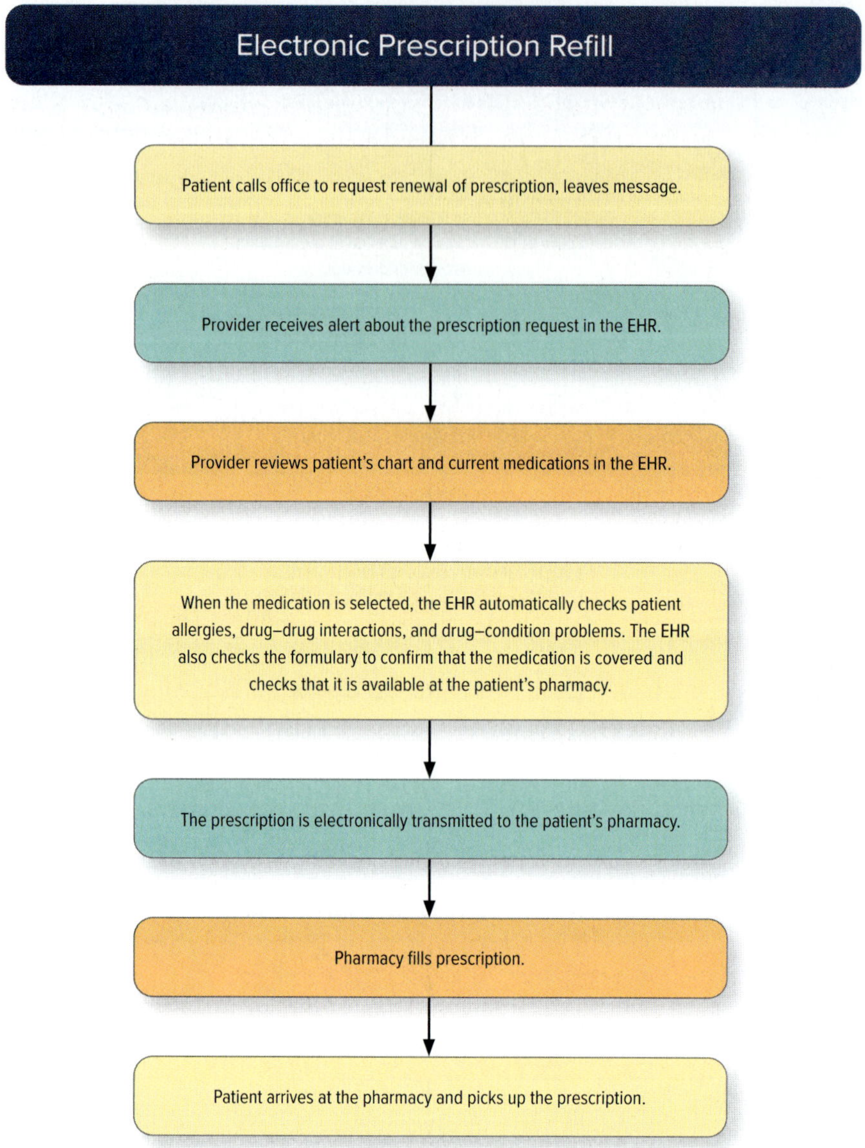

Figure 8.4 Medication Section of the Face Sheet

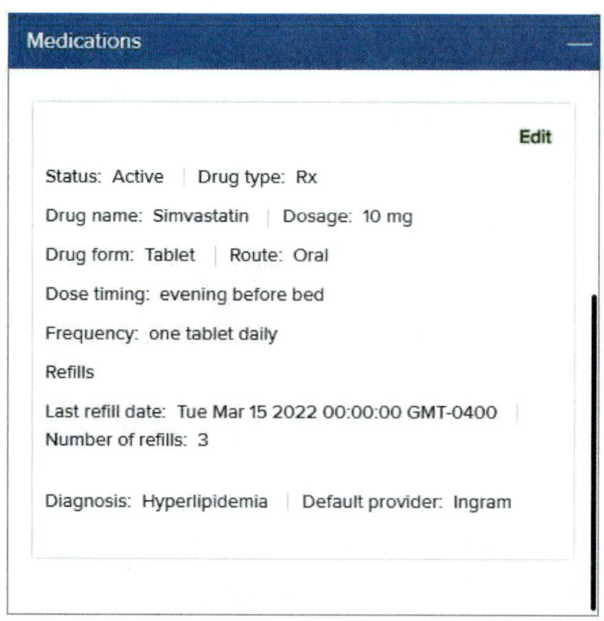

PIN signature To prevent unauthorized personnel from writing prescriptions, a **personal identification number (PIN)** that serves as a special electronic signature is required to transmit prescriptions to the pharmacy. When a signature is required, the prescription cannot be transmitted until the PIN is provided.

personal identification number (PIN) unique number that is assigned to or selected by an individual; in EHRs, the use of a PIN often serves as an electronic signature

point-of-care (POC) ability of providers to document clinical information while interacting with the patient during the patient encounter

Drug database Medications prescribed by a practice are typically managed in the practice's drug database. In EHRclinic, the drug database is found by accessing the practice Tools and then clicking on "Manage practice data." Drugs can be searched, stored, edited, added, or deleted in the database. The advantages to storing drug information in a database are that drugs are easily accessible for prescribing and multiple dosage options can be added to each. The EHRclinic drug database will be discussed in greater detail in Chapter 18.

EXERCISE 8.1

Utilize E-Prescribing EHRclinic

As you are rooming a patient, she mentions that she will need medication refills. Prepare the refill requests for the provider to approve in EHRclinic so they can be electronically transmitted to the patient's pharmacy.

Your instructor may assign this exercise to you in Connect. Exercise steps and EHRclinic Help Guides can be downloaded at http://www.mhhe.com/pmehr2.

8.2 Electronic Order Entry

Once a physician is finished examining a patient, it may be necessary to order tests or procedures as part of diagnosing or treating the patient's condition. EHRs allow providers to order tests without the use of traditional paper forms. Some EHRs include built-in standard order sets based on the provider's specialty or on specific diseases.

Benefits of Electronic Order Entry

Electronic order entry is designed to reduce errors associated with handwritten and paper orders. It is, however, more than a replacement for a paper order system; it provides numerous safety and cost-control benefits. For example, the software can incorporate the rules of different insurance carriers, making it easy to determine whether a test requires preauthorization and whether it is limited to specified diagnoses. The software can delay sending out these orders until approval is received. In addition, some EHR systems are capable of checking orders against information specific to the patient, such as whether the order would be inappropriate based on a patient's medications, lab tests, diagnoses, allergies, or other factors.

In an office with an EHR, the provider enters the orders for a test directly in the program, which is known as **point-of-care** order entry. Once the order has been entered, a staff member receives and processes the order. Orders can then be printed or transmitted electronically.

Figure 8.5 Flowchart of Order Entry in a Paper-Based Office

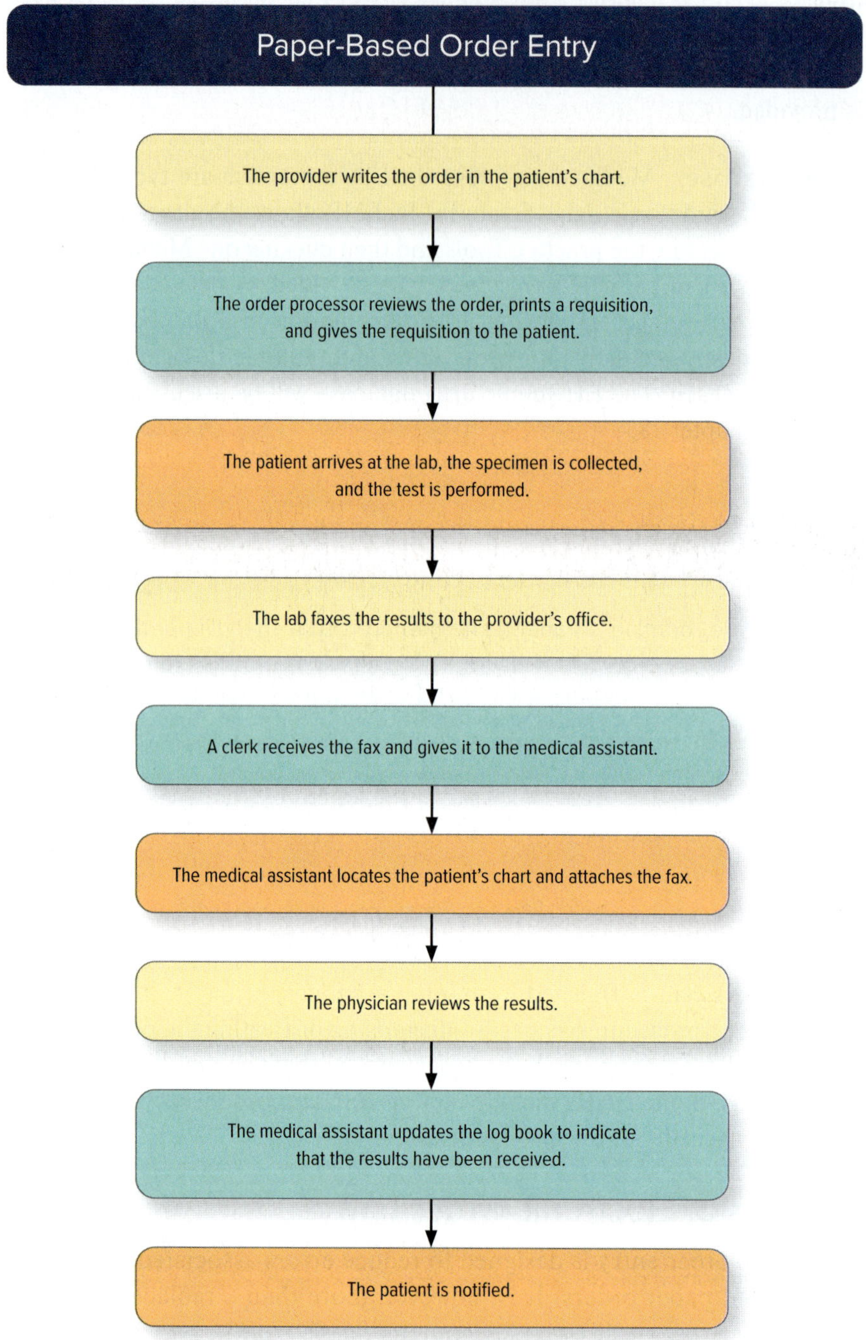

Figures 8.5 and 8.6 illustrate the steps required to send and receive a lab test in a paper-based office and in an office with an EHR.

THINKING IT THROUGH 8.2

When an order is entered in an EHR, the program can check whether the test requires preauthorization and delay the order until that authorization is received. Obviously this is a benefit to the patient, who will not have to pay for a test that was performed prior to authorization. How does this also benefit the medical practice?

Figure 8.6 Flowchart of Order Entry in an Office with an EHR

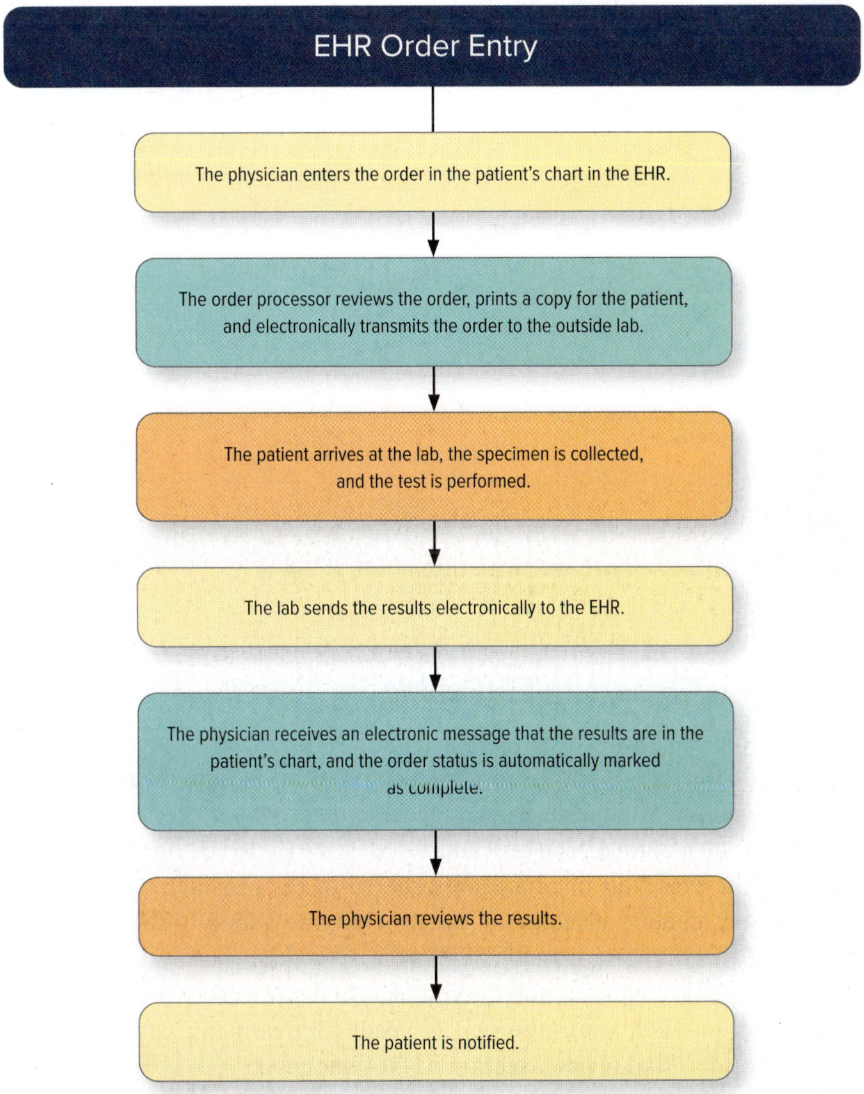

Types of Electronic Orders

Creating electronic orders within an EHR requires interoperability with other systems, meaning that a practice's EHR must be able to communicate with the computer system of the facility receiving the lab order. For example, an order for an MRI can be electronically sent to an MRI facility if each system is set up to send and receive the orders. This interoperability is not limited to submitting orders; the testing facility can also send electronic results back to the provider.

Each EHR is set up differently in terms of facility partnerships and the delivery of electronic orders. The types of orders, however, are common to most practices. They include the following (with examples):

- Laboratory testing (bloodwork, urinalysis, cultures, cytology)
- Radiology (X-rays, MRIs, CT scans, ultrasounds, mammography)
- Cardiac testing (stress testing, nuclear cardiac testing, echocardiography, Holter monitors)
- Procedures (colonoscopies, biopsies, EGDs)
- Referrals (specialists, therapeutic, dietary, weight management, speech pathology)

Figure 8.7 Electronic Order Entry in an EHRclinic Encounter

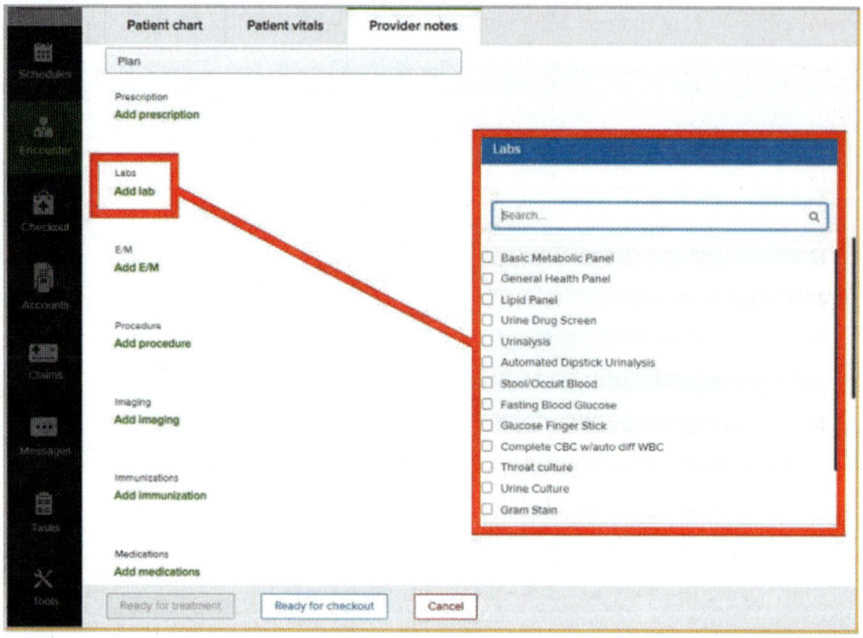

Electronic Orders in EHRclinic

In EHRclinic, electronic orders are generated within the patient's encounter, as shown in Figure 8.7. This is a convenient place to initiate the order while also documenting that it has been done. As orders are selected, their procedure codes are assigned. The procedure codes, added to the order, will communicate the exact test or procedure ordered by the provider. Additionally, the diagnosis code(s) selected by the provider are added to the electronic order so the facility can properly bill for the procedure.

Once an EHRclinic encounter is complete and any tests or procedures are ordered, the provider marks the visit as "ready for treatment," at which point it is sent to the "Plan review" section of the encounter.

EXERCISE 8.2

Create Electronic Orders in an OV

EHRclinic

You are assisting the provider with point-of-care documentation. Complete the patient's encounter and create electronic orders for any tests and procedures that are needed.

Your instructor may assign this exercise to you in Connect. Exercise steps and EHRclinic Help Guides can be downloaded at http://www.mhhe.com/pmehr2.

8.3 Monitoring Order Status

Although creating and transmitting electronic orders is the most efficient method of order entry, it is still necessary for a practice to develop workflow procedures to monitor the status of those orders. Monitoring order status will ensure that results were obtained for any completed tests, and it will identify any patients who failed to complete a test or procedure.

Plan Review in EHRclinic

After completion of the patient encounter, the office visit documentation is sent to "Plan review." This is the area of the EHR that is used to monitor the status of treatment and orders and, in some cases, enter results. As shown in Figure 8.8, "Plan review" has tabs to access the patient chart, patient vitals, provider notes, and treatment status. This allows providers to easily toggle back and forth to review the chart and the office visit notes as the treatment results are documented.

Each item (lab, imaging, procedure, immunization, or E/M) that was selected during the encounter is displayed in the Treatment tab. As each item is completed, its status is updated by the medical assistant. Some procedures may be started and completed at the end of the encounter. For example, if the provider orders an ECG to be complete before the patient leaves the clinic, the status can be updated to Complete when the medical assistant has finished performing the test. In other cases, the patient may need to wait for an appointment with an outside facility or may have pending test results, in which cases the status would be marked as "In progress" until they are complete.

EXAMPLES

Etta Ingersol made an appointment with Dr. McGrath because she felt a small lump in her left breast. Dr. McGrath ordered a mammogram, which Mrs. Ingersol completed within a few days after her appointment.

A week later, the medical assistant reviewed outstanding orders and identified that Mrs. Ingersol's mammogram was marked as being in progress, but the results were never received.

Because Trilogy Family Care Center has a procedure for monitoring the status of orders, this lost test result did not fall through the cracks. It could have been potentially dangerous for the patient if it was never identified that the results were missing.

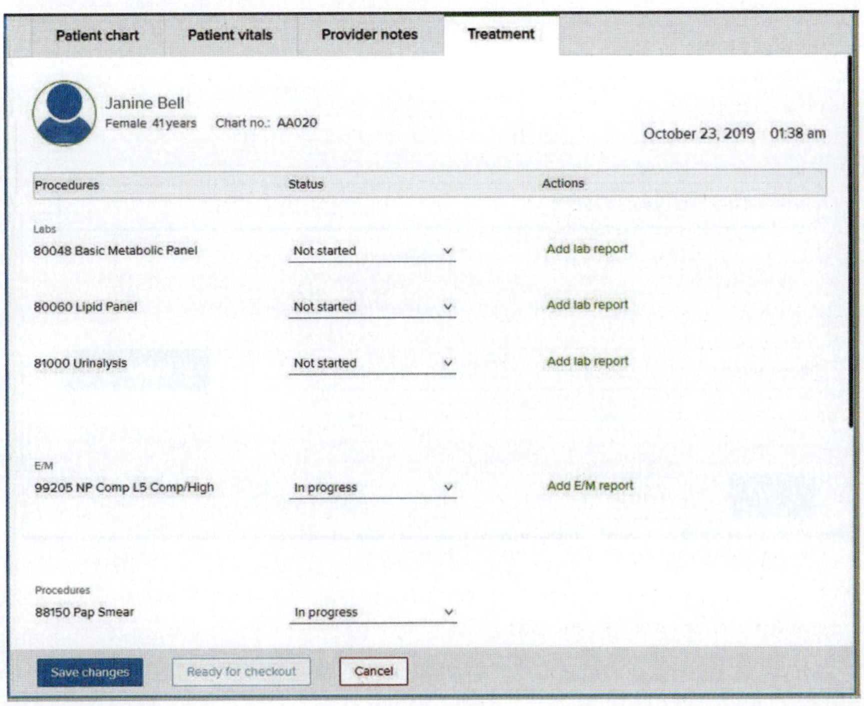

Figure 8.8 Example Result Entry in Plan Review

Receiving Results

Physician practices vary in regard to whether tests and procedures are performed in-house or by an outside facility. Very small practices may use outside labs for almost all tests, while larger group practices may have their own in-house lab facilities. If an outside facility is used, an EHR can receive the results electronically. In-house tests and procedure results can either be uploaded electronically or documented in the patient's chart at the point of care.

In EHRclinic, the results for any procedures can be added directly to the patient's chart. This occurs in either the Treatment tab of the Plan review section of the encounter (shown in Figure 8.8) or by uploading them to the Lab or Imaging report areas in the patient's face sheet, as shown in Figure 8.9.

EXERCISE 8.3 Add Test Results to a Patient's Chart

Each day, the Trilogy Family Care Center assigns a medical assistant to monitor the status of orders by reviewing charts and attaching reports for the providers to review. Today, you are assigned to this task. Add test results to a patient's chart, and identify any missing items for the provider.

Your instructor may assign this exercise to you in Connect. Exercise steps and EHRclinic Help Guides can be downloaded at http://www.mhhe.com/pmehr2.

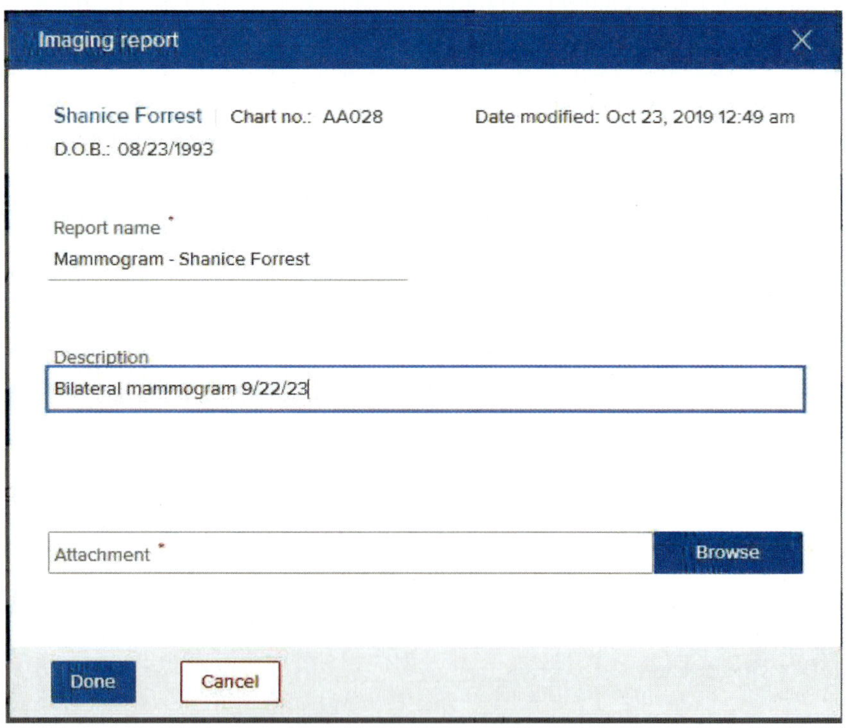

Figure 8.9 Example of Image Report Entry

chapter 8 summary

KEY TERMS

controlled substance
drug-diagnosis warning
drug-drug interaction
drug interaction checker
formulary
medication reconciliation
personal identification number (PIN)
point-of-care (POC)

LEARNING OUTCOME	KEY CONCEPTS/EXAMPLES
8.1 Explain why E-Prescribing reduces some medical errors.	In E-Prescribing, the EHR checks for drug allergies, drug-drug interactions, and other potential conflicts using information in the patient's medical record, including past history, allergies, and a complete medication list. The EHR also checks that the medication is in the formulary of the patient's health plan. If a medication is not in the formulary, the EHR can suggest an alternative drug. The EHR can also check to make sure the patient's pharmacy has the medication in stock.
8.2 Explain why ordering and receiving test results electronically is more efficient than paper methods.	Electronic order entry is designed to reduce errors associated with handwriting and paper orders. It also provides numerous safety and cost-control benefits. It can incorporate the rules of different insurance carriers, making it easy to determine whether a test requires preauthorization and whether it is limited to specified diagnoses. It can delay sending orders until approval is received. In addition, it is capable of checking orders against information specific to the patient, such as whether the order would be inappropriate based on a patient's medications, lab tests, diagnoses, allergies, or other factors.
8.3 Explain how orders are processed in an EHR.	Despite the efficiency of using electronic orders in an EHR, it is necessary for a practice to develop workflow procedures to monitor order status. This ensures that test results are received by the provider and that patients who failed to complete their testing are identified for follow-up. In most EHR systems, results can be entered directly into a patient's chart or uploaded.

chapter 8 review

MATCHING QUESTIONS

Match the key terms with their definitions.

_____ 1. *[LO 8.1]* drug-diagnosis warning

_____ 2. *[LO 8.1]* formulary

_____ 3. *[LO 8.1]* drug-drug interaction

_____ 4. *[LO 8.1]* controlled substance

_____ 5. *[LO 8.1]* E-Prescribing

_____ 6. *[LO 8.1]* medication reconciliation

_____ 7. *[LO 8.2]* interoperability

_____ 8. *[LO 8.2]* point-of-care

_____ 9. *[LO 8.1]* drug interaction checker

_____ 10. *[LO 8.1]* PIN

a. Electronic transmission of prescriptions to pharmacies.

b. List of a plan's selected drugs and their proper dosages.

c. Tool used to identify potentially harmful combinations of prescription medications.

d. Reaction between two or more drugs.

e. Unique number assigned to an individual that is often used as an electronic signature.

f. Documentation of clinical information during a patient encounter.

g. Allows computer applications or software to share and exchange information.

h. Identification and review of the most current list of medications taken by a patient.

i. Notice that a patient's reported diagnosis does not support a specific medication being prescribed.

j. Drug whose use and possession are regulated by law.

MULTIPLE-CHOICE QUESTIONS

Select the letter that best completes the statement or answers the question.

1. *[LO 8.1]* What feature of an E-Prescribing system provides the most common prescribing information to providers?
   a. Clinical decision support
   b. Drug interaction checker
   c. Drug-diagnosis warning
   d. Formulary

2. *[LO 8.1]* Why is it a benefit that E-Prescribing helps providers to monitor controlled substances?
   a. They are only prescribed to elderly patients.
   b. There is a high incidence of drug interactions when taken with other medications.
   c. Their use and possession are regulated by law.
   d. They can only be prescribed for a duration of two weeks or less.

3. *[LO 8.1]* E-Prescribing systems within EHRs have built-in safety checks for ______.
   a. lab reporting
   b. drug allergies
   c. vital sign monitoring
   d. insurance coverage

4. *[LO 8.1]* A list of drugs that are approved as being the most effective and economical for the treatment of specific conditions is known as a(n) ______.
   a. charge schedule
   b. formulary
   c. monograph
   d. superbill

5. *[LO 8.2]* It is known as ______ order entry when the provider inputs a test or procedure order during the patient's encounter.
   a. E-Orders
   b. point-of-care
   c. real-time
   d. time-specific

6. *[LO 8.2]* Interoperability refers to ______.
   a. multiple departments working together in the same medical practice
   b. electronic scheduling of surgical procedures
   c. the practice's ability to directly bill the insurance carriers
   d. two or more software systems that can communicate with each other

7. *[LO 8.3]* When using electronic orders in an EHR, it is important for a practice to ______.
   a. create a cover letter for the receiving facility
   b. print a copy of each order
   c. monitor order status
   d. report the order to the insurance carrier

8. *[LO 8.3]* What area of EHRclinic is used to monitor the status of treatment and orders?
   a. Provider encounter
   b. Accounts
   c. Patient intake
   d. Plan review

9. *[LO 8.2]* Electronic order entry and E-Prescribing are made possible because of ______ between software systems.
   a. interoperability
   b. accessibility
   c. reconciliation
   d. adaptability

10. *[LO 8.3]* Which of the following is an example of a drug-diagnosis warning?
    a. A blood pressure drug decreases the effectiveness of a thyroid drug.
    b. A patient with pancreatitis should avoid taking a specific drug.
    c. A drug may cause an allergic reaction in patients who are allergic to a specific food.
    d. An immunization should be avoided for patients who cannot eat eggs.

SHORT-ANSWER QUESTIONS

Define the following abbreviations.

1. *[LO 8.1]* ERX ____________________
2. *[LO 8.1]* PIN ____________________
3. *[LO 8.2]* POC ____________________

APPLYING YOUR KNOWLEDGE

8.1 *[LO 8.1]* A patient is out of town on a family vacation. After unpacking her suitcase, she realizes that she left her bag of blood pressure and diabetes medications on her bed at home. She calls her doctor and asks what can be done. How can E-Prescribing help a patient in this situation?

____

____

8.2 *[LO 8.2]* An MRI and blood work were ordered for a patient, but he called and stated that he lost the orders that were printed for him.

a. How would this situation be handled if electronic orders were used?

____

____

b. What is the process for replacing paper orders if they are lost?

____

____

c. How can using electronic orders benefit patients? Providers?

____

____

8.3 *[LO 8.3]* A patient had blood work done at an outside lab, but she had to reschedule her follow-up appointment. At her next appointment two months later, it was discovered that the results of the lab work were never received by the ordering provider.

a. What are the potential consequences in this scenario?

____

____

b. How could these issues have been avoided?

____

____

chapter 9

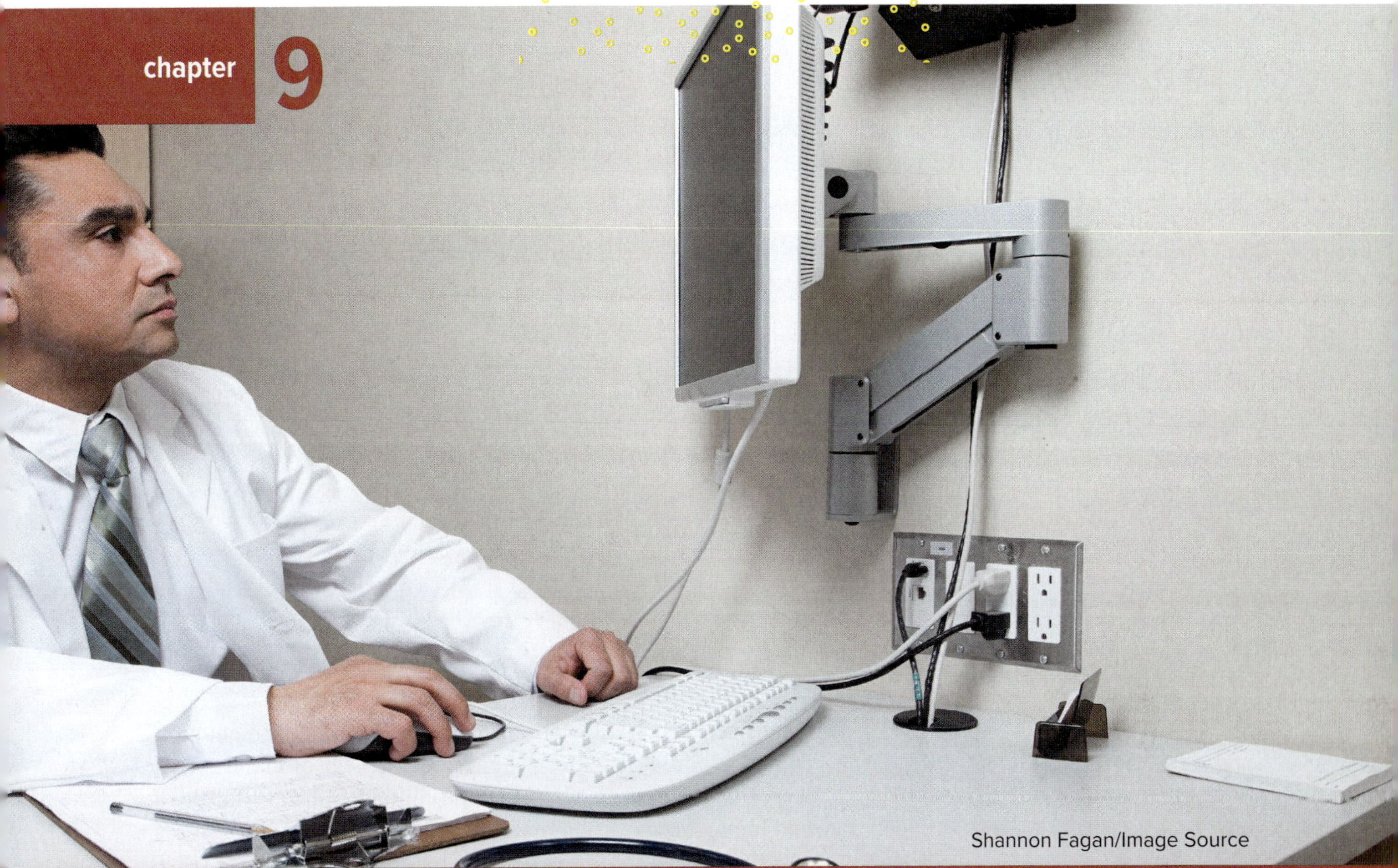
Shannon Fagan/Image Source

Office Visit: Coding

LEARNING OUTCOMES

When you finish this chapter, you will be able to:

- **9.1** Describe the role of EHR in reimbursement.
- **9.2** Explain the relationship between documentation and coding.
- **9.3** Describe the HIPAA-required code sets.
- **9.4** Describe the use of procedure coding.
- **9.5** Explain the use of E&M coding and its documentation requirements.
- **9.6** Describe the use of diagnosis coding.
- **9.7** Explain the medical necessity requirements in coding.
- **9.8** Describe the electronic signature as it relates to coding.

Documentation Matters

Elrene Harrison is the new revenue cycle manager at Trilogy Family Care Center. She is having a staff meeting to get to know the staff and to learn the clinic's revenue processes.

One of the coders, Aiden West, mentioned that Dr. Martinez documents using code words to identify the procedures that were performed and need to be charged for billing. An example he gave was that a "New patient female PE with the works" meant that the patient had a new patient physical exam, an ECG, a specific blood panel, and a Pap smear. When the coders see Dr. Martinez's notes, they know the procedures that need to be captured based on these descriptions in the medical record. Aiden even showed Elrene a cheat sheet that listed the descriptions and how to code for each. He mentioned that Dr. Martinez is much more efficient once he adopted this system.

How should Elrene respond after learning Dr. Martinez's process? Is this an acceptable system to use for coding? Why or why not?

9.1 The Role of EHR in Reimbursement

Electronic health records (EHRs) produce more accurate documentation, leading to complete coding and accurate reimbursement of claims. They offer many benefits, including saving time, prompting clinicians for documentation, and improving consistency and completeness in medical records. EHRs are now the driving force to a clinic's reimbursement. The EHR is used throughout the patient's encounter, including the coding and billing, leading to reimbursement.

Using EHRs: Integrated Medical Documentation and Billing Cycle

The increased use of electronic health records in physician practices has changed the office workflow. A medical office needs a flow of work that provides medical care to patients and collects payment for these services. When EHRs are used, previous paper-based tasks, such as pulling file folders and making photocopies, are replaced by efficient electronic processes. The medical documentation and **billing cycle** explains how the use of EHRs is integrated with practice management programs as the ten-step billing process is performed. This cycle is illustrated in Figure 9.1.

billing cycle steps that establish financial responsibility, check-in, checkout, and coding, the professional medical staff gathering clinical information

Following the billing steps that establish financial responsibility, check-in, checkout, and coding, the professional medical staff gathers clinical information. Often a medical assistant inputs vital signs (temperature, pulse, respiration, blood pressure) and measurements (height and weight) in the EHR. The physician then documents the results of the physical examination, relevant history, and planned treatments.

As the medical documentation and billing cycle continues, so does the interaction between the two types of information. The physician or a medical coder assigns medical codes to the patient's diagnosis and procedures, and the charges for those procedures are determined. Based on this information, the biller/coder reviews coding and billing compliance and checks out

Medical Documentation and Billing Cycle

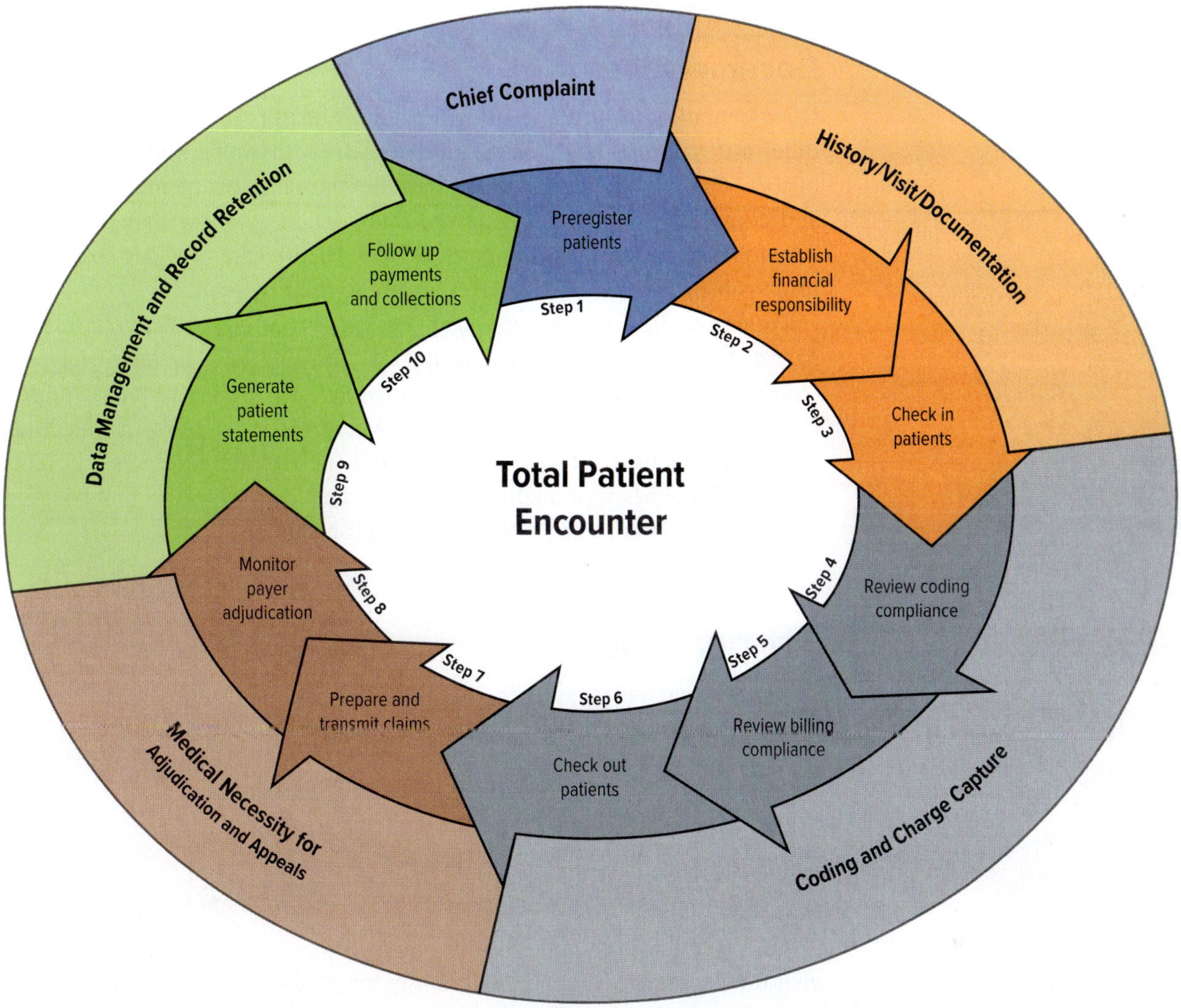

Figure 9.1 The Medical Documentation and Billing Cycle

the patient. When the biller then prepares and transmits claims, documentation may be studied to support medical necessity during claim creation and later during adjudication, if a payer requires it. During the steps of claim follow-up, patients' statements and payment and collections are documented, and the process of managing and retaining patient data according to regulations is carried out, all within the EHR.

Medical billers and coders should be knowledgeable about this EHR cycle so that they can access the clinical information they need to complete claims and provide documentation to support the medical necessity of a service.

9.2 Relationship Between Documentation and Coding

Although physicians are ultimately responsible for proper documentation and correct coding, administrative staff members help ensure maximum appropriate reimbursement by auditing medical coding. The staff member must work with the physician to ensure that the codes that have been assigned are supported in the documentation. This process takes place after a patient encounter, but before the charges are billed.

Documentation

Documentation means organizing a patient's health record in chronological order using a systematic, logical, and consistent method. A patient's health history, exam, tests, and results of treatment are all documented. Complete and comprehensive documentation is important to show that physicians have followed the medical standards of care. Health care providers are legally responsible for providing this level of care to their patients.

Patient medical records are legal documents. Good medical records are part of the physician's defense against accusations that patients were not treated correctly or for services not provided. They clearly state who performed what service and describe why, where, when, and how it was done. Physicians document the rationale behind their treatment decisions. This rationale is the basis for medical necessity–the clinically logical link between a patient's conditions and a treatment or procedure.

> **CODING TIP**
>
> **Documenting Services**
>
> The connection between documentation and coding is essential: If a service is not documented, it cannot be coded.

9.3 HIPAA-Required Code Sets

Once the patient examination is complete, the information recorded in the visit documentation becomes the basis for medical billing in the practice management program. The procedures that were performed, as well as the patient's diagnosis, must be submitted to the patient's insurance carrier for reimbursement. Before the information is transmitted to the practice management program within the EHR, it must be coded.

medical coding the process of applying the HIPAA-mandated code sets to assign codes to diagnoses and procedures

Medical coding is the process of applying the HIPAA-mandated code sets (under the HIPAA Electronic Health Care Transactions and Code Sets Rule) to assign codes to diagnoses and procedures. In the outpatient setting, the required code sets are:

- CPT (*Current Procedural Terminology*)
- HCPCS (Healthcare Common Procedure Coding System)
- ICD-10-CM (*International Classification of Diseases,* Tenth Revision, *Clinical Modification*)

These code sets are used to report the diagnostic and procedural information in the medical record on health care claims. Whether physicians are reimbursed for the services they provide is directly linked to the codes submitted to the payer on the insurance claim. When a payer receives a claim, the codes are reviewed. Payers want to know whether the service provided was appropriate for the patient's condition and whether the treatment was necessary. If an asthmatic patient diagnosed with an upper respiratory infection receives a chest X-ray to rule out pneumonia, the payer probably will not question the claim. If the same patient receives an ankle X-ray, the claim will probably be rejected, since there is not a clear relationship between the diagnosis and the service provided. And while a chest X-ray would be common for the asthmatic patient, its medical necessity might be questioned if it was performed on a twenty-year-old with the same symptoms but no asthma. Since the codes assigned to diagnoses and services play a major role in whether a physician is paid, it is important to document and code the information as accurately as possible.

9.4 Procedure Coding

Procedure codes, like diagnosis codes, are an important part of medical billing. Standard procedure codes are used by physicians in medical practices to report the medical, surgical, and diagnostic services they provide. These codes are used by payers to determine payments. Accurate procedural coding ensures that providers receive the maximum appropriate reimbursement for services.

Procedure codes are also used to establish guidelines for the delivery of the best possible care for patients. Medical researchers track various treatment plans for patients with similar diagnoses and evaluate patients' outcomes. The results are shared with physicians and payers so that best practices can be implemented. For example, this type of analysis has shown that patients who have had heart attacks can reduce the risk of another attack by taking a class of drugs called beta blockers.

CPT and HCPCS

The procedure codes for physicians' and other health care providers' services are selected from the **Current Procedural Terminology** data set, called **CPT,** which is owned and maintained by the American Medical Association (AMA).

CPT lists the procedures and services that are commonly performed by physicians across the country. There was also a need for codes for items that are used in medical practices but not listed in CPT, like supplies and equipment. These codes are found in the **Healthcare Common Procedure Coding System,** referred to as **HCPCS** (pronounced 'hick-picks'). Officially, CPT is the first part (called Level I) of HCPCS, and the supply codes are the second part (Level II). Most people, though, call the codes in the CPT book "CPT codes" and the Level II codes "HCPCS codes."

Current Procedural Terminology (CPT) the standardized classification system for reporting medical procedures and services

Healthcare Common Procedure Coding System (HCPCS) procedure codes and supplies for Medicare claims

Category I codes procedure codes found in the main body of CPT

There are three categories of CPT codes:

1. Category I codes
2. Category II codes
3. Category III codes

Category I Codes

CPT **Category I codes** –which are the majority–have five digits (with no decimals) followed by a descriptor, which is a brief explanation of the procedure:

EXAMPLES

99204	Office visit for evaluation and management of a new patient
00730	Anesthesia for procedures on upper posterior abdominal wall
24006	Arthrotomy of the elbow, with capsular excision for capsular release
70100	Radiologic examination of the mandible
80400	ACTH stimulation panel; for adrenal insufficiency
93000	Electrocardiogram, routine ECG with at least 12 leads; with interpretation and report

TIP

Mandated Use of CPT

CPT is the mandated code set for physicians' work under HIPAA's Electronic Health Care Transactions and Code Sets. Codes must be current as of the date of service.

Although the codes are grouped into sections, such as Surgery, codes from any section can be used by all types of physicians. For example, a family practitioner might use codes from the Surgery section to describe an office procedure such as the incision and drainage of an abscess.

Category II Codes

Category II codes optional CPT codes that track performance measures

Category III codes temporary codes for emerging technology, services, and procedures

Category II codes are used to track performance measures for a medical goal, such as reducing tobacco use. These codes are optional; they are not paid by insurance carriers. They help in the development of best practice care and improve documentation. These codes have an alphabetic character for the fifth digit:

EXAMPLES

0002F	Tobacco use, smoking, assessed
0004F	Tobacco use cessation intervention, counseling

Category III Codes

Category III codes are temporary codes for emerging technology, services, and procedures. These codes also have an alphabetic character for the fifth digit:

EXAMPLES

0001T	Endovascular repair of infrarenal abdominal aortic aneurysm or dissection
0041T	Urinalysis infectious agent detection

A temporary code may become permanent and part of the regular codes if the service it identifies proves effective and is widely performed.

THINKING IT THROUGH 9.1

Which category of procedure codes—I, II, or III—do you think is most important for physician reimbursement? Why are three different categories necessary?

CPT Organization and Format

The CPT manual is made up of the main text–sections of codes–followed by appendixes and an index. The main text has the following six sections of Category I procedure codes:

1. Evaluation and Management	Codes 99201–99499
2. Anesthesia	Codes 00100–01999
3. Surgery	Codes 10040–69990
4. Radiology	Codes 70010–79999
5. Pathology and Laboratory	Codes 80047–89398
6. Medicine	Codes 90281–99607

Each section begins with section guidelines for the use of its codes. The guidelines also include special notes about the structure or rules for use. The guidelines must be carefully followed in order to correctly assign codes from the section. In general, the steps for assigning correct codes are shown in Figure 9.2.

Figure 9.2 Procedure Code Assignment Flowchart

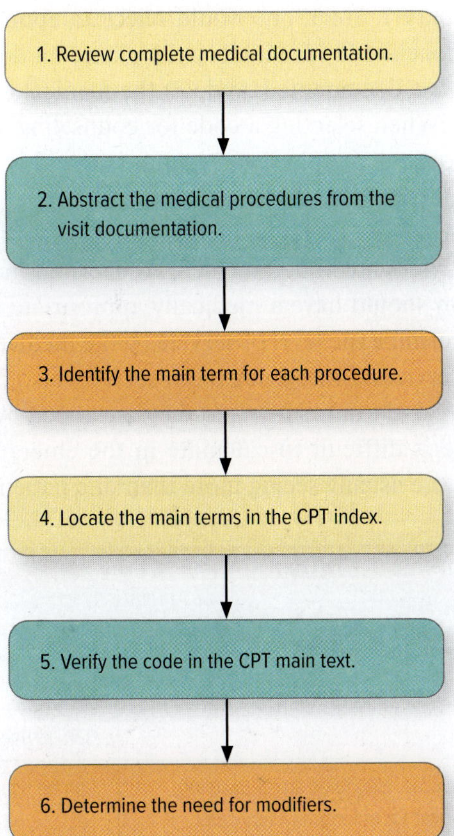

9.5 Documentation and E/M Coding

When billing for a patient visit, the provider must submit a procedure code that represents the work done by the physician. Often, the service involves a process physicians use to collect and analyze information about a patient's condition and to make decisions about the best treatment, rather than surgery or a specialized service like X-rays or laboratory testing. The CPT codes that represent the thought process that the physician follows to determine the best course of care are known as **evaluation and management (E/M) codes.**

evaluation and management (E/M) codes codes that cover physicians' services performed to determine the optimum course for patient care

key components factors documented for various levels of evaluation and management services

Patients' conditions require different levels of information gathering, analysis, and decision making by physicians. Consider that a patient with a mild case of poison ivy might be on the low end of the range. On the opposite end is a patient with a life-threatening condition. The E/M codes reflect these different levels. For example, there are four codes for an office visit with a new patient, and another five for an office visit with an established patient. A financial value is assigned by payers to each code in a range. To justify the use of a higher-level code in the range—one that is tied to a higher value—physicians must perform and document specific clinical facts about patient encounters.

E/M Code Selection Process

Codes in the E/M section are organized by the place of service, such as the office, the hospital, or a patient's home. A few (for example, consultations) are grouped by type of service. Some have different code ranges for new and established patients, such as the office visits described above. Others have a single range of codes, such as hospital inpatient services.

For coding observation, inpatient, emergency, and nursing facility services prior to January 1, 2023, one would select an appropriate code based on three **key components:** (1) the history the physician documented, (2) the examination that was documented, and (3) the medical decisions the physician documented. When selecting a code for counseling, or coordination of care, the amount of time the physician spends is the only key component to determine the level (see Table 9.1).

After January 1, 2023, coding guidelines for observation, inpatient, and nursing facility services are coded by medical decision making or time, and the documentation should have a medically appropriate history and exam. The coder will determine the level of service by the medical decision making or time for these services. Emergency room services also require a medically appropriate history and exam. However, they are coded by medical decision making only; time is difficult to calculate in the emergency room setting because providers are usually seeing more than one patient at a time.

TABLE 9.1 E/M Code Selections Comparison Prior to January 1, 2023

Component	Counseling, Observation, Inpatient, Consults, Nursing Facilities, Emergency Services	Office Outpatient
History and Exam	Used in code selection	Not used in code selection
Medical Decision Making	Used in code selection	Can be used in code selection
Time	Used for some of the other services. Examples are counseling and/or coordination of care. Never for emergency services.	Can be used in code selection

Figure 9.3 Selecting an Evaluation and Management Code

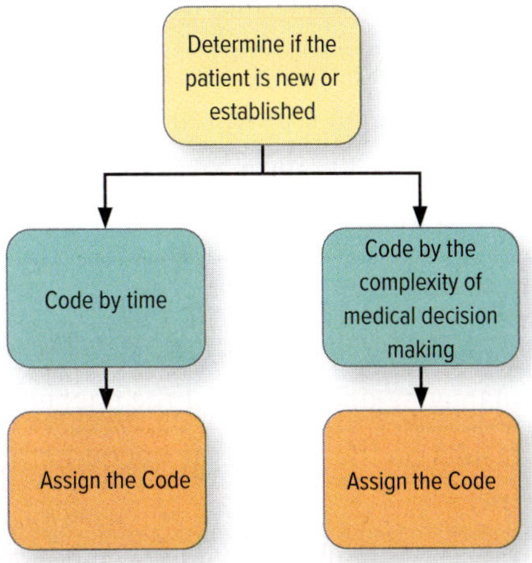

These changes have streamlined the coding process and help the providers focus on patient care. Instead of documenting to code, they can now focus on documenting for patient care.

Medical assistants and office billers/coders typically work in outpatient settings, so we will take a deeper dive into how to select the correct E/M code for these services. Outpatient service codes are selected by time or by the complexity of the medical decision making (see Figure 9.3).

The following coding guidelines will focus on how to select an outpatient/office.

Determine if the Patient Is New or Established

The list of E/M categories, such as office visits, is used to locate the appropriate place or type of service in the index. In the main text of the selected category, the subcategory–such as new or established patient–is then chosen. Emergency room visits do not have a new or established preference. It is determined that all patients in the ER are considered new.

EXAMPLES

Documentation: office visit to established patient

Index: Office Visit

  Office or Other Outpatient Services

  Established Patient

Code Ranges: 99211-99215

Determine if Coding by Time or Complexity of the Medical Decision Making

The compliance department and revenue cycle leaders will determine if the office is going to base coding on the amount of time spent with the patient or by determining the complexity of medical decision making (MDM). A determination can also be made stating that the coder can determine how to code the encounter; either by time or by the complexity of the MDM. The coder will look at which method will provide the highest level, as long as documentation is provided to support the coding. Whichever determination the office chooses should be in the compliance plan of coding.

Code by Time

The provider must document time in the medical record or provider note. The provider calculates time using these guidelines:

- Face-to-face
  - During the exam
  - Obtaining the history and review of systems
- Assessing and managing on the date of the encounter
- Review of test results on the date of the encounter (prior or during seeing the patient)
- Review of prior history obtained by others in the medical record
- Ordering medications, tests, or procedures
- Documenting in the EHR
- Independently interpreting results (not separately reported)
- Care coordination

The provider's documentation needs to justify the time spent for the visit. It should support medical necessity for the level of service that is being coded. The documentation cannot simply state the amount of time spent with the patient. The provider should still document a history, exam, and an assessment and plan, along with the time documented as shown below.

EXAMPLE

A total of 25 minutes was spent on this visit, with 20 minutes spent reviewing previous notes, counseling the patient on DM and HTN, ordering tests, refilling meds, and documenting the findings in the note.

Selection of the E/M level will be based on the time documented, which correlates with the E/M code description.

EXAMPLE

99213 **Office or other outpatient visit** for an established patient that requires an appropriate history and/or examination with a low level of medical decision making. When using time for coding, 20–29 minutes of total time is documented.

Code by the Complexity of Medical Decision Making

The complexity of the medical decisions that the physician makes involves the number of possible diagnoses and treatment options that are considered, how much information (test results or previous records reviewed or ordered) was considered in analyzing the patient's problem, and how serious the illness is, meaning how much risk there is for significant complications, advanced illness, or death.

The decision-making process that the physician documents is categorized as one of four types on a scale from lesser to greater complexity:

1. **Straightforward** Minimal diagnosis options, a minimal amount of data, and minimum risk
2. **Low complexity** Limited diagnosis options, a low amount of data, and low risk
3. **Moderate complexity** Multiple diagnosis options, a moderate amount of data, and moderate risk
4. **High complexity** Extensive diagnosis options, an extensive amount of data, and high risk

EXAMPLES

99203 **Office or other outpatient visit** for a new patient that requires an appropriate history and/or examination with a low level of medical decision making. When using time for coding, 30–44 minutes of total time is documented.

CODING TIP

99203 Office or other outpatient visit

This means that to select code 99203, the medical record must show that a history and examination were taken, and that medical decision making was at least at the level of low complexity. Or that 30–44 minutes was spent working on the patient's care and treatment.

Assign the Code

After reviewing the documentation and confirming that the documentation supports medical necessity, the E/M code is assigned. The patient's medical record must contain the clinical details to support it.

THINKING IT THROUGH 9.2

Evaluation and management (E/M) codes have separate codes for new and established patients. Most insurance carriers reimburse the codes for a new patient's visit at a higher level than a similar visit for an established patient. Why do you think there is a difference in reimbursement rates between new and established patient visits?

9.6 Diagnosis Coding

In physicians' practices, diagnosis codes are used to report patients' conditions on claims. Physicians determine the diagnosis, both the **primary diagnosis**—the diagnosis that relates to the patient's stated reason for the visit—and secondary

primary diagnosis the patient's major illness or condition for an encounter

or additional problems. The physicians, medical coders, insurance/billing specialists, or medical assistants may be responsible for assigning the codes for those diagnoses. Expertise in diagnostic coding requires knowledge of medical terminology, pathophysiology, and anatomy, as well as experience in correctly applying the guidelines for assigning codes.

As of October 1, 2015, the United States uses the *International Classification of Diseases (ICD),* 10th Revision, for diagnosis coding. The ICD-10 lists diseases and codes according to a system copyrighted by the World Health Organization of the United Nations. ICD has been revised a number of times since the coding system was first developed more than 100 years ago.

The federal government has used ICD-10 to categorize mortality data from death certificates since 1999. An expanded version of this tenth revision was published prior to the mandated compliance date for the health care community to review. A committee of health care professionals from various organizations and specialties prepared this version, which is called the ICD-10's *Clinical Modification,* or **ICD-10-CM.** It is used to code and classify morbidity data from patient medical records, physician offices, and surveys conducted by the National Center for Health Statistics (NCHS). Codes in ICD-10-CM describe conditions and illnesses more precisely than does the World Health Organization's ICD-10 because the codes are intended to provide a more complete picture of patients' conditions.

International Classification of Disease 10th Revision, Clinical Modification (ICD-10-CM) the source of the codes used for reporting diagnoses since October 1, 2015

Code Makeup

In ICD-10-CM, a code is a three- to seven-character alphanumeric representation of a disease or condition. The system is built on categories for diseases, injuries, and symptoms. A category has three characters. Most categories have subcategories of either four- or five-character codes. Valid codes themselves are either three, four, five, six, or seven characters in length, depending on the number of subcategories provided. For example, the code for the first visit for a closed and displaced fracture of the right tibial spine requires seven characters:

EXAMPLES

- Category S82 **Fracture of lower leg, including ankle**
  - Subcategory S82.1 **Fracture of upper end of tibia**
    - Subcategory S82.11 **Fracture of tibial spine**
      - Code S82.111 **Displaced fracture of right tibial spine**
      - Code S82.111A **Displaced fracture of tibial spine, closed fracture, initial encounter**

This variable structure enables coders to assign the most specific diagnosis that is documented in the patient medical record. A sixth character code is more specific than one with fourth or fifth characters, and the seventh character extension can provide additional specific information about the health-related condition. When they are available for assignment in the ICD-10-CM code set, sixth and seventh characters are not optional but must be used. For example, Centers for Medicare and Medicaid Services (CMS) rules state that a Medicare claim will be rejected when the most specific code available is not used.

Organization of ICD-10-CM

ICD-10-CM has two major parts:

- *ICD-10-CM Index to Diseases and Injuries:* The major section of this part, known as the **Alphabetic Index,** provides an index of the disease descriptions in the second major part, the Tabular List. Many descriptions are listed in more than one manner.
- *ICD-10-CM Tabular List of Diseases and Injuries:* The **Tabular List** is made up of twenty-one chapters of disease descriptions and their codes.

Alphabetic Index section of ICD-10-CM alphabetically listing diseases and injuries with corresponding diagnosis codes

Tabular List section of ICD-10-CM listing diagnosis codes numerically

diagnostic statement the medical term describing the condition for which a patient is receiving care

ICD-10-CM's first part also has three additional sections that provide resources for researching correct codes:

- *ICD-10-CM Neoplasm Table:* The Neoplasm Table provides code numbers for neoplasms by anatomical site and divided by the description of the neoplasm.
- *ICD-10-CM Table of Drugs and Chemicals:* The Table of Drugs and Chemicals provides in table format an index of drugs and chemicals that are listed in the Tabular List.
- *ICD-10-CM Index to External Causes:* The Index to External Causes provides an index of all the external causes of diseases and injuries that are listed in the related chapter of the Tabular List.

The process of assigning ICD-10-CM codes begins with the physician's **diagnostic statement,** which contains the medical term describing the condition for which a patient is receiving care. For each encounter, this medical documentation includes the main reason for the patient encounter. It may also provide descriptions of additional conditions or symptoms that have been treated or that are related to the patient's current illness.

In each part of ICD-10-CM, conventions–which are typographic techniques that provide visual guidance for understanding information–help coders to understand the rules and select the right code. The primary rule is that both the Alphabetic Index and the Tabular List are used sequentially to pick a code. The coder first locates the description/code in the Alphabetic Index and then verifies the proposed code selection by turning to the Tabular List and studying its entries.

This process must be followed when assigning all codes. A code followed by a hyphen in the Alphabetic Index is a clear reminder of this rule. The hyphen means that the coder will need to drill down to select the right code. For example, the index entry for otitis media is H66.9-. The coder turns to the Tabular List and reviews these entries:

- H66.90 Otitis media, unspecified, unspecified ear
- H66.91 Otitis media, unspecified, right ear
- H66.92 Otitis media, unspecified, left ear
- H66.93 Otitis media, unspecified, bilateral

Based on the documentation, one of these must be selected for compliant coding; H66.9 alone is not sufficient.

ICD-10-CM Official Guidelines for Coding

Assigning HIPAA-mandated diagnosis codes follows both the conventions that are incorporated in the Alphabetic Index/Tabular List and a separate set

ICD-10-CM Official Guidelines for Coding and Reporting American Hospital Association publication that provides rules for selecting and sequencing diagnosis codes

of rules called **ICD-10-CM** *Official Guidelines for Coding and Reporting.* Known as the "*Official Guidelines,*" these rules are developed by a group known as the four cooperating parties made up of CMS advisers and participants from the American Hospital Association (AHA), the American Health Information Management Association (AHIMA), and the NCHS.

ICD-10-CM OFFICIAL GUIDELINES

www.cdc.gov/nchs/icd/icd10cm.htm

The *Official Guidelines* has sections for general rules, inpatient (hospital) coding, and outpatient (physician office/clinic) coding:

- Section I, *Conventions, general coding guidelines, and chapter-specific guidelines,* first reviews the Alphabetic Index and Tabular List conventions and broad coding rules and then discusses key topics affecting the use of codes in each of the twenty-one chapters.
- Section II, *Selection of Principal Diagnosis,* and Section III, *Reporting Additional Diagnoses,* explain the guidelines for establishing the diagnosis or diagnoses for inpatient cases.
- Section IV, *Diagnostic Coding and Reporting Guidelines for Outpatient Services,* explains the guidelines for establishing the diagnosis or diagnoses for all outpatient encounters. The key points from this section can be summarized as follows:

  1. Code the primary diagnosis first, which is the first-listed diagnosis, followed by current coexisting conditions.
  2. Code to the highest level of certainty.
  3. Code to the highest level of specificity.

Coding Steps

The correct procedure for assigning accurate diagnosis codes has five steps, as shown in Figure 9.4.

Step 1: Review Complete Medical Documentation

In outpatient settings, diagnosis coding begins with the patient's chief complaint (CC). The chief complaint is the medical reason that the patient presents for the visit. This is documented in the patient's medical record. The physician then examines the patient and evaluates the condition or complaint, documenting the diagnosis, condition, problem, or other reason that the documentation shows as being chiefly responsible for the services that are provided. This primary diagnosis provides the main term to be coded first. Documentation will also mention any coexisting complaints that should be coded.

Step 2: Abstract the Medical Conditions from the Visit Documentation

The code will be assigned based on the physician's diagnosis or diagnoses. This information may be located on the encounter form or elsewhere in the patient's medical record, such as in a progress note. For example, a medical record reads:

Figure 9.4 Diagnosis Code Assignment Flowchart

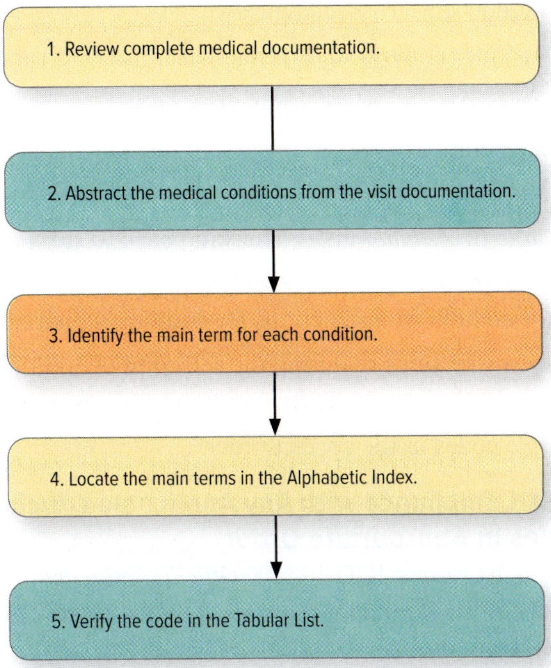

- CC: Chest and epigastric pain; feels like a burning inside. Occasional reflux. Abdomen soft, flat without tenderness. No bowel masses or organomegaly.
- Dx: Peptic ulcer.

The diagnosis is peptic ulcer.

Step 3: Identify the Main Term for Each Condition

If needed, decide which is the main term or condition of the diagnosis. For example, in the diagnosis above, the main term or condition is *ulcer.* The word *peptic* describes what type of ulcer it is. Here are other examples:

- Dx: Complete paralysis.

The main term is *paralysis,* and the supplementary term is *complete.*

- Dx: Heart palpitation.

The main term is *palpitation,* and the supplementary term is *heart.*

- Dx: Panner's disease.

This condition can be found in either of two ways: by looking up the main term *disease,* followed by *Panner's,* or by looking up *Panner's disease.*

Step 4: Locate the Main Terms in the Alphabetic Index

The main term for the patient's primary diagnosis is located in the Alphabetic Index. These guidelines should be observed in choosing the correct term:

- Use any supplementary terms in the diagnostic statement to help locate the main term.
- Read and follow any notes below the main term.

- Review the subterms to find the most specific match to the diagnosis.
- Read and follow any cross-references.
- Note a two-code (etiology and/or manifestation) indication.

Step 5: Verify the Code in the Tabular List

The code for the main term is then located in the Tabular List. These guidelines are observed to verify the selection of the correct code:

- Read *includes* or *excludes* notes, checking back to see if any apply to the code's category, section, or chapter.
- Be alert for and follow instructions for additional digit requirements.
- Follow any instructions requiring the selection of additional codes (such as "code also" or "code first underlying disease").
- List multiple codes in the correct order.

Step 6: Check Compliance with Any Applicable *Official Guidelines* and List Codes in Appropriate Order

The final step is to review ICD-10-CM *Official Guidelines for Coding and Reporting* to check for applicable points. Coders should be sure not to include suspected conditions (for outpatient settings) and to report the primary diagnosis as the first-listed code followed by any coexisting conditions and external source codes.

9.7 Medical Necessity

code linkage clinically appropriate connection between a provided service and a patient's condition or illness

The diagnosis and the medical services that are documented in the patient's medical record should be logically connected so that the medical necessity of the charges is clear to the health plan. Health plans require reported services to be consistent with the diagnosis and meet generally accepted professional medical standards of care. The term **code linkage** describes the connection between a procedure code and the related diagnosis code. Procedures must be:

- In accordance with generally accepted standards of medical practice
- Clinically appropriate in terms of type, frequency, extent, site, and duration
- Not primarily for the convenience of the patient, physician, or other health care provider

If medical necessity is not met, the physician will not receive payment from the health plan. In general, codes that support medical necessity meet these conditions:

- The CPT procedure codes match the ICD-10-CM diagnosis codes.

EXAMPLE

A procedure to drain an abscess of the external ear or auditory canal should be supported by a diagnosis of disorders of the external ear or an ear carbuncle or cyst.

- The procedures are not elective, experimental, or nonessential.

EXAMPLE

Cosmetic nasal surgery performed to improve a patient's appearance is typically excluded. However, a cosmetic procedure may be considered medically necessary when it is performed to repair an accidental injury or to improve the functioning of a malformed body member. A diagnosis of deviated septum, nasal obstruction, acquired facial deformity, or late effects of facial bone fracture supports medical necessity for cosmetic nasal surgery.

- The procedures are furnished at an appropriate level.

EXAMPLE

A high-level evaluation and management code for an office visit (such as 99204/99205 and 99214/99215) must be matched by a serious, complex condition such as a sudden, unexplained large loss of weight.

THINKING IT THROUGH 9.3

In your opinion, is each of the following procedures likely to be considered medically necessary by a payer's health care claim examiner? Why?

- Diagnosis: deviated septum; procedure: nasal surgery _____
- Diagnosis: mole on a female patient's cheek, questionable nature; procedure: surgical removal and biopsy _____
- Diagnosis: male syndrome hair loss; procedure: implant hair plugs on scalp _____
- Diagnosis: probable broken wrist; procedure: comprehensive full-body examination, with complete set of lab tests, chest X-ray, and ECG _____

EXERCISE 9.1

Perform Code Linkage

EHRclinic

You are preparing a patient's encounter for claim submission. Perform code linkage by identifying and linking the diagnosis codes that support each procedure that was documented.

Your instructor may assign this exercise to you in Connect. Exercise steps and EHRclinic Help Guides can be downloaded at www.mhhe.com/pmehr2.

9.8 Electronic Signature

In the past, the act of manually signing a provider note was authentication of the truth of what was done during the encounter. However, this definition of signing a provider's note has evolved with electronic medical records.

Signatures, like medical records, can be either manual, known as **analog** (e.g., stored on paper and unable to be read by a computer) or **digital** (e.g., stored on electronic media that can be read by a computer). The term

analog stored on paper and unable to be read by a computer

digital stored on electronic media that can be read by a computer

electronic signature symbols or other data in a digital form attached to an electronically transmitted document as verification of the sender's intent to the document

electronic signature is used in reference to signatures in a digital format. An **electronic signature** refers to symbols or other data in a digital form attached to an electronically transmitted document as verification of the sender's intent to the document.

An electronic signature serves three main purposes in coding and documentation:

- **Intent** Confirmation that the signer reviewed and approved the content, or the signer authored the document and approves the content.
- **Identity** The signature identifies the person signing.
- **Integrity** The signer claiming the entry is valid or alteration of the document is valid.

The provider's full printed name should appear at the end of the document with the date and time, the digitized signature, or a signature statement with the author's credentials.

EXAMPLE

"Electronically signed by Dr. Jane Doe on 10/1/2020 at 01:15am" or an abbreviation such as "/es/Dr. Jane Doe, 10/1/2020; 01:15am."

We cannot code any services unless we have documentation and an electronic signature by the provider.

chapter 9 summary

KEY TERMS

Alphabetic Index
analog
billing cycle
Category I codes
Category II codes
Category III codes
code linkage
Current Procedural Terminology (CPT)
diagnostic statement
digital
electronic signature
evaluation and management coding (E/M)
Healthcare Common Procedure Coding System (HCPCS)
International Classification of Disease 10th Revision, Clinical Modification (ICD-10-CM)
key components
medical coding
primary diagnosis
Tabular List

LEARNING OUTCOME	KEY CONCEPTS/EXAMPLES
9.1 Describe the role of EHR in reimbursement.	The EHR plays a role in reimbursement because it is part of the billing cycle. We use the EHR to pull data to help support the medical necessity of a service.
9.2 Explain the relationship between documentation and coding.	The connection between documentation and coding is essential: If a service is not documented, it cannot be coded.
9.3 Describe the HIPAA required code sets.	Medical coding is the process of applying the HIPAA-mandated code sets (under the HIPAA Electronic Health Care Transactions and Code Sets Rule) to assign codes to diagnoses and procedures. In the outpatient setting, the required code sets are: • CPT (*Current Procedural Terminology*) • HCPCS (Healthcare Common Procedure Coding System) • ICD-10-CM (*International Classification of Diseases,* Tenth Revision, *Clinical Modification*)
9.4 Describe the use of procedure coding.	Procedure codes are an important part of medical billing. Standard procedure codes are used by physicians in medical practices to report the medical, surgical, and diagnostic services they provide. These codes are used by payers to determine payments and to establish guidelines for the delivery of the best possible care for patients.

LEARNING OUTCOME	KEY CONCEPTS/EXAMPLES
9.5 Explain the use of E&M coding and its documentation requirements.	The CPT codes that represent the thought process that the physician follows to determine the best course of care are known as evaluation and management (E/M) codes. Patients' conditions require different levels of information gathering, analysis, and decision making by physicians. The E/M codes reflect the different levels, calculated by the three key components, the complexity of medical decision making, or by time.
9.6 Describe the use of diagnosis coding.	Physicians determine the diagnosis, both the primary diagnosis and secondary or additional problems. The process of assigning ICD-10-CM codes begins with the physician's diagnostic statement, which contains the medical term describing the condition for which a patient is receiving care. For each encounter, this medical documentation includes the main reason for the patient encounter. It may also provide descriptions of additional conditions or symptoms that have been treated or that are related to the patient's current illness. The diagnosis helps establish medical necessity.
9.7 Explain the medical necessity requirements in coding.	The diagnosis and the medical services that are documented in the patient's medical record should be logically connected so that the medical necessity of the charges is clear to the health plan. Health plans require reported services to be consistent with the diagnosis and meet generally accepted professional medical standards of care. Code linkage describes the connection between a procedure code and the related diagnosis code.
9.8 Describe the electronic signature as it relates to coding.	An electronic signature serves three main purposes in coding and documentation: • Intent: confirmation that the signer reviewed and approved the content, or the signer authored the document and approves the content. • Identity: the signature identifies the person signing. • Integrity: the signer claiming the entry is valid or alteration of the document is valid.

chapter 9 review

MATCHING QUESTIONS

Match the key terms with their definitions.

_____ 1. *[LO 9.1]* billing cycle

_____ 2. *[LO 9.5]* key components

_____ 3. *[LO 9.3]* medical coding

_____ 4. *[LO 9.7]* code linkage

_____ 5. *[LO 9.8]* analog signature

_____ 6. *[LO 9.6]* diagnostic statement

_____ 7. *[LO 9.6]* primary diagnosis

_____ 8. *[LO 9.5]* evaluation and management coding (E&M)

_____ 9. *[LO 9.4]* Current Procedural Terminology (CPT)

_____ 10. *[LO 9.4]* Healthcare Common Procedure Coding System (HCPCS)

a. Stored on paper and unable to be read by a computer.

b. Factors documented for various levels of evaluation and management services.

c. The process of applying the HIPAA-mandated code sets to assign codes to diagnoses and procedures.

d. The medical term describing the condition for which a patient is receiving care.

e. Codes that cover physicians' services performed to determine the optimum course for patient care.

f. The patient's major illness or condition for an encounter.

g. Steps that establish financial responsibility and communication from patient to provider to insurance company.

h. Procedure codes and supplies for Medicare claims.

i. The standardized classification system for reporting medical procedures and services.

j. The clinically appropriate connection between a provided service and a patient's condition or illness.

MULTIPLE CHOICE QUESTIONS

Select the letter that best completes the statement or answers the question.

1. *[LO 9.2]* Which of the following is NOT an advantage of documenting in an EHR?
   a. immediate access to health information
   b. clinical decision support
   c. manual reporting
   d. error reduction

2. *[LO 9.3]* What are the three code sets mandated by HIPAA for medical coding for outpatient services?
   a. CPT, HCPCS, ICD-10-CM
   b. OPT, HCPCS, ICD-9-CM
   c. CPT, HCPCS, ICD-9-PCS
   d. CPT, CPC, ICD-10-CM

3. *[LO 9.4]* In which category are most of the CPT codes found?
   a. Category II
   b. Category III
   c. Category I
   d. Category IV

4. *[LO 9.7]* ________ describes the connection between a procedure code and the related diagnosis code(s).
   a. Charge capture
   b. Code linkage
   c. Unbundling
   d. Compliant billing

5. *[LO 9.4]* Which category is used for tracking performance measures for a medical goal?
   a. Category I
   b. Category II
   c. Category III
   d. Category IV

6. *[LO 9.5]* An office visit E/M code can be selected by calculating time or by the ________.
   a. complexity of the history
   b. complexity of the exam
   c. complexity of the ROS
   d. complexity of medical decision making

7. *[LO 9.5]* Prior to January 1, 2023, ________ are the factors that determine the inpatient levels of E&M services.
   a. digital factors
   b. analog factors
   c. diagnostic statements
   d. key components

8. *[LO 9.6]* How many times has the ICD been revised?
   a. 10
   b. 9
   c. 8
   d. 7

9. *[LO 9.8]* The electronic signature has three main purposes. What are they?
   a. Intent, Identity, Fraud
   b. Intent, Identity, Integrity
   c. Intent, Integrity, Value
   d. Intent, Integrity, Reimbursement

10. *[LO 9.1]* ________ is the steps that establish financial responsibility, check-in procedures, and coding to request payment from a payer.
    a. Code linkage
    b. Medical necessity
    c. Billing cycle
    d. Medical coding

SHORT ANSWER QUESTIONS

Define the following abbreviations.

1. *[LO 9.3]* CPT ____________________
2. *[LO 9.3]* HCPCS ____________________
3. *[LO 9.3]* ICD-10-CM ____________________
4. *[LO 9.4]* AMA ____________________
5. *[LO 9.5]* E/M ____________________
6. *[LO 9.6]* AHIMA ____________________
7. *[LO 9.6]* CC ____________________

APPLYING YOUR KNOWLEDGE

Answer the questions below in the space provided.

9.1 *[LO 9.1]* List the ten steps in the billing cycle process in order.

____

____

9.2 *[LO 9.2]* Explain documentation as it relates to coding.

____

____

9.3 *[LO 9.5]* List what a provider can use to calculate time to determine an E/M level.

____

____

9.4 *[LO 9.7]* Why is code linkage important when supporting medical necessity?

____

____

part three

Charge Capture and Billing Patient Encounters

chapter 10

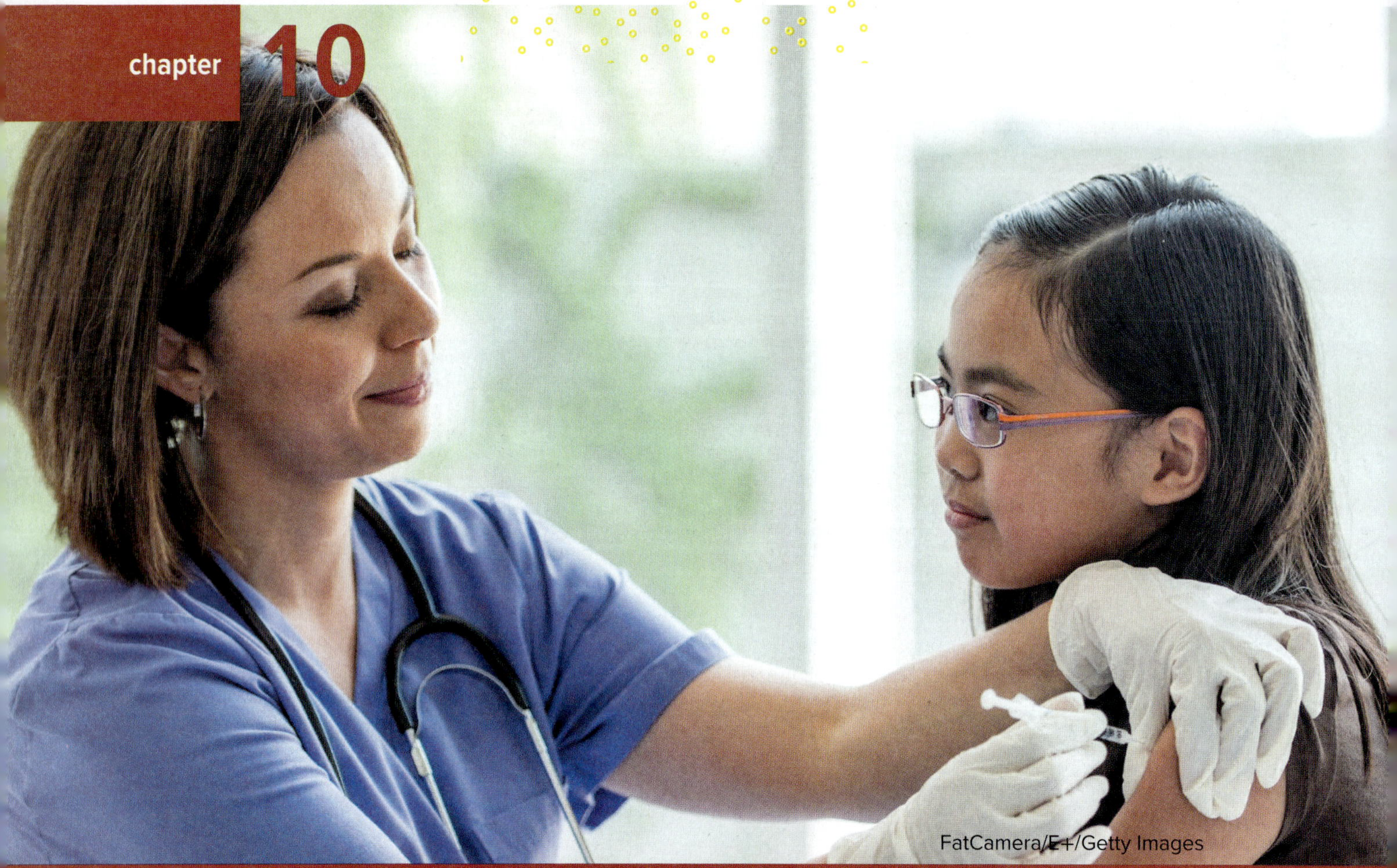
FatCamera/E+/Getty Images

Office Visit: Clinical Check-Out Procedures

LEARNING OUTCOMES

When you finish this chapter, you will be able to:

10.1 Explain order processing in the flow of clinical check-out procedures.

10.2 Discuss encounter follow-up, including patient referrals and patient education.

10.3 Identify the purpose of a clinical visit summary.

Just a Few More Steps

Nadia Abdalla has an appointment with Dr. Cheng to follow up her new diagnosis of type 2 diabetes. After the examination, Dr. Cheng informs the medical assistant, Derek, that Nadia needs blood work, an ECG, a flu vaccine, and a referral to an endocrinologist. She will also need some patient education about diabetes and diabetic nutrition.

Think about what happens after a provider finishes a patient's examination. What actions might Derek need to take to complete Nadia Abdalla's encounter during the clinical check-out process?

10.1 Order Processing

As discussed in Chapter 8, orders are entered electronically during or just after the patient encounter. Once an order has been entered by a provider, it is received by the staff member responsible for processing orders, and it becomes a part of the **clinical check-out** procedures. For example, after an office visit, a provider may order blood work and an ECG. In this case, the medical assistant may be responsible for completing these procedures before the patient leaves the office. In EHRclinic, order processing begins when the order is entered into the office visit encounter. When the office visit is signed and marked "Ready for treatment," the order goes to "Plan review" to be processed for clinical check-out.

clinical check-out performing the final steps of a patient's encounter or office visit; includes initiating orders such as lab work or radiology, providing referrals, administering in-office medications, and any other task designated by the provider as part of the encounter

status relates to the progress of a patient's orders

Treatment in Plan Review

After an encounter is documented in EHRclinic, the patient's **status** is moved from the "Provider encounter" area to "Plan review," as shown in Figure 10.1.

When a provider has completed the office visit and moved the patient to "Plan review," the medical assistant will then begin the clinical check-out procedures by selecting the patient's name. The patient's Treatment area is then shown, which identifies any testing, procedures, or other follow up that the provider ordered during the encounter (see Figure 10.2).

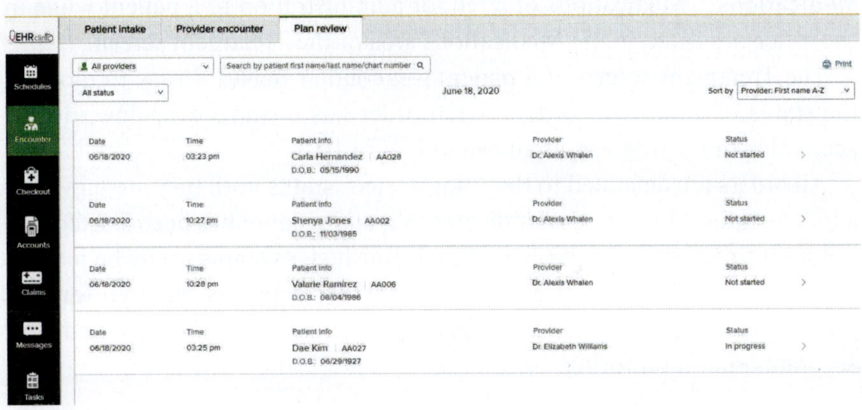

Figure 10.1 Patients Moved from Provider Encounter to Plan Review in EHRclinic

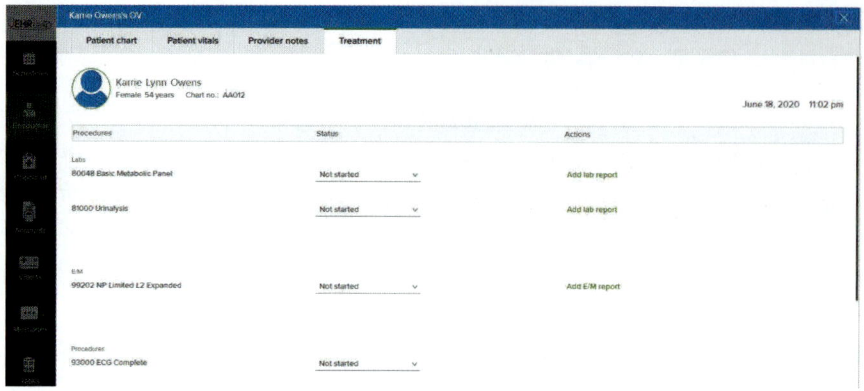

Figure 10.2 Treatment Screen in EHRclinic

The patient's chart, vital signs, and office visit notes can also be accessed here, in tabs along the top of the screen. These sections are helpful to reference when needed. For example, a medical assistant may need to make note of a patient's allergies on a procedure order form. Having the chart available is the most efficient way to access this information.

In the Treatment area, orders are shown and are broken down into types of procedures. Each of the procedures listed in Treatment was ordered by the provider within the encounter notes. They directly correspond to the CPT procedure codes that will be used to bill for the encounter.

Labs Includes blood work, urinalysis, and other lab tests.

E/M E/M procedures correlate to the E/M code selected by the provider. This indicates how the office visit is coded for billing.

Procedures Non-lab procedures such as ECGs, mole removals, and ear irrigations are listed under Procedures in EHRclinic.

Imaging Radiology tests such as mammograms, X-rays, ultrasounds, CT scans, and MRIs are ordered in the Imaging section.

Immunizations Immunizations and other injections, including the administration of immunizations, are reported in this section.

Medications Medications ordered for administration to a patient while in the office are listed in the Medications area of the Treatment screen.

The Treatment screen of a patient's encounter makes it easy to monitor the status of a patient's orders. Each order has a status drop-down list to keep track of its progress, as shown in Figure 10.3.

All orders are defaulted to the "Not started" status until they are moved to another status. "In progress" indicates that a procedure has been started and is not yet finished. Once the procedure is finished, its status would be marked as "Completed." This indicates that no further action is required for that procedure. Utilizing the order status drop-down is essential for efficient and accurate order monitoring.

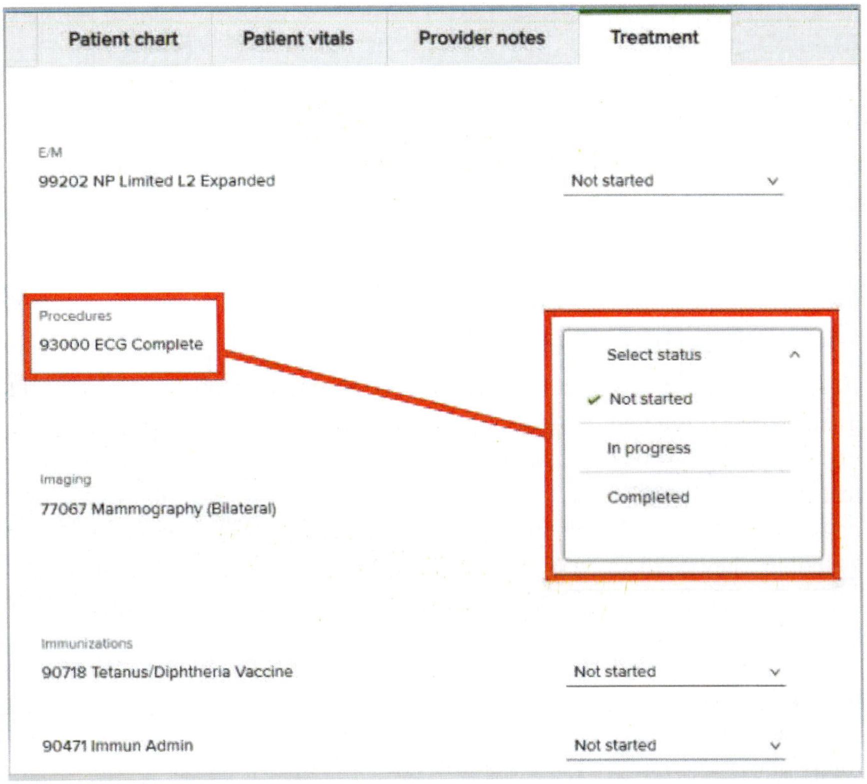

Figure 10.3 The Order Status Drop-Down

EXAMPLES

Orders will have varying statuses depending on their type and when they are completed. For example:

E/M—The E/M code is determined by the level and complexity of the patient's office visit. During the check-out procedures, the E/M code would be marked as "Completed" because the encounter with the provider has ended.

Blood work—A medical assistant draws blood and sends it to the lab for testing. This would be marked "In progress" until the results are returned, at which time it would be marked as "Completed."

Imaging—A provider orders a mammogram, and the medical assistant marks the status as "In progress." When the results are sent to the provider, they are added to the patient's chart and the status is marked as "Completed."

Procedures—A medical assistant performs an ECG on a patient and uploads the results to the patient's chart for the provider's review. The status would then be marked as "Completed" because the test and results were complete before the patient left the office.

Once all of the orders are marked as completed, the encounter is closed by marking it as "Ready for check-out."

EXERCISE 10.1

Mark Order Status

EHRclinic

You have completed a patient's clinical check-out. Mark the order statuses in the Treatment area of the encounter.

Your instructor may assign this exercise to you in Connect. Exercise steps and EHRclinic Help Guides can be downloaded at http://www.mhhe.com/pmehr2.

Documenting Order Completion

It is necessary to document lab and imaging, procedures, and immunizations as they are completed, as discussed in Chapter 8. In some cases, this will occur at the point of care, such as documenting the results of a rapid strep test that was performed in the office. In other cases, the results will be sent at a later date, such as when a mammogram is ordered. When results are available, they need to be uploaded to the patient's chart for the provider's review. For efficiency and convenience, this can be done in the encounter's Treatment area as the status is being updated in EHRclinic.

Point of Care

Point-of-care (POC) tests and procedures are those that occur at the time of the patient's encounter. Some examples of POC tests include:

- ECGs
- Rapid tests, such as for mono or strep
- Urinalysis dipstick
- Vision or hearing tests
- Glucometer testing
- Pregnancy testing
- Fecal occult blood testing (FOBT) sample that is obtained in the office

In EHRclinic, most POC test results are recorded in the Notes section of the patient's facesheet, as shown in Figure 10.4.

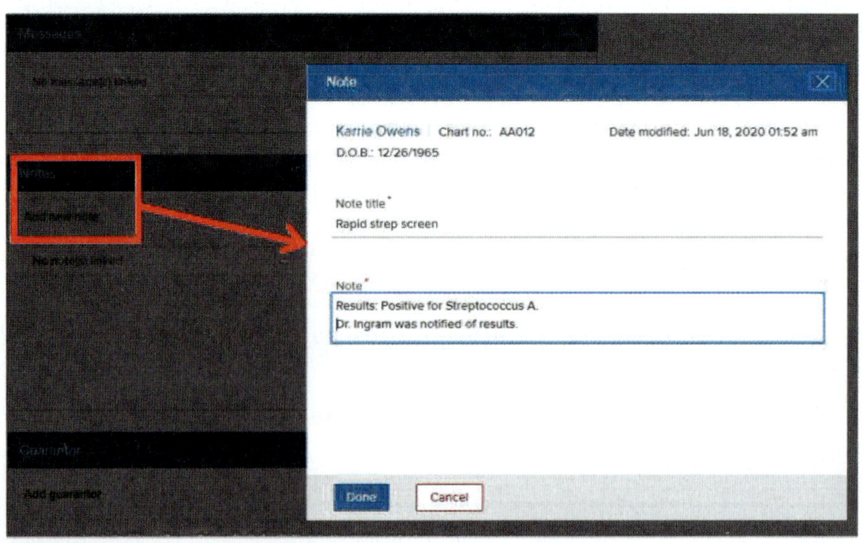

Figure 10.4 Documenting Test Results in a Patient's Notes

EXERCISE 10.2

Document Point-of-Care Results

EHRclinic

You completed an ECG and a vision test for a patient's physical. Record the results of the test in the patient's EHR.

Your instructor may assign this exercise to you in Connect. Exercise steps and EHRclinic Help Guides can be downloaded at http://www.mhhe.com/pmehr2.

Printed or Recorded Results

Tests or procedures that provide printouts or recorded results can be uploaded directly into EHRclinic. These include POC ECG tracings and results that are received from labs, radiologists, or pathologists. They can be uploaded within the facesheet or in the "Treatment" area of the encounter. To upload results when updating the status of an order, click "Add report" next to the order's status. A dialog box will pop up, as shown in Figure 10.5. The report is then named and a description is added. It is a best practice to provide a detailed description, including the test date, so providers can easily identify test results within patients' charts. In EHRclinic, incoming lab results are uploaded to the system every morning. To attach them to a patient's chart, click the Browse button, then select the correct file.

> **TIP**
>
> **Accuracy in Results**
>
> Care must be taken to accurately identify and attach patient results to their electronic health records. Always use two patient identifiers, such as name and date of birth, to ensure that the right results are being saved to the correct patient's chart.

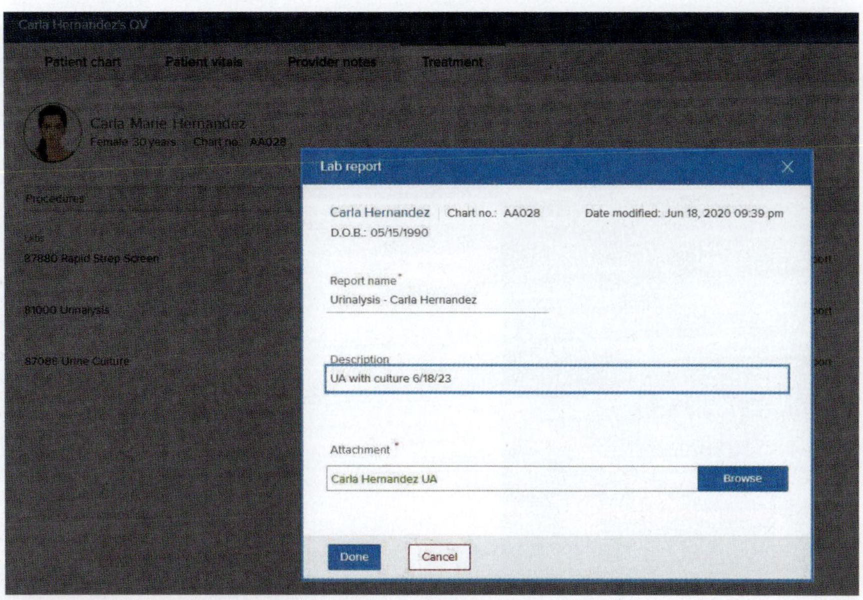

Figure 10.5 Attaching Test Results to a Patient's Chart

Immunizations

Immunizations and injectable medications are also administered at the time of the patient's encounter. Most health care practices charge a fee for the administration of an injection. This is a procedure charge, and the order status can be marked as "Completed" when the injection has been administered because no further action is required.

After administration of the drug or immunization, the status can be updated to "Completed" as well. However, the administration must also be documented at the point of care. In EHRclinic, immunizations and injectable medications can be documented within the patient's facesheet or by clicking the "Add immunization report" button next to the order's status in the Treatment area. A dialog box will pop up so details can be entered (see Figure 10.6).

As discussed in Chapter 6, the fields in the Immunization dialog box include:

Immunization type Select the immunization type from the drop-down list.

Ordering physician Enter the name of the ordering provider.

Follow-up directions Enter follow-up directions, if given.

Dosage Enter the dosage, including units of measurement. If the immunization is a one-dose unit, enter the total volume of medication. For example, 0.5 mL.

manufacturer a company that makes drugs or vaccines

lot number a number given to a specific batch of drug or vaccine as it was manufactured; used for identification of a drug or vaccine

expiration date date after which a drug or vaccine should not be administered

Manufacturer Enter the **manufacturer** of the immunization.

Lot number Enter the **lot number** listed on the immunization packaging. This is important in case there is a recall.

Expiration date Enter the **expiration date** listed on the packaging. Always check the expiration date before administering a drug or immunization. If it is expired, discard the medication according to the practice's protocol.

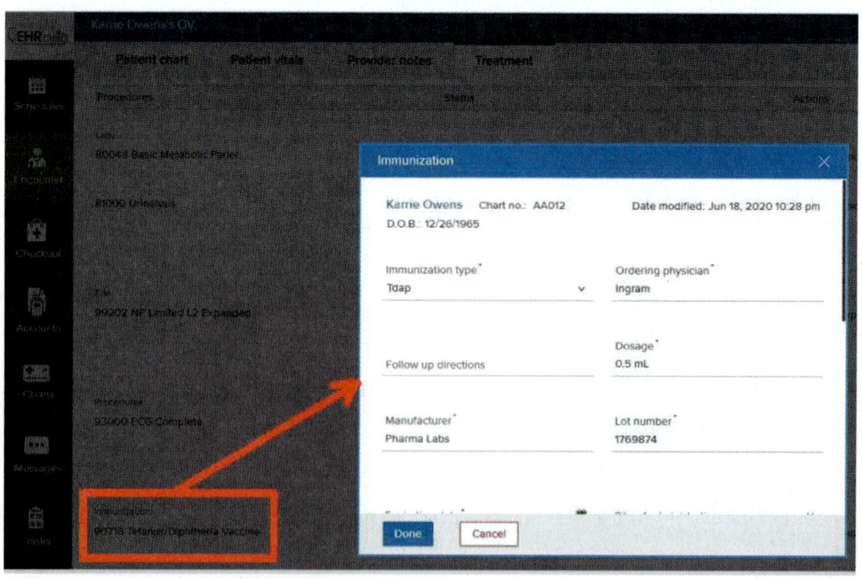

Figure 10.6 Documenting an Immunization

Site of administration If the immunization is injected, select the side of the site of administration, such as left or right.

Site If the immunization is injected, select the location from the drop-down menu.

Adverse effects Note any **adverse effects** that the patient experienced after administration of the immunization. If no adverse effects were observed or reported, enter None.

adverse effects undesired harmful effects resulting from a medication

Vaccine Information Statement (VIS) information sheets produced by the Centers for Disease Control and Prevention (CDC) that explain both the benefits and risks of a vaccine to vaccine recipients

VIS given Select whether a **Vaccine Information Statement (VIS)** was given. In real-world EHR software, the version of the VIS used would also be recorded.

Follow-up directions provided Enter any follow-up directions, such as "Return in 48–72 hours to have PPD skin test read."

Patient instructed to return on Select the date the patient should return if a follow-up visit to the provider is necessary.

Immunization start date Select the date of the first immunization in a series or the date of administration for a single-dose immunization.

Next dose due date Select the approximate date of return, indicated by when the next immunization is due. For example, a hepatitis B vaccine is given in a series of three immunizations over six months or a tetanus booster is due after 10 years.

EXERCISE 10.3

Document Administration of an Immunization

EHRclinic

You administered an immunization to a patient, per Dr. Ingram's orders. Document the details of the immunization in the patient's EHR.

Your instructor may assign this exercise to you in Connect. Exercise steps and EHRclinic Help Guides can be downloaded at http://www.mhhe.com/pmehr2.

10.2 Encounter Follow-Up

In addition to ordering tests, imaging, procedures, and immunizations, providers may recommend other types of patient follow-up. This may include ordering prescriptions, referring patients to other providers or facilities, and providing patient education. An example of ordering patient education and referrals in EHRclinic is shown in Figure 10.7. During the clinical check-out process, medical assistants are responsible for ensuring that the patient has the necessary information to complete this follow-up.

Prescriptions

During patient intake (see Chapter 6), the medical assistant performs medication reconciliation, in which the drugs documented in the EHR are compared with the drugs the patient is taking. Any medications that are discontinued are archived, and any new medications, such as those prescribed by another provider, are added to the medication list. This process

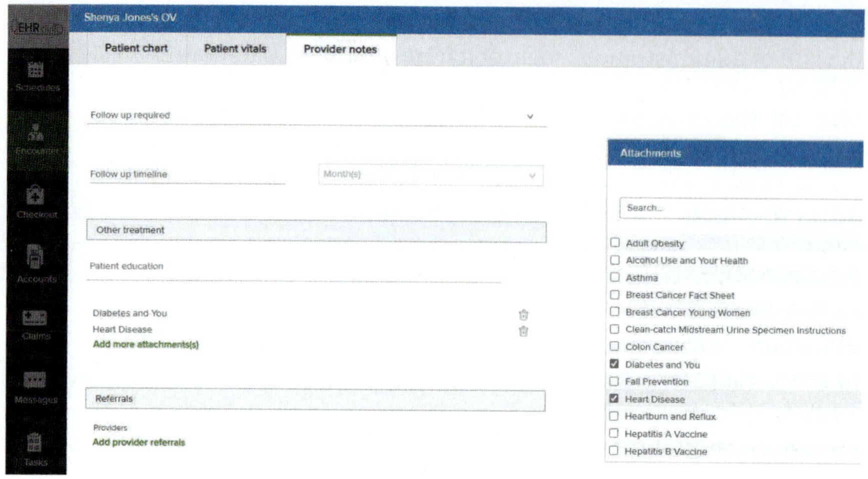

Figure 10.7 Follow-up Patient Education and Order Entry in an EHRclinic Office Visit

ensures that the provider is working from the most current and accurate medication list possible. At the time of the patient's office visit, however, the provider may determine that there should be a change to the patient's medications. For example, an antihypertensive drug would be prescribed for a patient newly diagnosed with hypertension.

Electronic health records have E-Prescribing functionality, as discussed in Chapter 8, This refers to the ability to send prescriptions to the pharmacy electronically. The benefits of E-Prescribing are improved patient safety, greater accuracy in prescribing, and convenience for the patient. Additionally, prescriptions that are sent via E-Prescribing are automatically documented in the patient's EHR.

In most cases, the ordering provider will send any new medications or refills to the pharmacy via E-Prescribing, but the medical assistant still needs to discuss this with the patient during the clinical check-out process. Any new medications should be identified and explained to the patient, and discontinued medications should also be reviewed. If the patient has additional questions, the provider can be brought back into the exam room to answer them.

Referrals

referral transfer of patient care from one provider to another

In some cases, patients may be given a **referral** to see another provider or seek care through a different type of service. Depending on the patient's insurance plan, some referrals need to be processed or approved through the insurance portal. In other cases, a referral may simply be providing a patient with another provider's contact information and the directive to call to schedule an appointment.

EXAMPLES

Patients often seek initial care through a primary care provider (PCP). These encounters may lead to referrals to other specialty providers or services. For example:

- A patient has an ECG during a routine physical. His ECG results indicate an irregular heart rhythm, so he is referred to cardiology for further evaluation.

(Continued)

(*Continued*)

- An elderly patient sees her PCP for hearing loss. She is referred to audiology for testing.
- A three-year-old child sees her pediatrician for a well-child visit. Her parents indicate that she is still not able to form many words clearly. She is referred to speech therapy for evaluation and treatment.
- A patient is newly diagnosed with diabetes. He is referred to an endocrinologist for diabetes management and a nutritionist for diet education.

Referrals can include, but are not limited to, the following specialists or services:

- **Specialty care** Non-primary care providers, such as orthopedics, dermatology, cardiology, pulmonology, gastroenterology, allergy, ENG, endocrinology, gynecology, and so on
- **Therapeutic services** Physical therapy, speech therapy, and occupational therapy
- **Procedural services** Tests or procedures, such as EMG, EGD, colonoscopy, hearing/vision testing, stress testing, and fertility testing
- **Behavioral and mental health services** Psychiatry/psychology, substance abuse/rehabilitation, mental health treatment (inpatient and outpatient), smoking cessation, behavioral therapy, and grief counseling
- **Nutritional services** (nutritionist, dietician, or weight loss)

If a patient is referred to another provider or service, the details of the referral should be discussed with the patient during check-out. Any relevant information, such as the reason for the referral, the other provider's contact information, and the insurance referral or pre-authorization numbers should also be provided to the patient.

Patient Education

If the physician has ordered patient education materials to be given to the patient, these items are handled during check-out. For example, it may be appropriate to provide materials to help patients better understand their diagnoses and treatments, or to provide instructions following an office procedure.

EXAMPLES

Most practices have a database of patient educational materials that are relevant to that practice or specialty. They often include education topics such as:

- **Nutrition**—Diets, diagnosis-related nutrition (such as diabetes and hypertension), and foods to avoid for specific conditions or prevention of symptoms (such as elevated cholesterol, low potassium, and heartburn)
- **Safety**—Fall prevention, child and elder safety, fire safety, and medication safety

(*Continued*)

(*Continued*)

- **Education**—Disease prevention, at-home exercises for treatment, and information about diseases or conditions, management of conditions, and overall health information
- **Procedures**—Procedure descriptions and expectations, preparation, post-procedure follow-up
- **Patient teaching**—Self breast or testicular examination, glucometer testing, insulin (or other) injections, and how to use assistive devices (crutches, walkers, canes)

The patient education feature of EHRclinic provides a built-in set of patient education articles that can be printed and given to patients. There are different sets of articles for pediatrics, adults, seniors, women, men, behavioral health, procedures, and other information. As discussed in Chapter 17, the articles are maintained in the practice's database to ensure that they are relevant and that they cover a variety of topics. During the office visit, the provider can select patient education for the patient by clicking the checkbox for each, as shown in Figure 10.7. If patient education is ordered during an office visit, it will print with the patient's clinical visit summary, which is covered later in this chapter. Otherwise, it can be emailed or printed separately for the patient.

TIP

Document Everything!

Be sure to document any referrals or patient education given to the patient to provide a record of care for reference and liability purposes.

EXERCISE 10.4 **Document Encounter Follow-Up**

EHRclinic

A patient calls Trilogy Family Care Center stating that she saw Dr. Ingram the week before and she lost the information for the specialist she needs to schedule an appointment with. Identify who Dr. Ingram referred the patient to, and document that you provided her with this information.

Your instructor may assign this exercise to you in Connect. Exercise steps and EHRclinic Help Guides can be downloaded at http://www.mhhe.com/pmehr2.

10.3 Clinical Visit Summary

clinical visit summary provides patients with relevant information and instructions pertaining to an encounter

The final piece to the clinical check-out procedures is to provide the patient with a **clinical visit summary.** Also known as a clinical summary, this is provided to patients after an encounter. It includes relevant and actionable information and instructions pertaining to the visit and the patient's overall health records.

Clinical Visit Summaries in EHRs

With the implementation of electronic health records came governance to ensure that they were used in a meaningful way. The Centers for Medicare and Medicaid Services (CMS) developed an EHR incentive program called *Meaningful Use,* in which achieving specific objectives was required for eligible providers and hospitals to participate in the programs. Essentially, Meaningful Use was developed to encourage the use of certified EHR software to improve efficiency in patient care, patient safety, and improved quality of care overall, thus ensuring its **meaningful use.**

The three primary stages of Meaningful Use included:

- Stage 1 (2011-2012): Data capturing and sharing
- Stage 2 (2014): Advanced clinical processes
- Stage 3 (2016): Improved outcomes

Each of these stages addressed specific goals and objectives for the widespread adoption of EHR use, as identified in the Meaningful Use Core Measures. Stage 1 promoted basic EHR adoption and data gathering; Stage 2 emphasized care coordination and exchange of patient information; and Stage 3 focused on improving health care outcomes. It is in Stage 3 of Meaningful Use that the CMS declared eight objectives for reporting. These include:

1. Protect patients' health information by maintaining secure EHR software.
2. Use E-Prescribing for more than 80% of all allowed prescriptions.
3. Implement at least five clinical decision support interventions that relate to at least four clinical quality measures (CQMs).
4. Use Computerized Provider Order Entry (CPOE) for medication, lab, and diagnostic image orders.
5. Enable patients to access their electronic health information, such as by using patient portals.
6. Demonstrate **coordination of care** through improved patient engagement, such as by using the patient portal to send secure messages.
7. Create electronic summary of care records.
8. Meet at least three of five public health and clinical registry report requirements (syndromes, immunizations, case reporting, clinical data registries, or public health registries).

The consistent use of clinical visit summaries was addressed in the Core Measures of Stages 1 and 2, but it also met the Stage 3 objectives related to enabling patients to access their health information, improving patient engagement, and creating electronic summaries of care records. Patients are typically provided with the clinical visit summary during their clinical check-out, and they can also access them electronically in their patient portals.

Since the implementation of these three stages, Meaningful Use has evolved. This program has now shifted to being one of the four components of the Merit-based Incentive Payment System (MIPS) (see Chapter 1), which is a part of the **Medicare Access and CHIP Reauthorization Act of 2015 (MACRA).** In its new format, it works together with other CMS quality programs, the Physician Quality Reporting System, and Value-Based Modifiers.

meaningful use the utilization of certified EHR technology to improve quality, efficiency, and patient safety in the health care system

coordination of care deliberate organization of patient care between a patient and at least one other participant, such as a health care provider

Medicare Access and CHIP Reauthorization Act (MACRA) legislation that created the Quality Payment Program that changes the way that Medicare rewards clinicians, streamlines quality programs under MIPS, and provides bonuses for participation in eligible alternative payment models

While there have been changes to the structure of the original Meaningful Use program, the goal remains the same–to improve the quality of care for patients. As a result, clinical visit summaries are still widely provided to patients after their outpatient encounters.

Components of a Clinical Visit Summary

Eligible providers (EPs) are required to include specific data elements in the clinical visit summaries they provide to patients. This information is typically populated into the visit summary template by the EHR technology, as shown in Figure 10.8.

The required information includes:

- Patient's full name (usually with the date of birth and medical record number listed)
- Provider's office contact information (practice name, address, and phone number)
- Date and location of the visit
- Updated medication list
- Allergy list
- Updated vital signs
- Reason(s) for the visit
- Procedures and instructions (based on discussions that took place during the office visit)
- Updated problem list
- Immunizations or medications administered during the visit
- Summary of topics covered during the visit
- Upcoming appointments (times and locations) or recommended follow-up timeline
- List of tests and procedures recommended, with contact information for scheduling
- Diagnostic test orders
- Patient decision aids, such as information about medications, diagnoses, or tests

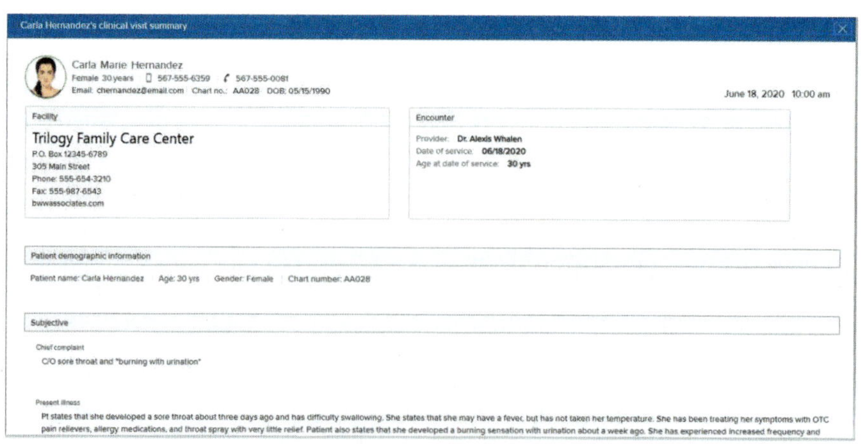
Carla Hernandez's clinical visit summary

Carla Marie Hernandez
Female 30 years 567-555-6359 567-555-0081
Email: chernandez@email.com Chart no.: AA028 DOB: 05/15/1990

June 18, 2020 10:00 am

Facility

Trilogy Family Care Center
P.O. Box 12345-6789
305 Main Street
Phone: 555-654-3210
Fax: 555-987-6543
bwwassociates.com

Encounter

Provider: **Dr. Alexis Whalen**
Date of service: **06/18/2020**
Age at date of service: **30 yrs**

Patient demographic information

Patient name: Carla Hernandez | Age: 30 yrs | Gender: Female | Chart number: AA028

Subjective

Chief complaint
C/O sore throat and "burning with urination"

Present illness
Pt states that she developed a sore throat about three days ago and has difficulty swallowing. She states that she may have a fever, but has not taken her temperature. She has been treating her symptoms with OTC pain relievers, allergy medications, and throat spray with very little relief. Patient also states that she developed a burning sensation with urination about a week ago. She has experienced increased frequency and

Figure 10.8 Excerpt of a Clinical Visit Summary from EHRclinic

THINKING IT THROUGH 10.1

What are the advantages to providing clinical visit summaries to patients after their office visits?

EXERCISE 10.5

Create a Clinical Visit Summary

You have completed a patient's clinical check-out procedures. Print a clinical visit summary for the patient's office visit.

Your instructor may assign this exercise to you in Connect. Exercise steps and EHRclinic Help Guides can be downloaded at http://www.mhhe.com/pmehr2.

chapter 10 summary

KEY TERMS

adverse effects
clinical check-out
clinical visit summary
coordination of care
expiration date
lot number
manufacturer
meaningful use
Medicare Access and CHIP Reauthorization Act (MACRA)
referral
status
Vaccine Information Statement (VIS)

LEARNING OUTCOME	KEY CONCEPTS/EXAMPLES
10.1 Explain order processing in the flow of clinical check-out procedures.	During a patient's encounter, a provider may order labs, tests, imaging, or other procedures. These orders become part of the clinical check-out procedure, in which the medical assistant processes them, such as by drawing blood to send to the lab, informing patients of electronic orders, or performing point-of-care (in-office) testing or procedures (ECGs, immunizations, urine dipstick testing, etc). Any treatment that is ordered must be monitored with status updates of *Not started, In progress,* or *Completed.* Upon completion, test results must be uploaded or documented in the patient's EHR.
10.2 Discuss encounter follow-up, including patient referrals and patient education.	During a patient encounter, other types of patient follow-up may be ordered by the provider. These include: 1. **Prescriptions**–Any prescriptions ordered should be explained to the patient. If the medications are E-Prescribed, then patients should be directed to the pharmacy to pick them up. Patients should have the opportunity to ask questions and should be informed of any changes to their medications. 2. **Referrals**–Providers may determine that a patient should be referred to a specialist for evaluation or treatment. These referrals can include specialty providers as well as therapeutic, behavioral/mental health, nutritional, or procedural services, 3. **Patient education**–Patient education may be provided for a variety of reasons, such as nutrition, safety, management of conditions, procedure preparation, and other types of instruction.

LEARNING OUTCOME	KEY CONCEPTS/EXAMPLES
10.3 Identify the purpose of a clinical visit summary.	Clinical visit summaries are provided to patients after office visit encounters. They include relevant and actionable information and instructions pertaining to the visit and the patient's overall health records. Information provided in a clinical visit summary includes: • Patient information (name, date of birth, and record number) • Provider contact information • Date and location of the visit • Updated medication and allergy lists • Vital signs • Reason(s) for the visit • Procedures and follow-up instructions • Problem list • Immunizations • Summary of topics discussed • Upcoming appointments • Lists of tests and procedures • Patient decision aids

chapter 10 review

MATCHING QUESTIONS

Match the key terms with their definitions.

_____ 1. *[LO 10.1]* clinical check-out

_____ 2. *[LO 10.1]* lot number

_____ 3. *[LO 10.1]* vaccine information statement

_____ 4. *[LO 10.1]* status

_____ 5. *[LO 10.3]* clinical visit summary

_____ 6. *[LO 10.2]* referral

_____ 7. *[LO 10.3]* patient portal

_____ 8. *[LO 10.1]* manufacturer

_____ 9. *[LO 10.3]* Meaningful Use

_____ 10. *[LO 10.1]* adverse effects

a. Provides patients with relevant information about an encounter.

b. Undesired and potentially harmful symptoms resulting from a medication.

c. Transfer of patient care from one provider to another.

d. Assigned to a specific batch of drug or vaccine for identification purposes.

e. Relates to the progress of a patient's orders.

f. The original utilization of certified EHR technology to improve quality, efficiency, and patient safety.

g. Information that explains the benefits and risks of an immunization.

h. Performing the final steps of a patient's encounter.

i. A company that makes drugs or vaccines.

j. Secure website that enables communication between providers and patients.

MULTIPLE-CHOICE QUESTIONS

Select the letter that best completes the statement or answers the question.

1. *[LO 10.1]* What codes indicate how office visits are coded for billing?
   a. Diagnostic codes
   b. E/M codes
   c. HCPCS codes
   d. Procedure codes

2. *[LO 10.1]* It is referred to as _____ when tests and procedures are completed at the time of the patient's encounter.
   a. aftercare
   b. ambulatory care
   c. point-of-care
   d. real-time services

3. *[LO 10.2]* Prescriptions sent by E-Prescribing are automatically ______ in a patient's EHR.
   a. approved
   b. denied
   c. documented
   d. renewed

4. *[LO 10.3]* What is the main benefit of a clinical visit summary?
   a. Includes relevant and actionable information related to the encounter
   b. Provides patients with past medical history records
   c. Includes a patient's entire record for continuity of care
   d. Lists community resources

5. *[LO 10.2]* When a provider directs a patient to see another provider or have services performed elsewhere, it is known as a(n) ______.
   a. authorization
   b. point-of-care service
   c. referral
   d. outbound request

6. *[LO 10.1]* Before administering a vaccine, a(n) ______ must be provided to the patient or patient's guardian.
   a. clinical visit summary
   b. electronic order
   c. lot number
   d. VIS

7. *[LO 10.3]* The Meaningful Use program has shifted to being one of the four components of ______.
   a. HIPAA
   b. MACRA
   c. MIPS
   d. PQRS

8. *[LO 10.3]* Stage 3 of Meaningful Use indicated that patients should have access to their electronic health information through the use of ______.
   a. clinical decision support
   b. computerized orders
   c. E-Prescribing
   d. patient portals

9. *[LO 10.3]* Using EHR software to improve the efficiency, safety, and quality of patient care ensures its ______.
   a. compliance
   b. meaningful use
   c. quality control
   d. retention

10. *[LO 10.1]* Which of the following is considered to be a point-of-care test or procedure?
   a. ECG
   b. EMG
   c. Treadmill stress test
   d. Urine culture

SHORT-ANSWER QUESTIONS

Define the following abbreviations.

1. *[LO 10.1]* POC ______________________
2. *[LO 10.1]* FOBT ______________________
3. *[LO 10.3]* CPOE ______________________
4. *[LO 10.3]* MIPS ______________________
5. *[LO 10.3]* MACRA ______________________

APPLYING YOUR KNOWLEDGE

Answer the questions below in the space provided.

10.1 *[LO 10.3]* What is the purpose of a clinical visit summary?

____

____

10.2 *[LO 10.3]* What benefits do clinical visit summaries have for patients? For providers?

____

____

10.3 *[LO 10.1]* Describe the clinical check-out process.

____

____

10.4 *[LO 10.2]* What information should be provided to patients about their medications and prescriptions during the clinical check-out process?

____

____

10.5 *[LO 10.2]* Why might patients need to be referred to other providers or services? Provide an example.

____

____

chapter 11

Office Visit: Billing Check-Out Procedures

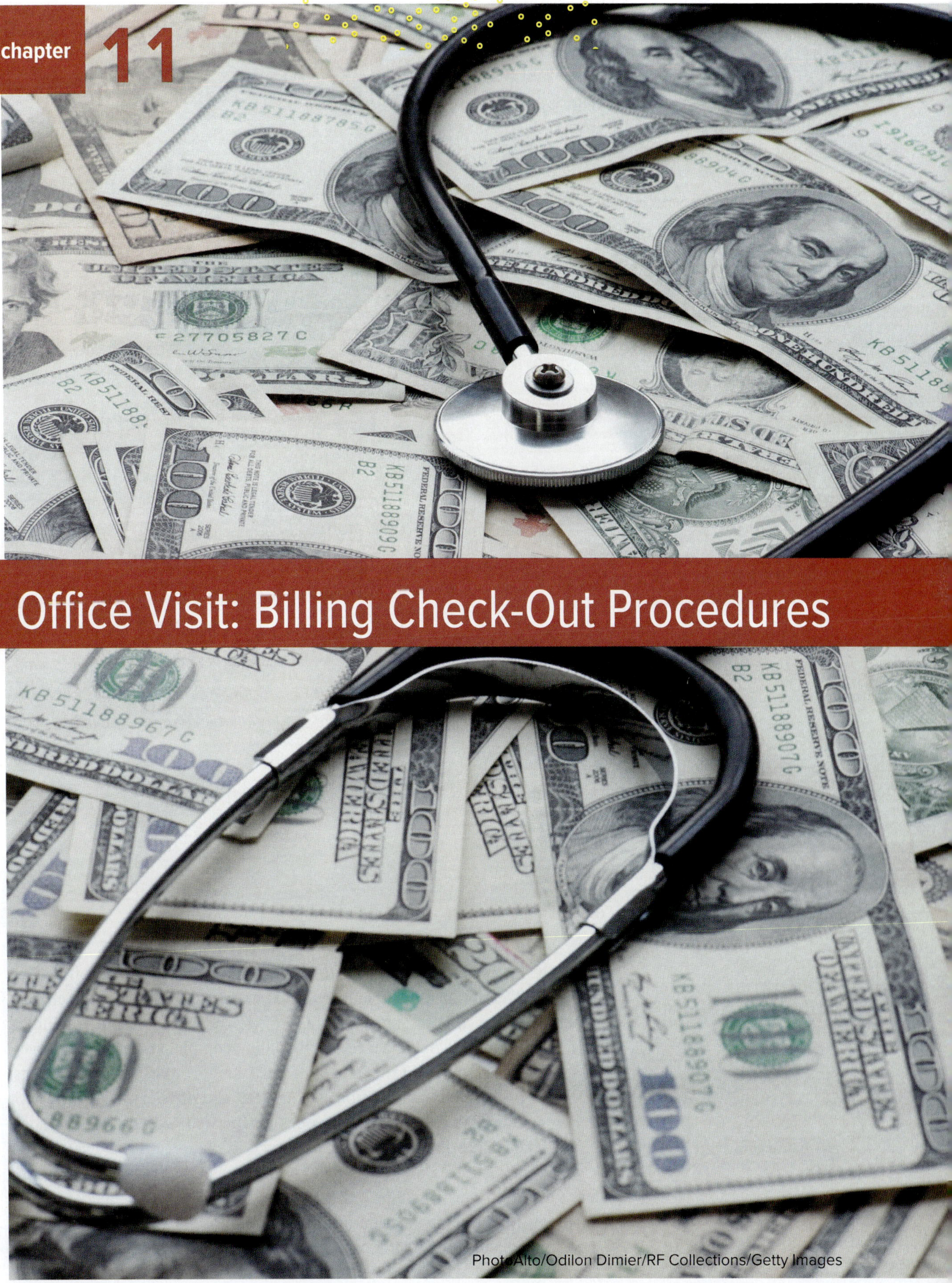

PhotoAlto/Odilon Dimier/RF Collections/Getty Images

LEARNING OUTCOMES

When you finish this chapter, you will be able to:

11.1 Explain the charge capture process.

11.2 Describe the electronic encounter form.

11.3 Explain coding compliance.

11.4 Explain billing compliance.

11.5 Discuss strategies to avoid common coding/billing problems.

11.6 Explain patient time of service payments.

11.7 Explain what walkout receipts are to a patient.

Consistency in Compliance

Trilogy Family Care Center's new revenue cycle manager, Elrene Harrison, is working to revise the clinic's billing and coding compliance plans. After reviewing the current process, she identifies several areas that can be improved to increase compliance and efficiency.

She developed and implemented a new process; however, she thinks that some of the billing staff are resistant to adopting the changes. She notices that they are following the new plan some of the time, but there are other times they are going back to the old process. Elrene thinks this might be contributing to a recent increase in claim denials.

Consider these factors. Why do you think there has been a recent increase in claim denials? How might an internal audit help Elrene identify the cause of the issues so she can address it with the staff?

11.1 Overview: Charge Capture Process

Other chapters in this textbook outlined the standard flow of an office visit from check-in until the completion of the patient examination. This chapter describes many of the steps that take place during check-out, including reviewing coding compliance, reviewing billing compliance, posting charges, posting payments made at the time of the visit, and printing payment receipts.

charge capture process of recording billable services

When the patient examination is complete, the physician signs the visit documentation, reviews procedure codes for the visit, and assigns diagnosis codes. The **charge capture** process, as shown in Figure 11.1, involves itemizing each medical treatment and service that was provided to determine the amounts to bill health plans and patients. The charges are also checked for accuracy. If all the information is correct, the transaction data are posted in a practice management software, usually within the EHR. If it is incorrect, the data are edited and then posted.

Figure 11.1 Electronic Charge Capture Process Flowchart

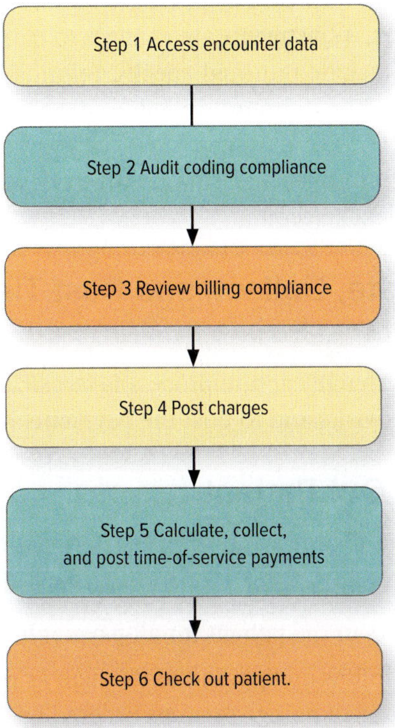

Step 1: Access Encounter Data

In the first step of the charge capture process, the procedure and diagnosis data from the patient visit are located.

Step 2: Audit Coding Compliance

In the second step of the charge capture process, all listed codes are checked to be sure that they are current and correct and that they are correctly linked to establish the medical necessity of the services the patient received. It is often necessary to also review and check documentation to be sure it supports the codes being reported.

In a PM/EHR, codes can be checked in the EHR before they are transmitted to the PM, or they can be reviewed in the PM before they are posted to a patient's account. If necessary, the patient's chart can be viewed from within the EHR.

Step 3: Review Billing Compliance

In the third step of the charge capture process, the billing rules of the particular health plan providing primary coverage for the visit are reviewed. Although the codes themselves may be current, correct, and properly linked, each service is not necessarily billable. For example, Medicare generally does not cover procedures considered experimental, and some private payers do not pay for two similar procedures on the same date of service. Following such rules when calculating charges results in billing compliance.

Step 4: Post Charges

In the fourth step of the charge capture process, the biller posts the visit charges in the PM. Three types of transactions are recorded in the PM/EHR:

charges amount a provider bills for performed health care services

payments money paid by patients and health plans

adjustments changes to a patient's account

electronic encounter form (EEF) an electronic version of the form that lists procedures and charges for a patient's visit

charges, payments, and adjustments. **Charges** are the amounts a provider bills for the services performed. **Payments** are monies received from patients and insurance carriers. **Adjustments** are changes to patients' accounts. Examples of adjustments include returned checks, refunds of overpayments, and differences between the amount billed and the amount allowed per contract.

In a PM/EHR, after codes and charges are reviewed, they are electronically posted to a patient's account.

Step 5: Calculate, Collect, and Post Time-of-Service (TOS) Payments

The fifth step of the charge capture process is to calculate the amounts that patients owe for their visits and to post the payments they make in the PM.

Step 6: Check Out Patient

The final step of the charge capture process is patient check-out, which involves:

- Providing receipts to the patient for all payments made
- Scheduling any follow-up appointments, such as return office visits, laboratory tests, or radiology services ordered by the provider
- Providing referrals as required
- Providing patient education materials ordered by the provider

In a PM/EHR, many of the check-out activities are completed electronically, such as printing receipts for payments and printing patient education handouts.

THINKING IT THROUGH 11.1

Assign the step number of the charge capture process to each of the following actions:

- _____ Provide patient with a booklet on controlling type II diabetes.
- _____ Receive the unprocessed transactions for yesterday's appointments.
- _____ Validate the connection between the diagnosis of a splinter and an incision/drainage procedure.
- _____ Send an email message to a payer to clarify the rule for billing out-of-network visits.
- _____ Answer the patient who asks, "How much do I owe for this visit?"
- _____ Post a patient's copayment of $5 to the appropriate account.

11.2 Electronic Encounter Form

An **electronic encounter form (EEF)** is an electronic version of the form that lists procedures and charges for a patient's visit. This form is used to post charges in the PM/EHR system for reimbursement. Some offices begin using electronic encounter forms right after they switch to a PM/EHR, while other offices continue to use paper encounter forms for posting charges.

Figure 11.2 Comparison of Paper and Electronic Encounter Forms

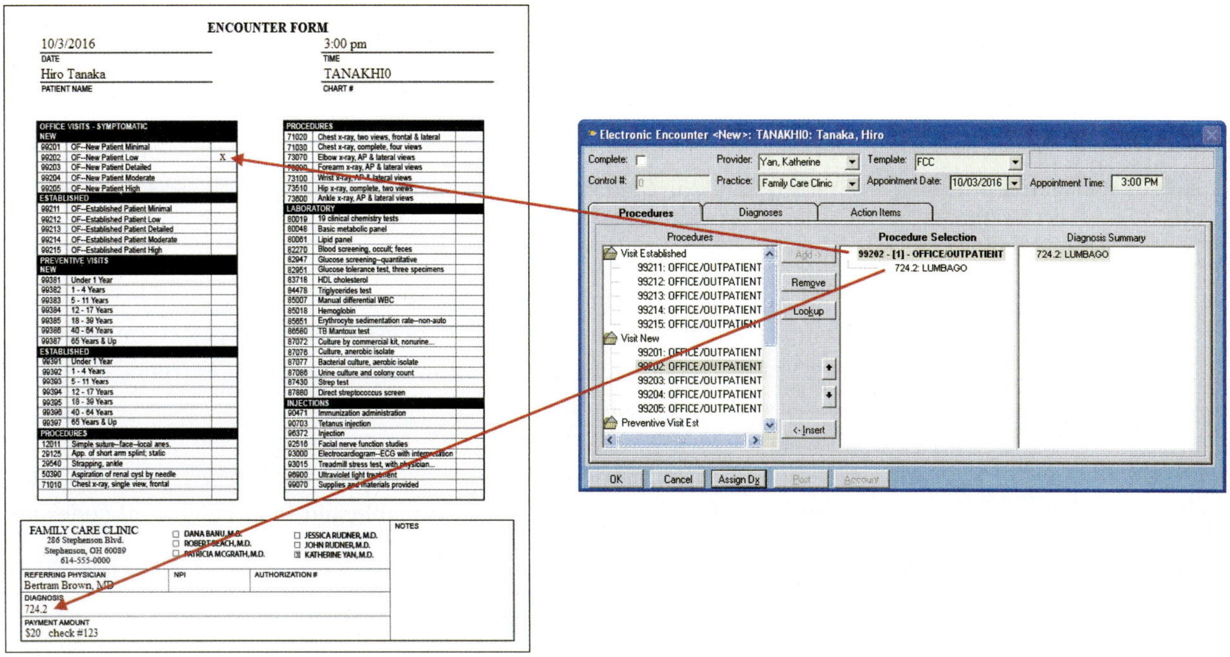

Microsoft Corporation

The process used to post charges differs depending on whether an office uses a paper encounter form or an electronic encounter form. When a paper encounter form is used, a member of the billing staff enters each procedure charge manually; when an electronic encounter form is used, the charges are reviewed and then the procedure charges are automatically posted in the PM/EHR.

Figure 11.2 shows a paper encounter form and an electronic encounter form for the same office visit. The red arrows show the location of the procedure and diagnosis codes on both forms.

When charges are posted in the PM/EHR, most of the fields listed in this section are completed by the program. A paper encounter form is filled in by the provider and/or medical assistant, then manually keyed into the system.

EXERCISE 11.1

Create an Electronic Routing Slip (Encounter Form)

EHRclinic

A new patient is being seen for a complete physical exam. Blood work and an ECG were ordered. Mark these procedures as complete, and perform code linkage in the electronic routing slip (encounter form) to prepare the charges for claim submission.

Your instructor may assign this exercise to you in Connect. Exercise steps and EHRclinic Help Guides can be downloaded at www.mhhe.com/pmehr2.

11.3 Coding Compliance

Although providers are ultimately responsible for proper documentation and correct coding, administrative staff members help ensure maximum appropriate reimbursement by auditing medical coding. The staff member must work with the physician to ensure that the codes that have been assigned are current and correct. This process takes place after a patient encounter, but before the charges are billed.

Current, Correct Diagnosis Codes

Centers for Medicare and Medicaid Services (CMS) federal agency in the Department of Health and Human Services that runs Medicare, Medicaid, clinical laboratories, and other government health programs; responsible for enforcing all HIPAA standards other than the privacy and security standards

claim scrubber software that checks claims to permit error correction

The ICD-10-CM code set is revised annually. The National Center for Health Statistics and the **Centers for Medicare and Medicaid Services (CMS)** release ICD-10-CM updates called the addenda twice a year. The changes take effect on October 1 and April 1. The October 1 changes are the major updates; April 1 is used to catch up on codes that were not included in the major changes. The major new, invalid, and revised codes are posted on the CDC (www.cdc.gov/nchs/icd.htm) and CMS (www.cms.gov) websites, usually in June for use as of October 1.

Current codes must be used for reporting encounters as of the date they go into effect, and invalid (deleted) codes must not be used. Practices must ensure that the current reference is available and that the current codes are in use.

Current, Correct Procedure Codes

CPT is a proprietary code set, meaning that it is not available for free to the public. Rather, the information must be purchased, either in print or electronic format, from the American Medical Association (AMA), which issues revised CPT codes each year.

During the year, practicing physicians, medical specialty societies, and state medical associations send their suggestions for revision to the AMA. This input is reviewed by the AMA's Editorial Panel, which includes physicians as well as representatives from the Health Insurance Association of America, CMS, the American Health Information Management Association (AHIMA), the American Hospital Association (AHA), and Blue Cross and Blue Shield. The panel decides what changes will be made in the annual revision.

The annual changes are released by the AMA on October 1 and are in effect for procedures and services provided after January 1 of the following year. The AMA also reports the new codes on its website. Unlike the ICD-10-CM codes, the new CPT code set has to be used for dates of service starting January 1.

Claim Scrubbing

PM/EHRs typically include a software feature known as a **claim scrubber.** This term comes from the phrase "clean claim," meaning an error-free claim submitted to a health plan that the health plan accepts for processing. The data reported in a claim can be made clean by scrubbing with the PM/EHR scrubber. This software tool analyzes medical codes for patient encounters and reports those that appear to be outdated or otherwise problematic. Reviewing this report gives billers an opportunity to research and revise the codes. If necessary, the PM/EHR must be updated to reflect code changes based on the scrubber's report before the claim is submitted.

11.4 Billing Compliance

Medical practices bill numerous health plans and government payers. The provider's fees for services are listed on the medical practice's fee schedule. Most medical practices have standard fee schedules listing their usual fees. Each charge, or fee, is related to a specific procedure code.

However, the fees listed on the master fee schedule are not necessarily the amount the provider will be paid. Instead, each health plan and government payer reimburses the practice according to its own negotiated or government-mandated fee schedule. For example, many providers enter into contracts with health plans that require a discount from standard fees. A single fee may be set for a number of related services, as is often done for obstetrical packages that set a fee that covers all of the mother's prenatal and birth services.

As a result, although there is a separate fee associated with each code, each code is not necessarily billable. Listing the correct individual codes on claims does not mean that each will be paid. Health plans issue many billing rules that govern what will and will not be covered. The term **compliant billing** refers to following these rules so that the practice and the health plan have the same expectations for the payment that will be made. Noncompliant billing, because it may appear to be intentional fraud, may have serious consequences:

compliant billing billing actions that satisfy official requirements

package combination of services included in a single procedure code

bundled code two or more related procedure codes combined into one

- Delays in processing claims and receiving payments
- Reduced payments
- Denied claims
- Fines and other sanctions
- Loss of hospital privileges
- Exclusion from health plans' programs
- Loss of the physician's license to practice medicine
- Prison sentences

Health plans' billing rules are stated in patients' medical insurance policies and in providers' participation contracts. Because contracts change and rules are updated, administrative staff members also rely on health plan bulletins, online billing manuals, websites, and regular communications with health plan representatives to stay current.

Package Codes and Global Periods

Many payer rules address typical surgical procedures that routinely involve a number of related procedural steps. A **package** is a group of related procedures and/or services included under a single code. As defined in CPT, a surgical package includes the operation itself, local anesthesia (injection of a metacarpal/digital block or topical anesthesia), and all routine follow-up services. The single code is called a **bundled code.** For example, in the musculoskeletal subsection, surgical package codes include the application and removal of the first cast or traction device. Health plans often add some preoperative services to their definition of a package.

global period days surrounding a surgical procedure when all services relating to the procedure are considered part of the surgical package

Correct Coding Initiative (CCI) computerized Medicare system that prevents overpayment

CCI edits CPT code combinations that are used by computers to check Medicare claims

unbundling incorrect billing practice of breaking a panel or package of services/procedures into component parts

Health plans set a **global period**–a certain length of time in which the expected services are to be provided–for each package. During a global period, no service that is part of the package is reimbursed in addition to the reimbursement for the package code. After the global period ends, all services that are provided can be reported.

Some types of services are not considered to be routine follow-up and are reported during the global period. For example, complications or recurrences that arise after therapeutic surgical procedures are reported with appropriate modifiers (such as for repeat or related surgical procedures). Care for other illnesses, injuries, or conditions that are unrelated to the surgical procedure are also separately reported. Following a diagnostic procedure, services not related to the recovery from that procedure may be reported, even though the care may be related to the patient's underlying condition.

Medicare National Correct Coding Initiative

The rules from CMS about billing Medicare often set the standard for the industry. Other health plans watch what CMS is doing and adopt similar rules. For this reason, two major Medicare reimbursement initiatives are discussed; other health plans can be expected to have similar programs in place that guide the practice's billing.

Especially important for billing is Medicare's national policy on correct coding, which is called the Medicare National **Correct Coding Initiative (CCI).** CCI controls improper coding that would lead to inappropriate payment for Medicare claims. It has coding policies that are based on:

- Coding conventions in CPT
- Medicare's national and local coverage and payment policies
- National medical societies' coding guidelines
- Medicare's analysis of standard medical and surgical practice

CCI, updated every quarter, has many thousands of CPT code combinations called **CCI edits** that are used by computers in the Medicare system to check claims. Examples of the CCI edits, which are available on a CMS website, are shown in Figure 11.3. CCI edits apply to claims that bill for more than one procedure performed on the same patient (Medicare beneficiary), on the same date of service, by the same performing provider. Claims are denied when codes reported together do not pass an edit.

CCI prevents billing for two procedures that, according to Medicare, could not possibly have been performed together, such as reporting the removal of an organ both through an open incision and with laparoscopy, or reporting female-specific and male-specific codes for the same patient.

CCI edits also test for **unbundling.** That is, a claim should report a bundled procedure code instead of multiple codes that describe parts of the complete procedure. For example, since a single code is available to describe removal of the uterus, ovaries, and fallopian tubes, physicians should not use separate codes to report the removal of the uterus, ovaries, and fallopian tubes individually. CCI requires physicians to report only the more extensive version of the procedure performed and disallows reporting of both extensive and limited procedures. For example, only a deep biopsy should be reported if both a deep biopsy and a superficial biopsy are performed at the same location.

Column 1/Column 2 Edits

Column 1	Column 2	* = In existence prior to 1996	Effective Date	Deletion Date * = no data	Modifier 0 = not allowed 1 = allowed 9 = not applicable
10021	19290		20020101	*	1
10021	36000		20021001	*	1
10021	36410		20021001	*	1
10021	37202		20021001	*	1
10021	62318		20021001	*	1
10021	62319		20021001	*	1
10021	64415		20021001	*	1
10021	64416		20030101	*	1
10021	64417		20021001	*	1
10021	64450		20021001	*	1
10021	64470		20021001	*	1
10021	64475		20021001	*	1
10021	76000		20030701	*	1
10021	76003		20030101	*	1
10021	76360		20030101	*	1
10021	76393		20030101	*	1
10021	76942		20030101	*	1

Mutually Exclusive Edits

Column 1	Column 2	* = In existence prior to 1996	Effective Date	Deletion Date * = no data	Modifier 0 = not allowed 1 = allowed 9 = not applicable
11010	21240		19980101	*	1
11010	21242		19980101	*	1
11010	21243		19980101	*	1
11010	21244		19980101	*	1
11010	21245		19980101	*	1
11010	21246		19980101	*	1
11010	21247		19980101	*	1
11010	21248		19980101	*	1
11010	21249		19980101	*	1
11010	21255		19980101	*	1
11010	21256		19980101	*	1
11010	21260		19980101	*	1
11010	21261		19980101	*	1
11010	21263		19980101	*	1
11010	21267		19980101	*	1
11010	21268		19980101	*	1
11010	21270		19980101	*	1

Figure 11.3 Examples of Medicare CCI Edits: Column 1/Column 2 Edits and Mutually Exclusive Edits

Organization of the CCI Edits

CCI edits are organized into the following categories:

- Column 1/column 2 code pair edits
- Mutually exclusive code edits
- **Modifier indicators**

CCI modifier indicator number showing whether the use of a modifier can bypass a CCI edit

CCI column 1/column 2 code pair edits Medicare code edit in which CPT codes in column 2 will not be paid if reported for same day of service, for the same patient, and by the same provider as the column 1 code

CCI mutually exclusive code (MEC) edits edits for codes for services that could not have reasonably been done during one encounter

Column 1/column 2 code pairs Two columns of codes are listed in the **CCI column 1/column 2 code pair edits.** Most often, one code is a component of the other. This means that the column 1 code includes all the services described by the column 2 code, so the column 2 code cannot be billed together with the column 1 code for the same patient on the same day of service. Medicare pays for the column 1 code only; the column 2 code is considered bundled into the column 1 code.

EXAMPLE

Column 1	*Column 2*
27370	20610, 76000, 76003

If 27370 is billed, neither 20610, 76000, nor 76003 should be billed with it because the payment for each of these codes is already included in the column 1 code.

Mutually exclusive code edits **CCI mutually exclusive code (MEC) edits** also list codes in two columns. According to CMS regulations, both services represented by these codes could not have reasonably been done during a single patient encounter, so they cannot be billed together. If the provider reports both codes from both columns for a patient on the same day, Medicare pays only the lower-paid code.

EXAMPLE

Column 1	*Column 2*
50021	49061, 50020

This means that a biller cannot report either 49061 or 50020 when reporting 50021.

THINKING IT THROUGH 11.2

What type of code edit could be used for the following rule?

Medicare Part B covers a screening Pap smear for women for the early detection of cervical cancer but will not pay for an E/M service for the patient on the same day.

Medicare Medically Unlikely Edits

Also important for Medicare billing and compliance, and thus for other health plans as well, are the unit of service (UOS) edits CMS uses, which are called **medically unlikely edits (MUEs).** An MUE is related to a specific CPT or HCPCS code and applies to the services that a single provider (or supplier, for supplies such as durable medical equipment) provides for a single patient on the same date of service. The MUE value is based on the maximum units of service that would be reported for a code on the vast majority of correct claims.

medically unlikely edits (MUEs) units of service edits used to lower the Medicare fee-for-service paid claims error rate

MUEs are designed to reduce errors on claims due to clerical entries, and scrubbers store these rules to check encounter data before claims are transmitted. MUEs check for and correct coding mistakes based on anatomic considerations, CPT/HCPCS code descriptors, CPT coding instructions, Medicare policies, or unlikely services. An example is an MUE edit that rejects a claim for a hysterectomy on a male patient. The goal is to reduce the number of health care claims that are sent back simply because of data-entry errors. The MUE system is set up to allow reporting of appropriate extra units of services when the situation warrants it.

11.5 Strategies to Avoid Common Coding/Billing Problems

Health plans often base their decisions to pay or deny claims only on the diagnosis and procedure codes. The integrity of the request for payment rests on the accuracy and honesty of the coding and billing. Incorrect work may simply be an error, or it may represent a deliberate effort to obtain fraudulent payment. Compliance errors can result from incorrect code selection or billing practices.

Errors Relating to the Coding Process

These coding problems may cause rejected claims:

- Truncated coding–using diagnosis codes that are not as specific as possible
- Mismatching between the gender or age of the patient and the selected code when the code involves selection for either criterion
- Assumption coding–reporting items or services that are not actually documented, but that the coder assumes were performed
- Altering documentation after services are reported
- Coding without proper documentation
- Reporting services provided by unlicensed or unqualified clinical personnel
- Failing to satisfy the conditions of coverage for a particular service, such as the physician's direct supervision of a radiologist's work
- Coding conditions that are present but were not addressed during the visit

Errors Relating to the Billing Process

A number of errors are related to the billing process. These are the most frequent errors:

- Billing noncovered services
- Billing overlimit services
- Unbundling
- Using an inappropriate modifier or no modifier when one is required
- Always assigning the same level of E/M service
- Billing a consultation instead of an office visit
- Billing invalid/outdated codes
- Either upcoding–using a procedure code that provides a higher reimbursement rate than the correct code–or downcoding–using a lower-level code. Some physicians downcode to be "safe," especially E/M codes
- Billing without proper signatures on file
- Billing a service with the incorrect **place of service (POS) code.** The POS indicates where services were performed. Since some places of service are paid at higher rates than others because more equipment and supplies have to be available, it is important to correctly assign POS codes. The standard numerical codes used for physician practices are:

  11 Provider's office
  21 Inpatient hospital
  22 Outpatient hospital
  23 Hospital emergency room

place of service (POS) code location where medical services were provided

query request for more information from a provider

Strategies for Compliance

Compliant billing can be difficult and complex; the strategies discussed in this section are helpful.

- **Carefully define bundled codes and know global periods** To avoid unbundling, coders and medical insurance specialists must be clear on which individual procedures are contained in bundled codes and what the global periods are for surgical procedures. Many practices use Medicare's CCI list of bundling rules and global periods for deciding what is included in a procedure code; they inform their other health plans that they are following this system of edits. If the health plan has a unique set of edits, coders and billers need access to it.
- **Use modifiers appropriately** CPT modifiers can eliminate the impression of duplicate billing or unbundling.
- **Follow the practice's compliance plan, especially the guidelines about physician queries** A **query** is a question transmitted to a provider to obtain additional clarifying documentation to improve the specificity and completeness of the data used to assign diagnosis and procedure codes in the patient's health record. Queries are used when there is conflicting, incomplete, or ambiguous information in the health record regarding a significant condition or procedure. For example, two

treating providers of a hospitalized patient might disagree with respect to a diagnosis, as in the case of a patient who has shortness of breath that a pulmonologist documents as caused by pneumonia but the attending physician documents as congestive heart failure.

Practices' compliance plans often provide for a query process. EHRs often provide electronic templates to generate and respond to electronic queries. Query guidelines must be followed in order to avoid leading the provider in any way.

THINKING IT THROUGH 11.3

Botox injections have been approved by the Food and Drug Administration (FDA) to treat spasms of the flexor muscles of the elbow, wrist, and fingers. Should a payer reject a claim for this use of Botox based on lack of medical necessity?

11.6 Patient Time of Service Payments

As discussed in Chapter 4, practices routinely collect payment for the following types of charges at the time of service:

- Previous balances
- Copayments or coinsurance
- Noncovered or overlimit fees
- Charges of nonparticipating providers
- Charges for self-pay patients
- Deductibles for patients with consumer-driven health plans (CDHPs)

Depending on the practice's financial procedures, some charges may be collected at check-in before the encounter, and others may be collected during patient check-out.

Previous Balances

Practices routinely check their patient financial records and, if a balance is due, collect it at the time of service.

Copayments

Copayments are always collected at the time of service. In some practices, they are collected before the encounter; in others, they are collected during check-out.

The amount of copayment that is due depends on the type of service and on whether the provider is in the patient's network. Copays for out-of-network providers are usually higher than for in-network providers. Specific copay amounts may be required for office visits to primary care providers or to specialists, and for lab work, radiology services such as X-rays, and surgery.

When patients receive more than one covered service in a single day, their health plan may permit multiple copayments. For example, copays for an annual physical exam and for lab tests may both be due from the patient. Review the terms of the policy to determine whether multiple copays should be collected on the same day of service.

EXERCISE 11.2

Post a Patient Copayment

EHRclinic

Trilogy Family Care Center's policy is that copayments are to be made at the time of service. Post a patient copayment in EHRclinic.

Your instructor may assign this exercise to you in Connect. Exercise steps and EHRclinic Help Guides can be downloaded at http://www.mhhe.com/pmehr2.

Coinsurance

As health care costs have risen, employers have to pay more for their employees' medical benefit plans. As a result, employers are requiring employees to pay a larger share of those costs. Annual health insurance premiums are higher, deductibles are higher, and many employers have stopped requiring small fixed-amount copayments and have replaced them with coinsurance payments that are often due at the time of service.

Charges for Noncovered/Overlimit Services

Health plans require patients to pay for noncovered (excluded) services under their policies, and they do not have any say about what the providers charge for the excluded services. Likewise, in managed care plans that set limits on the usage of certain covered services, patients are responsible for paying for visits beyond the allowed number. For example, if five physical therapy visits are permitted annually, the patient must pay for any additional visits. For this reason, practices usually collect these fees at the time of service.

Charges of Nonparticipating Providers

A patient who has an encounter with a provider who participates in the plan under which he or she has coverage—such as a Medicare participating (PAR) provider—signs an assignment of benefits statement. This authorizes the provider to accept assignment for the patient; that is, to file claims for the patient and receive payment directly from the health plan.

If the provider is a nonparticipating (nonPAR) provider, the procedure is usually different. To avoid problems collecting later on, most practices require the patient to pay in full at the time of services. If the patient does not wish to do this, the practice often requires the patient to assign benefits so that payment can be collected directly from the insurance plan by filing a claim.

Charges for Services to Self-Pay Patients

Patients who do not have insurance coverage are called **self-pay patients.** Since not all Americans have health insurance, self-pay patient office visits are a regular occurrence in most practices. Billers follow the practice's procedures for informing patients of their responsibility for paying their bills.

self-pay patients patients with no medical insurance

real-time claim adjudication (RTCA) process used to contact health plans electronically to determine visit charges

walkout receipt report that lists the diagnoses, services provided, fees, and payments received and due after an encounter

Deductibles for Patients with Consumer-Driven Health Plans (CDHPs)

Patients who have consumer-driven health plans must meet large deductibles before the health plans make payments. The practice is responsible for finding out whether the deductible has been met and, if not, for collecting the fee at the time of service.

Real-Time Claim Adjudication

The ideal tool for collecting at the time of service is known as **real-time claim adjudication (RTCA).** Offered by major health plans, RTCA is an Internet-based service that allows the practice to transmit the facts of the patient's visit, such as the demographics, the diagnosis and procedure codes, dates of service, and the provider's charges. The health plan transmits a response immediately (the meaning of "real time"), indicating the amount that the health plan will pay and the amount for which the patient is responsible.

The information transmitted by the health plan allows the practice to:

- Verify that the services are covered under the policy
- Learn whether the patient has met the annual deductible and, if not, collect it (if that is the policy)
- Know the patient's financial responsibility for the visit and collect it
- Provide the patient with an explanation of benefits from the health plan so that any questions the patient has about denial of coverage or payment history can be resolved immediately

Note that the RTCA does not generate a real-time payment; the payment usually follows within twenty-four hours.

11.7 Walkout Receipts

After a patient payment has been entered in the PM/EHR, a walkout receipt is printed and given to the patient before he or she leaves the office. A **walkout receipt,** also known as a walkout statement, includes information on the procedures, diagnosis, charges, and payments for a visit. This receipt is similar to the encounter form, but it is for the patient's use.

If there is a balance due, the receipt reminds the patient about the amount owed. See Figure 11.4 for a sample of a walkout receipt a patient will receive after services are rendered.

Figure 11.4 Sample Walkout Receipt

Facility	Receipt information	
Trilogy Family Care Center	Patient name:	Janine Bell
P.O. Box 48094 43514 Bridgewater Ave Phone: 586-555-4100 Fax: +1-586-5554110 trilogyfamilycarexy.com	Chart number:	AA010

Charges and payments

Date	Description	Procedure	Modifier	Units	Charge in USD
01/20/2022	Basic Metabolic Panel	80048		1	$68
01/20/2022	Lipid Panel	80060		1	$64
01/20/2022	Pap Smear	88150		1	$29
01/20/2022	EKG (tracing only)	93005		1	$30
01/20/2022	Check	COPAY		1	-$20.00

Total charges:	$191
Total payments:	-$20
Total account balance:	$171

EXERCISE 11.3 Print a Patient Receipt

Post a patient payment and print a walkout receipt.

Your instructor may assign this exercise to you in Connect. Exercise steps and EHRclinic Help Guides can be downloaded at http://www.mhhe.com/pmehr2.

chapter 11 summary

KEY TERMS

adjustments
bundled code
Centers for Medicare and Medicaid Services (CMS)
CCI column 1/column 2 code pair edits
CCI edits
CCI modifier indicator
CCI mutually exclusive code (MEC) edits
charge
charge capture
claim scrubber
compliant billing
Correct Coding Initiative (CCI)
electronic encounter form (EEF)
global period
medically unlikely edits (MUEs)
package
payments
place of service (POS) code
query
real-time claim adjudication (RTCA)
self-pay patients
unbundling
walkout receipt

LEARNING OUTCOME	KEY CONCEPTS/EXAMPLES
11.1 Explain the charge capture process.	1. Access encounter data 2. Audit coding compliance 3. Review billing compliance 4. Post charges 5. Calculate, collect, and post time-of-service (TOS) payments 6. Check out patients
11.2 Describe the electronic encounter form.	An electronic encounter form (EEF) is an electronic version of the form that lists procedures and charges for a patient's visit. This form is used to post charges in the PM/EHR system for reimbursement.
11.3 Explain coding compliance.	Staff members must work with the providers to ensure that the codes that have been assigned are current and correct. CPT and ICD-10-CM codes should be updated yearly to stay compliant with appropriate reporting. Claim scrubbers should be used to submit clean claims.
11.4 Explain billing compliance.	The term *compliant billing* refers to following these rules so that the practice and the health plan have the same expectations for the payment that will be made. Noncompliant billing, because it may appear to be intentional fraud, may have serious consequences: • Delays in processing claims and receiving payments • Reduced payments • Denied claims • Fines and other sanctions • Loss of hospital privileges • Exclusion from health plans' programs • Loss of the physician's license to practice medicine • Prison sentences

LEARNING OUTCOME	KEY CONCEPTS/EXAMPLES
11.5 Discuss strategies to avoid common coding/billing problems.	Compliance errors can result from incorrect code selection or billing practices. • Carefully define bundled codes and know global periods. • Use modifiers appropriately. • Follow the practice's compliance plan.
11.6 Explain patient time of service payments.	Practices routinely collect payment for the following types of charges at the time of service: • Previous balances • Copayments or coinsurance • Noncovered or overlimit fees • Charges of nonparticipating providers • Charges for self-pay patients • Deductibles for patients with consumer-driven health plans (CDHPs)
11.7 Explain what walkout receipts are to a patient.	After a patient payment has been entered in the PM/EHR, a walkout receipt is printed and given to the patient before he or she leaves the office. A walkout receipt, also known as a walkout statement, includes information on the procedures, diagnosis, charges, and payments for a visit. It is similar to the encounter form, but it is for the patient's use.

chapter 11 review

MATCHING QUESTIONS

Match the key terms with their definitions.

_____ 1. *[LO 11.4]* CCI mutually exclusive code (MEC) edits

_____ 2. *[LO 11.4]* Correct Coding Initiative (CCI)

_____ 3. *[LO 11.1]* charge capture

_____ 4. *[LO 11.5]* query

_____ 5. *[LO 11.4]* compliant billing

_____ 6. *[LO 11.7]* walkout receipt

_____ 7. *[LO 11.4]* unbundling

_____ 8. *[LO 11.4]* global period

_____ 9. *[LO 11.6]* real-time claim adjudication (RTCA)

_____ 10. *[LO 11.1]* charges

a. A process of recording billable services.

b. Billing actions that satisfy official requirements.

c. Edits for codes for services that could not have reasonably been done during one encounter.

d. A report that lists the diagnoses, services provided, fees, and payments received and due after an encounter.

e. Incorrect billing practice of breaking a panel or package of services/procedures into component parts.

f. Amount a provider bills for performed health care services.

g. A process used to contact health plans electronically to determine visit charges.

h. A request for more information from a provider.

i. Days surrounding a surgical procedure when all services relating to the procedure are considered part of the surgical package.

j. Computerized Medicare system that prevents overpayment.

MULTIPLE CHOICE QUESTIONS

Select the letter that best completes the statement or answers the question.

1. *[LO 11.2]* _________ is an electronic version of the form that lists procedures and charges for a patient's visit.
   a. PM/EHR
   b. Medical record
   c. Global period
   d. Electronic encounter form

2. *[LO 11.1]* How many steps does the electronic charge capture process have?
   a. 6
   b. 5
   c. 4
   d. 3

3. *[LO 11.3]* How often is ICD-10-CM revised?
   a. every other year
   b. annually
   c. once a quarter
   d. every ten years

4. *[LO 11.4]* A(n) ________ is a group of related procedures and/or services included under a single code.
   a. package
   b. bundled code
   c. global period
   d. unbundling

5. *[LO 11.5]* Which one does NOT cause errors relating to the coding process?
   a. truncated coding
   b. coding without documentation
   c. CCI edits
   d. assumption coding

6. *[LO 11.6]* Practices routinely collect payment for all but one of the following. Which one is NOT collected at the time of service?
   a. deductibles for patients
   b. global package billing
   c. noncovered fees and/or services
   d. previous balances

7. *[LO 11.6]* What is it called when a provider is Medicare participating (PAR)?
   a. unbundling codes
   b. bundling codes
   c. accepting assignment
   d. patient self-pay

8. *[LO 11.7]* A(n) ________ includes information on the procedure, diagnosis, charges, and payments for a visit.
   a. walkout receipt
   b. explanation of benefits (EOB)
   c. standard statement
   d. remainder statement

9. *[LO 11.4]* ________ are edits listed in two columns that cannot be done during a single patient encounter.
   a. CCI edits
   b. Mutually exclusive code edits
   c. CCI column1/column 2 pair edits
   d. Unbundlings

10. *[LO 11.6]* Patients who do not have insurance coverage are called ________.
    a. assignments
    b. PARs
    c. non-PARs
    d. self-pay patients

SHORT ANSWER QUESTIONS

Define the following abbreviations.

1. *[LO 11.2]* EEF ____________________
2. *[LO 11.4]* CCI ____________________
3. *[LO 11.4]* MEC ____________________
4. *[LO 11.4]* MUEs ____________________
5. *[LO 11.5]* POS ____________________

APPLYING YOUR KNOWLEDGE

Answer the questions below in the space provided.

11.1 *[LO 11.1]* List the six steps of the charge capture process in order.

____

____

11.2 *[LO 11.2]* What is the difference between a paper encounter form and an EEF?

____

____

11.3 *[LO 11.3]* What is the importance of using a claim scrubber?

____

____

11.4 *[LO 11.4]* Explain the importance of understanding the global period.

____

____

11.5 *[LO 11.5]* Why is having a strategy for compliance important?

____

____

____

____

chapter 12

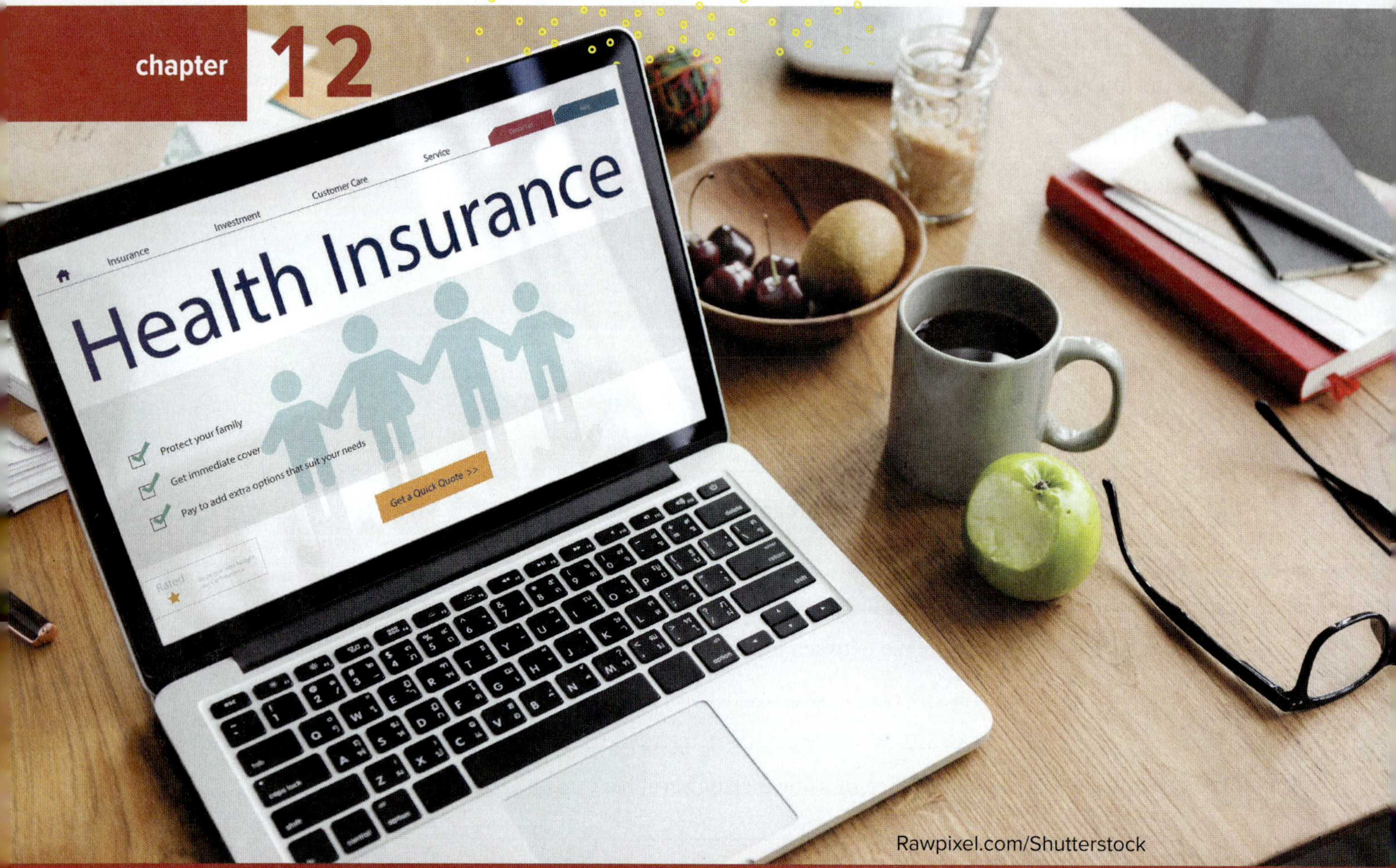

Rawpixel.com/Shutterstock

Third-Party Payers

LEARNING OUTCOMES

When you finish this chapter, you will be able to:

12.1 Compare the major features of health plans.

12.2 Discuss third-party payment methods.

12.3 Discuss the organization and regulation of employer-sponsored group health plans and self-insured plans.

12.4 Explain the purpose of government-sponsored insurance programs, workers' compensation, and disability plans.

12.5 Identify the three methods most payers use to pay providers.

A Patient with an HMO Plan

Cassidy Nichols is a new patient to Trilogy Family Care Center. She has an HMO insurance plan and has selected Dr. Kumar to be her primary care physician.

During Cassidy's new patient physical, Dr. Kumar orders blood work, an ECG, and a chest X-ray. She also refers Cassidy to a dermatologist to evaluate a suspicious-looking mole.

What is Dr. Kumar's role as a primary care physician? Why did Cassidy need a referral from Dr. Kumar to see a specialist? How would Cassidy's insurance carrier likely reimburse the services performed as part of her physical exam?

12.1 Types of Health Plans

Insured patients have medical coverage under either managed care or indemnity (fee-for-service) plans. The type of health plan affects the payments that patients must make for medical services, so it is important for medical office administrative staff to understand the plans' key features.

Third-Party Relationship

There are three participants in the medical insurance relationship. The patient (policyholder) is the first party, and the physician is the second party. In legal terms, a patient-physician contract is created when a physician agrees to treat a patient who is seeking medical services. Through this unwritten contract, the patient is legally responsible for paying for services.

When the patient has a policy with a health plan, the plan is a third party. The plan agrees to carry some of the risk of paying for the services and therefore is called a **third-party payer.**

third-party payer private or government organization that insures or pays for health care on behalf of beneficiaries

preferred provider organization (PPO) managed care network of health care providers who agree to perform services for plan members at discounted fees

Preferred Provider Organizations

The most popular type of health plan, as shown in Figure 12.1, is the **preferred provider organization (PPO),** which contracts with physicians, hospitals, clinics, and pharmacies to provide a network of care providers for its beneficiaries.

Under a PPO, the policyholder pays an annual premium and a yearly deductible to pay out of pocket. A PPO plan may offer either a low

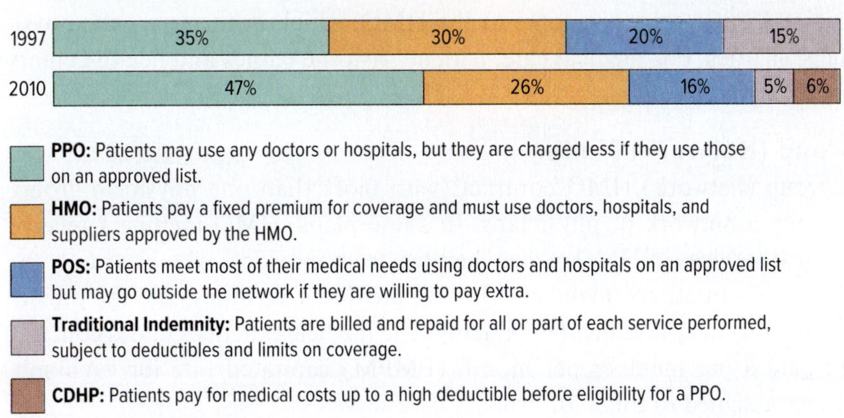

Figure 12.1 Employer-Sponsored Health Plans Source: www.Kaiserhealthnews.org.

deductible with a higher premium or a high deductible with a lower premium. The insured member typically pays a copayment at the time of each medical service, and coinsurance may also be charged for in-network providers. A patient may see an out-of-network doctor without a referral or preauthorization, but the deductible, copayment, and/or coinsurance for out-of-network services may be higher, and the amount the plan will pay may be lower. In other words, the patient will be responsible for more of the fee. This encourages the people insured with a PPO to use the physicians, other medical providers, and hospitals in their network.

Advantages of a PPO include the flexibility of seeking care with an out-of-network provider if desired, even though doing so is more expensive for the patient. PPO networks also have prescription services that provide prescription drugs at a reduced cost. A PPO plan often includes more covered medical services than do other types of plans. PPOs have large networks of medical providers representing large geographic areas.

Health Maintenance Organizations

health maintenance organization (HMO) managed health care system in which providers offer health care to members for fixed periodic payments

primary care physician (PCP) physician in a managed care organization who directs all aspects of a patient's care

Health maintenance organizations (HMOs) are licensed by the state. They have the most stringent guidelines and the narrowest choice of providers. Their members are assigned to **primary care physicians (PCPs)** and must use the network except in emergencies or pay a penalty. HMOs have traditionally emphasized preventive and wellness services as well as disease management, although PPOs and other plans now also often include many of these services.

HMOs were originally designed to cover all basic services at a cost to patients of an annual premium and visit copayments. This arrangement is called "first-dollar coverage," because patients who received treatment were not required to pay deductibles before the plan started covering services. However, HMOs may now apply deductibles to family coverage, and employer-sponsored HMOs are also beginning to replace copayments with coinsurance for some services.

An HMO is organized around one of three business models: the staff model, the group or network model, and the independent practice association model. Each model is based on the way the terms of the agreement connect the provider and the plan. In all, however, enrollees must see HMO providers in order to be covered.

Staff Model

In a staff HMO, physicians are employed by the organization. All the premiums and other revenues come to the HMO, which in turn pays the physicians' salaries. For medical care, patients visit the clinics and health centers owned by the HMO.

Group (Network) Model

A group (network) HMO contracts with more than one physician group, creating a network of physicians. In some plans, HMO members receive medical services in HMO-owned facilities from providers who work only for that HMO. In others, members visit the providers' facilities, and the providers can also treat nonmember patients. The medical practices under contract are paid a per member per month (PMPM) capitated rate for each subscriber assigned to them for primary care services.

Independent Practice Association Model

An independent practice association (IPA) type of HMO is an association formed by physicians with separately owned practices who contract together to provide care for HMO members. An HMO pays negotiated fees for medical services to the IPA. The IPA, in turn, pays its physician members, either by a capitated rate or a fee. A provider may join more than one IPA and usually also sees nonmember patients.

THINKING IT THROUGH 12.1

If PPO patients use out-of-network rather than participating providers, what is the effect on the payments they are responsible for?

Point-of-Service (POS) Plans

A **point-of-service (POS) plan** is a hybrid of HMO and PPO networks. Members may choose from a primary or secondary network. The primary network is HMO-like, and the secondary network is often a PPO network. Like HMOs, POS plans charge annual premiums and copayments for office visits. Monthly premiums are slightly higher than for HMOs, but POS plans offer some coverage for visits to non-network physicians for specialty care. A POS may be structured as a tiered plan, for example, with different rates for specially designated providers, regular participating providers, and out-of-network providers.

point-of-service (POS) plan managed care plan that permits patients to receive medical services from non-network providers

fee-for-service health plan that repays the policyholder for covered medical expenses

Indemnity Plans

Indemnity or **fee-for-service** plans require premium, deductible, and coinsurance payments. They typically cover 70 to 80 percent of the costs of covered benefits after the deductible is met. Some plans are structured with high deductibles, such as $5,000 to $10,000, in order to offer policyholders relatively lower premiums. Many have some managed care features, as payers compete for employers' contracts and try to control costs.

EXERCISE 12.1

Add an Insurance Carrier to the EHR Database

EHRclinic

A patient who is checking in presents an insurance card for a carrier that is not in the system. Add the new insurance carrier to the EHRclinic database.

Your instructor may assign this exercise to you in Connect. Exercise steps and EHRclinic Help Guides can be downloaded at www.mhhe.com/pmehr2.

EXERCISE 12.2

Edit Insurance Database Information

EHRclinic

Edit the address and phone number for an insurance carrier in the EHRclinic database.

Your instructor may assign this exercise to you in Connect. Exercise steps and EHRclinic Help Guides can be downloaded at www.mhhe.com/pmehr2.

12.2 Third-Party Payment Methods

The plan type for the charges listed on a claim affects the way physicians are paid for providing those services. Table 12.1 reviews the payment methods of the types of health plans. Payers use one of three main methods of paying providers: allowed charges, contracted fee schedules, and capitation.

Allowed Charges

allowed charge maximum charge a plan pays for a service or procedure

Many payers set an **allowed charge** for each procedure or service. This amount is the most the payer will pay any provider for that CPT code. Whether a provider actually receives the allowed charge depends on three things:

1. **The provider's usual charge for the procedure or service** The usual charge on the physician's fee schedule may be higher than, equal to, or lower than the allowed charge.
2. **The provider's status in the particular plan or program** The provider is either participating or nonparticipating. Participating (PAR) providers agree to accept allowed charges that are lower than their usual fees. In return, they are eligible for incentives, such as quicker payments of their claims and more patients.
3. **The payer's billing rules** These rules govern whether the provider can bill a patient for the part of the charge that the payer does not cover.

When a payer uses an allowed charge method, it never pays more than the allowed charge to a provider. If a provider's usual fee is higher, only the allowed charge is paid. If a provider's usual fee is lower, the payer reimburses that lower amount. The payer's payment is always the lower of the two amounts: the provider's charge or the allowed charge.

TIP

Other Terms for Allowed Charge

The allowed charge is also called a maximum allowable fee, maximum charge, allowed amount, allowed fee, and allowable charge.

TABLE 12.1 Health Plan Payment Methods

Plan Type	Participating Provider Payment Method
Preferred provider organization (PPO)	Discounted fee-for-service
Staff health maintenance organization (HMO)	Salary
Group HMO	Salary or contracted capitation rate or discounted fee-for-service
Independent practice association (IPA)	PCP: Contracted capitation rate Specialist: Fee-for-service
Point-of-service (POS) plan	Contracted capitation rate or discounted fee-for-service
Indemnity	Fee-for-service
Consumer-directed health plan (combined HDHP and funding option)	Up to deductible: Payment by patient After deductible: Discounted fee-for-service

EXAMPLE

The payer's allowed charge for a new patient's evaluation and management (E/M) service (CPT 99204) is $160.

Provider	Usual Charge	Payment
A	$180	$160
B	$140	$140

Whether a participating provider can bill the patient for the difference between a higher physician fee and a lower allowed charge– called **balance billing**–depends on the terms of the contract with the payer. Payers' rules may prohibit participating providers from balance billing the patient. Instead, the provider must write off the difference, meaning that the amount of the difference is subtracted from the patient's bill and never collected.

balance billing collecting the difference between a provider's usual fee and a payer's lower allowed charge

For example, Medicare-participating providers may not receive an amount greater than the Medicare allowed charge from the Medicare Physician Fee Schedule. Medicare is responsible for paying 80 percent of this allowed charge (after patients have met their annual deductible). Patients are responsible for the other 20 percent.

EXAMPLE

A Medicare PAR provider reports a usual charge of $200 for a diagnostic flexible sigmoidoscopy (CPT 45330), and the Medicare allowed charge is $84. The provider must write off the difference between the two charges. The patient is responsible for 20 percent of the allowed charge, not of the provider's usual charge:

Provider's usual fee	$.200.00
Medicare allowed charge	$ 84.00
Medicare pays 80 percent	$ 67.20
Patient pays 20 percent	$ 16.80

The total the provider can collect is $84. The provider must write off the difference between the usual fee and the allowed charge, $116.

A provider who does not participate in a private plan can usually balance bill patients. As shown in the following example, in this situation, if the provider's usual charge is higher than the allowed charge, the patient must pay the difference. (Note, however, that Medicare and other government-sponsored programs often have different rules for nonparticipating providers.)

EXAMPLE

Payer policy: There is an allowed charge for each procedure. The plan provides a benefit of 100 percent of the provider's usual charges, up to this maximum fee. Provider A is a participating provider; Provider B does not participate and can balance bill. Providers A and B both perform abdominal hysterectomies (CPT 58150). The policy's allowed charge for this procedure is $2,880.

Provider A (PAR)	
Provider's usual charge	$3,100.00
Policy pays its allowed charge................	$2,880.00
Provider writes off the difference	$ 220.00
Provider B (nonPAR)	
Provider's usual charge	$3,000.00
Policy pays its allowed charge................	$2,880.00
Provider bills patient for the difference.........	$ 120.00 ($3,000.00–$2,880.00)
There is no write-off	

Coinsurance provisions in many private plans provide for patient cost-sharing. Rather than paying the provider the full allowed charge, for example, a plan may require the patient to pay 25 percent, while the plan pays 75 percent. In this case, if a provider's usual charges are higher than the plan's allowed charge, the patient owes more for a service from a nonparticipating provider than from a participating provider. The calculations are explained below.

EXAMPLE

Payer policy: A policy provides a benefit of 75 percent of the provider's usual charges, and there is a maximum allowed charge for each procedure. The patient is responsible for 25 percent of the maximum allowed charge. Balance billing is not permitted for plan participants.

Provider A is a participating provider, and Provider B is a nonparticipant in the plan. Providers A and B both perform total abdominal hysterectomies (CPT 58150). The policy's allowed charge for this procedure is $2,880.00.

Provider A (PAR)	
Usual charge............................	$3,100.00
Policy pays 75 percent of its allowed charge....	$2,160.00 (75% of $2,880.00)
Patient pays 25 percent of the allowed charge ..	$ 720.00 (25% of $2,880.00)
Provider writes off the difference	$220.00
Provider B (nonPAR)	
Usual charge............................	$3,000.00
Policy pays 75 percent of its allowed charge....	$2,160.00 (75% of $2,880.00)
Patient pays for:	
(1) 25 percent of the allowed charge + ...	$ 720.00 (25% of $2,880.00)
(2) the difference between the usual charge and the allowed charge........	$ 120.00 ($3,000.00 - $2,880.00)
Patient pays	$ 840.00 ($720.00 + $120.00)
The provider has no write-off	

THINKING IT THROUGH 12.2

In a CDHP, why is the patient's payment after meeting the deductible based on a discounted fee?

Contracted Fee Schedule

Some payers, particularly those that contract directly with providers, establish fixed fee schedules with participating providers. They first decide what they will pay in particular geographic areas and then offer participation contracts with those fees to physician practices. If the practice chooses to join, it agrees by contract to accept the plan's fees for its member patients.

The plan's contract states what percentage of the charges, if any, its patients owe, and what percentage the payer covers. These fee schedules are often called **discounted fee-for-service** arrangements, since they are based on a reduction from the physician's usual fee schedule. Participating providers can typically bill patients their usual charges for procedures and services that are not covered by the plan.

discounted fee-for-service payment schedule for services based on a reduced percentage of usual charges

capitation a prepayment covering provider's services for a plan member for a specified period

capitation (cap) rate periodic prepayment to a provider for specified services to each plan member

Capitation

The fixed prepayment for each plan member in **capitation** plans, called the **capitation rate,** is determined by the managed care organization that contracts with providers. To determine the cap rate, the plan first decides on the allowed charges for the contracted services and then analyzes the health-related characteristics of the plan's members. The plan calculates the number of times each age group and gender group of members is likely to use each of the covered services. For example, if the primary care provider (PCP) contract covers obstetrics and a large percentage of the group's members are young women who are likely to require services related to childbirth, the cap rate is higher than for a group of members containing a greater percentage of men or of women in their forties or fifties who are not as likely to require obstetrics services.

12.3 Private Insurance Payers and Blue Cross Blue Shield

> **TIP**
>
> **Know Your Terms!**
>
> Payers' rules and interpretations may vary. The definitions of basic terms (for example, the age range for "neonate") differ, as do preauthorization requirements. Billers must research each payer's rules for correct billing and reimbursement.

The major payers of medical insurance are either private payers or government-sponsored programs. Private insurance payers include:

- Employer-sponsored medical insurance
- The Federal Employees Health Benefits Program
- Self-insured health plans
- Individual health plans
- The Blue Cross Blue Shield Association

group health plan (GHP) plan of an employer or employee organization to provide health care to employees, former employees, and/or their families

Employer-Sponsored Medical Insurance

Many employees have medical insurance coverage under **group health plans (GHPs)** that their employers sponsor. Human resource departments manage these health care benefits, negotiating with insurance carriers and managed care organizations and selecting one or more plans to offer employees. Both basic plans and riders that employees may buy and add to their policies may be offered. Riders, also called options, are often offered for vision and dental services. Another popular rider is for complementary health care, covering treatments such as chiropractic or manual manipulation, acupuncture, massage therapy, dietetic counseling, and vitamins and minerals.

During specified periods (usually once a year) called open enrollment periods, employees choose the plans they prefer for the coming benefit period. The employer provides tools (often Internet-based) and information to help employees match their personal and family needs with the best-priced plans. Employees can customize their policies by choosing to accept various levels of premiums, deductibles, and other costs.

Regulation and Eligibility for Benefits

Employer-sponsored group health plans must follow federal and state laws that mandate coverage of specific benefits or treatments and access to care. When a state law is more restrictive than the related federal law, the state law is followed.

The group health plan specifies the rules for eligibility and the process of enrolling and disenrolling members. Rules cover employment status, such as full-time, part-time, disabled employees, and laid-off or terminated employees, as well as the age and the conditions for enrolling a dependent.

- Many plans have a waiting period, an amount of time that must pass before a newly hired employee or a dependent is eligible to enroll. The waiting period usually begins on the date of hire and continues until the date the insurance is effective.
- The plan may impose different eligibility rules on a late enrollee, a person who enrolls in a plan after the earliest possible enrollment date or other than on a special enrollment date. For example, special enrollment may occur when a person becomes a dependent of a covered employee through marriage.
- Most plans require annual premiums. Although employers used to pay the total premium as a benefit for employees, currently they pay an average of 80 percent of the cost.
- Each health plan also has a deductible that is due per time period. Noncovered services under the plan that the patient must pay out-of-pocket do not count toward satisfying a deductible. Some plans require an individual deductible that must be met for each person—whether the policyholder or a covered dependent—who has an encounter. Others have a family deductible that can be met by the combined payments to providers for any and all covered members of the insured's family.

> **TIP**
>
> **Group Health Plans and PHI**
>
> Both employer-sponsored health plans and self-insured health plans are group health plans (GHPs) under HIPAA and are subject to HIPAA regulations, including the use of HIPAA-compliant claims and provision of the Notice of Privacy Practices.

Federal Employees Health Benefits Program

The largest employer-sponsored health program in the United States is the **Federal Employees Health Benefits (FEHB)** program, which covers more than 8 million federal employees, retirees, and their families through over 250 health plans from a number of carriers. FEHB is administered by the federal government's Office of Personnel Management (OPM), which receives and deposits premiums and remits payments to the carriers. Each carrier is responsible for furnishing identification cards and benefits brochures to enrollees, adjudicating claims, and maintaining records.

Federal Employees Health Benefits (FEHB) health care program that covers federal employees

self-insured health plans health insurance plans paid for directly by the organization, which sets up a fund from which to pay

Employee Retirement Income Security Act of 1974 (ERISA) law providing incentives and protection for companies with employee health and pension plans

individual health plan (IHP) medical insurance plan purchased by an individual

Self-Insured Health Plans

To save money, some large employers cover the costs of employee medical benefits themselves, rather than buying insurance from carriers or managed care organizations. They create **self-insured health plans** that do not pay premiums to insurance carriers or managed care organizations. Instead, employers with self-insured health plans "insure themselves" and assume the risk of paying directly for medical services, setting aside funds with which to pay benefits. The employer establishes the benefit levels and the plan types offered to employees.

Self-insured health plans may set up their own provider networks or, more often, lease the use of managed care organizations' networks. Self-insured health plans (in contrast to employer-sponsored fully insured plans) are regulated by the federal **Employee Retirement Income Security Act of 1974 (ERISA)** instead of by state laws.

Individual Health Plans

Individual health plans (IHPs) are also available for purchase; almost 10 percent of people with private health insurance have individual plans. People often elect to enroll in individual plans, although coverage is expensive, in order to continue their health insurance between jobs. Purchasers also include self-employed entrepreneurs, students, recent college graduates, and early retirees. Individual insurance plans have basic benefits without the riders or additional features associated with group health plans.

> **TIP**
>
> **Timely Payments**
>
> Group health plans must follow states' clean claims and/or prompt payment acts and must pay claims they accept for processing on a timely basis. ERISA (self-insured) plans are obligated to follow similar rules from the federal Department of Labor.

Major Private Payers and Blue Cross Blue Shield

A small number of large insurance companies dominate the national market and offer all types of health plans to employers and to self-insured plans. Local or regional payers are often affiliated with national plans or with the Blue Cross Blue Shield Association (discussed below). Some carriers offer health insurance to individuals and to small businesses. The law in a few states, such as Maryland, requires major insurance carriers to provide limited health plans that small businesses can afford.

Major Private Payers

Private payers supply complete insurance services, such as:

- Contracting with employers and with individuals to provide insurance benefits
- Setting up physician, hospital, and pharmacy networks
- Establishing fees
- Processing claims
- Managing the insurance risk

The leading national payers are:

- WellPoint, Inc.
- UnitedHealth Group
- Aetna
- CIGNA
- Kaiser Permanente
- Health Net
- Humana, Inc.
- Coventry

Blue Cross Blue Shield

Blue Cross Blue Shield Association (BCBS) licensing agency of Blue Cross Blue Shield plans

The **Blue Cross Blue Shield Association (BCBS),** founded in the 1930s to provide low-cost medical insurance, is a national organization of independent companies called Member Plans that insure over 90 million people. About half of the plan subscribers (policyholders) join PPOs; a quarter are in indemnity plans, about 20 percent in HMOs, and 8 percent in point-of-service plans. All BCBS Member Plans offer a full range of health plans, including consumer-driven health plans, to individuals, small and large employer groups, senior citizens, federal government employees, and others. In addition to major medical and hospital insurance, the "Blues" also have freestanding plans for dental, vision, mental health, prescription, and hearing coverage.

THINKING IT THROUGH 12.3

How would payments toward an individual deductible versus a family deductible be totaled, assuming a time period of one year? Do payments for noncovered services count toward meeting the deductible?

12.4 Government-Sponsored Insurance Programs, Worker's Compensation, and Disability Plans

Many patients of medical practices are insured under one of the four major government-sponsored insurance programs:

- Medicare
- Medicaid
- TRICARE
- CHAMPVA

Two other types of coverage, workers' compensation and disability plans, help people pay for losses from accidents and lost wages.

Medicare

Medicare federal health insurance program for people sixty-five or older and some people with disabilities

Medicare is a federal medical insurance program established in 1965 under Title XVIII of the Social Security Act. The Medicare program is managed by the Centers for Medicare and Medicaid Services (CMS) under the Department of Health and Human Services (HHS). Although it has just four parts, it is arguably the most complex program that medical practices deal with, involving numerous rules and regulations that must be followed.

Medicare benefits are controlled by federal statute. To be covered, an item or service must be in a benefit category established by law and not otherwise excluded. To receive benefits, individuals must be eligible under one of six beneficiary categories:

1. **Individuals age sixty-five or older** Persons age sixty-five or older who have paid FICA taxes or Railroad Retirement taxes for at least forty calendar quarters (ten years).
2. **Disabled adults** Individuals who have been receiving Social Security disability benefits or Railroad Retirement Board disability benefits for more than two years. Coverage begins five months after the two years of entitlement.
3. **Individuals disabled before age eighteen** Individuals under age eighteen who meet the disability criteria of the Social Security Act.
4. **Spouses of entitled individuals** Spouses of deceased or disabled individuals who are or were entitled to Medicare benefits.
5. **Retired federal employees enrolled in the Civil Service Retirement System (CSRS)** Retired CSRS employees and their spouses.
6. **Individuals with end-stage renal disease (ESRD)** Individuals of any age who receive dialysis or renal transplants for ESRD. Coverage typically begins on the first day of the month following the start of dialysis treatments. In the case of a transplant, entitlement begins the month the individual is hospitalized for the transplant, and the transplant must be completed within two months. The donor is covered for services related to the donation of the organ only.

Medicare Part A program that pays for hospitalization, care in a skilled nursing facility, home health care, and hospice care

Medicare Part B program that pays for physician services, outpatient hospital services, durable medical equipment, and other services and supplies

Supplementary Medical Insurance (SMI) also known as Medicare Part B; program that pays for physician services, outpatient hospital services, durable medical equipment, and other services and supplies

Original Medicare Plan Medicare fee-for-service plan

Medigap plan offered by a private insurance carrier to supplement Medicare coverage

Medicare Part C (Medicare Advantage) managed care health plans under the Medicare program

Medicare Part A

Medicare Part A pays for inpatient hospital care, skilled nursing facility care, home health care, and hospice care. Anyone who paid Medicare taxes while working is eligible for Part A at age sixty-five. Those who are receiving Social Security benefits automatically receive Part A coverage; others have to enroll. Eligible beneficiaries do not pay premiums. Individuals age sixty-five or older who are not eligible for Social Security benefits may enroll in Part A, but they must pay premiums for the coverage, and most are also required to take and pay for Part B coverage.

Medicare Part B

Medicare Part B, which is also called **Supplementary Medical Insurance (SMI),** helps beneficiaries pay for physician services, outpatient hospital services, medical equipment, and other supplies and services. Individuals entitled to Part A benefits are automatically qualified to enroll in Part B. United States citizens and permanent residents over the age of sixty-five are also eligible. (People eligible for this coverage can choose either the Original Medicare Plan or a Medicare Advantage plan, also known as Medicare Part C, both of which are explained below.)

Part B is a voluntary program; eligible persons do not have to take part in it. People who are receiving Social Security benefits are automatically signed up for Part B and must opt out if they do not want to take part. Others desiring Part B coverage must enroll; coverage is not automatic. If enrollment takes place more than twelve months after a person's initial enrollment period, there is a permanent 10 percent increase in the premium for each year the beneficiary failed to enroll.

Beneficiaries pay monthly premiums for Part B. They are also subject to annual deductibles and coinsurance, which are established by federal law.

Original Medicare Plan

The Medicare fee-for-service plan, referred to by Medicare as the **Original Medicare Plan,** allows the beneficiary to choose any licensed physician certified by Medicare. Each time the beneficiary receives services, a fee is billable. Part of this fee is generally paid by Medicare, and part is paid by the beneficiary or sometimes by a secondary policy.

Original Medicare Plan patients are responsible for an annual deductible. They are also responsible for the portion of the bill that Medicare does not pay (coinsurance), typically 20 percent of allowed charges. Patients receive a Medicare Summary Notice (MSN) that details the services they were provided over a thirty-day period, the amounts charged, and the amounts they may be billed.

Medigap Insurance

Medigap is private insurance that Original Medicare Plan beneficiaries may purchase to fill in some of the gaps–unpaid amounts–in Medicare coverage. These gaps include the annual deductible, any coinsurance that is required, and payment for some noncovered services. Even though private insurance carriers offer Medigap plans, coverage and standards are regulated by federal and state law.

Medicare Part C (Medicare Advantage Plans)

Medicare Part C (Medicare Advantage) is a program that permits private insurance carriers to contract with CMS to offer Medicare benefits under a managed care option. A Medicare Advantage organization (MAO) is responsible for providing all Medicare-covered services other than hospice care in return for a predetermined capitated payment. Medicare Advantage plans include fee-for-service and other types of plans, and some cover vision, dental, and other services.

Medicare Part D

Medicare Part D provides voluntary Medicare prescription drug plans that are open to people who are eligible for Medicare. All Medicare prescription drug plans are private insurance plans that are approved by Medicare, and most participants pay monthly premiums to access discounted prices. There are two types of plans. The prescription drug plan covers only drugs and can be used with an Original Medicare Plan and/or a Medicare supplement plan. The other type combines a prescription drug plan with a Medicare Advantage plan that includes medical coverage for doctor visits and hospital expenses. This kind of plan is called Medicare Advantage Plus Prescription Drug. A Medicare prescription drug plan has a list of drugs it covers, often structured in payment tiers.

Medicare Part D Medicare prescription drug reimbursement plans

Medicaid federal and state assistance program that pays for health care services for people who cannot afford them

Medi-Medi beneficiary person eligible for both Medicare and Medicaid

dual-eligible Medicare-Medicaid beneficiary

Medicaid

The **Medicaid** program covers more than 50 million low-income people. In 2018, Medicaid was the source of payment for 42.3% of births that year. Medicaid also paid 30.2% of expenditures for nursing care facilities and continuing care retirement communities in 2017. The program was established under Title XIX of the Social Security Act of 1965 to pay for the health care needs of individuals and families with low incomes and few resources.

Medicaid is jointly funded by the federal and state governments. The federal government makes payments to states under the Federal Medicaid Assistance Percentage (FMAP). The amount of the payment is based on the state's average per capita income in relation to the national income average.

Because Medicaid is run by states rather than by the federal government, billers refer to the laws and regulations of their state Medicaid programs to correctly process claims for these patients. Although the federal government sets broad standards for Medicaid coverage, there is variation among the states. States establish their own eligibility standards; the type, amount, duration, and scope of services; and payments to providers. States' income limits usually consider the applicant's income relative to the federal poverty level (FPL), taking household size into account. Most states also provide Medicaid coverage to medically needy individuals—people with high medical expenses and low financial resources (but not low enough to receive cash assistance). States may choose their own names for these programs.

Medi-Medi

Some individuals, called **Medi-Medi beneficiaries** or **dual-eligibles,** are eligible for both Medicaid and Medicare benefits. In many instances, Medicare requires payment of a deductible or coinsurance. When an individual has Medi-Medi coverage, such payments are sometimes paid by Medicaid. The total amount paid by Medicare and Medicaid is subject to a maximum allowed limit. In most states, Medicaid plans do not pay if Medicare does not.

TRICARE

TRICARE government health program serving dependents of active-duty service members, military retirees and their families, some former spouses, and survivors of deceased military members

Civilian Health and Medical Program of the Department of Veterans Affairs (CHAMPVA) health care plan for families of veterans with 100 percent service-related disabilities and the surviving spouses and children of veterans who die from service-related disabilities

TRICARE is the Department of Defense health insurance plan for military personnel and their families. TRICARE, which includes managed care options, replaced the program known as CHAMPUS, the Civilian Health and Medical Program of the Uniformed Services.

TRICARE is a regionally managed health care program that brings the resources of military hospitals together with a network of civilian facilities and providers to offer increased access to health care services. All military treatment facilities, including hospitals and clinics, are part of the TRICARE system. TRICARE also contracts with civilian facilities and physicians to provide more extensive services to beneficiaries.

TRICARE offers beneficiaries access to three different health care plans.

1. TRICARE Standard is a fee-for-service program that replaces the CHAMPUS program, which was also fee-for-service. The program covers medical services provided by a civilian physician when the individual cannot receive treatment from a military treatment facility (MTF). Military families may receive services at an MTF, but the services offered vary by facility, and first priority is given to service members on active duty. When service is not available, the individual seeks treatment from a civilian provider, and TRICARE Standard benefits go into effect.
2. TRICARE Prime is a managed care plan similar to an HMO. After enrolling in the plan, individuals are assigned a Primary Care Manager (PCM) who coordinates and manages their medical care. The PCM may be a single military or civilian provider or a group of providers. In addition to most of the benefits offered by TRICARE Standard, TRICARE Prime offers preventive care, including routine physical examinations. Active-duty service members are automatically enrolled in TRICARE Prime. TRICARE Prime enrollees receive the majority of their health care services from military treatment facilities and receive priority at these facilities.
3. TRICARE Extra is an alternative managed care plan for individuals who want to receive services primarily from civilian facilities and physicians rather than from military facilities. Since it is a managed care plan, individuals must receive health care services from a network of health care professionals. They may also seek treatment at military facilities, but active-duty personnel and other TRICARE Prime enrollees receive priority at those facilities, so care may not always be available. TRICARE Extra is more expensive than TRICARE Prime, but less costly than TRICARE Standard.

CHAMPVA

The **Civilian Health and Medical Program of the Department of Veterans Affairs (CHAMPVA)** is the government's health insurance program for veterans with a 100 percent service-related disability and their families. Under the program, health care expenses are shared between the Department of Veterans Affairs (VA) and the beneficiary.

The Veterans Health Care Eligibility Reform Act of 1996 requires veterans with a 100 percent disability to be enrolled in the program as CHAMPVA sponsors. The VA is responsible for determining eligibility for the CHAMPVA program. Eligible beneficiaries include:

- Dependents of a veteran who is totally and permanently disabled due to a service-connected injury
- Dependents of a veteran who was totally and permanently disabled due to a service-connected condition at the time of death
- Survivors of a veteran who died as a result of a service-related disability
- Survivors of a veteran who died in the line of duty

Note that eligible CHAMPVA sponsors may be entitled to receive medical care through the VA health care system based on their own veteran status. Additionally, if the eligible CHAMPVA sponsor is the spouse of another eligible CHAMPVA sponsor, both may now be eligible for CHAMPVA benefits. In each case where the eligible spouse requires medical attention, that person may choose the VA health care system or coverage under CHAMPVA for their health care needs.

Workers' Compensation

When someone is injured accidentally while performing work or a work-related duty or becomes ill as a result of the employment environment, the cost of medical care for the injury or illness is covered by a federal or state plan known as **workers' compensation insurance.** These plans also provide benefits for lost wages and permanent disabilities.

workers' compensation insurance state or federal plan that covers medical care and other benefits for employees who suffer accidental injury or become ill as a result of employment

Workers' compensation covers two kinds of situations that require medical care. A traumatic injury is caused by a specific event or series of events within a single workday or shift. An example is a broken leg caused by a fall from a catwalk in a warehouse. Occupational disease or illness (also known as nontraumatic injury) is caused by the work environment over a longer period of time. An example of an occupational disease is a lung condition caused by repeated exposure to fumes in the workplace.

Workers' compensation includes five types of payments for work-related illnesses and injuries:

1. For medical treatment
2. To replace lost wages (temporary disability)
3. As permanent disability payments (either partial or full disability)
4. As compensation for dependents of employees who are fatally injured
5. For vocational rehabilitation

Work-related illnesses or injuries suffered by civilian (nonmilitary) employees of most federal agencies are covered under the Federal Employees' Compensation Act (FECA) and administered by the Office of Workers' Compensation Programs (OWCP). Injured employees can choose a physician from among those who are authorized by the OWCP. When such a patient requests treatment, the biller should verify that the selected physician is authorized to administer medical care under the patient's workers' compensation coverage. If the patient later wants to change physicians, the

OWCP must approve the change. A patient who seeks care from an unauthorized physician may be responsible for the cost of that treatment.

State programs cover traumatic and nontraumatic injuries to state and private business employees within each state, although there are some exceptions. Eligibility and exceptions vary from state to state. A state compensation board or commission administers workers' compensation laws for employees eligible under state laws. The state board or commission handles employee appeals and provides information to employers and health care providers about regulations. Compliance with state laws is important.

Disability

disability compensation programs programs that provide partial reimbursement for lost income when a disability prevents an individual from working

fee schedule document that specifies the amount the provider bills for services

usual fees normal fees charged by a provider

Most of the insurance and compensation plans pay for health care costs resulting from illnesses or injuries. By comparison, **disability compensation programs** pay benefits for lost income when an illness or injury prevents a person from working. Unlike workers' compensation programs, which also include compensation for lost income, the illness or injury does not have to be work-related.

The federal government, some states, and many private insurance companies offer disability compensation programs and policies. Eligibility and benefits vary. However, they all require the insured to provide convincing medical evidence that the condition resulting from the illness or injury satisfies the criteria of the program or policy.

THINKING IT THROUGH 12.4

Why is it important to understand which services are and are not covered under patients' insurance plans?

12.5 Fee Schedules

Given all the possible types of health plans and payers, billers must often handle questions from patients about their fees. The answers are based on knowledge of the practice's charges and on estimates of what patients' insurance plans will pay.

Physicians have **fee schedules,** lists of fees for the procedures and services they frequently perform. These fees are called **usual fees,** meaning that the physicians charge them to most of their patients most of the time under typical conditions. Payers, too, set the fees that they pay providers. Most payers use one of three methods to set the fees that the health plan will pay physicians: (1) usual, customary, and reasonable; (2) relative value scale; and (3) resource-based relative value scale.

Usual, Customary, and Reasonable Payment Structure

Some health plans take the physicians' usual charges into account when they set their fee structures. A plan studies what many physicians have charged for similar services over a period of time. The fee that is set for each service is an average of the usual fee an individual physician charges for the service, the customary fee charged by most physicians in the community, and the reasonable fee for the service. This approach is called **usual, customary, and reasonable (UCR).**

UCR fees, for the most part, accurately reflect the charges of most physicians. However, fees may not be available for new or rare procedures. Lacking better information, a payer may set too low a fee for such procedures.

usual, customary, and reasonable (UCR) fees set by comparing usual fees, customary fees, and reasonable fees

relative value scale (RVS) system of assigning unit values to medical services based on their required skill and time

resource-based relative value scale (RBRVS) relative value scale for establishing Medicare charges

Relative Value Scale

Another method payers use to establish fees is the **relative value scale (RVS)** approach. Based on nationwide research, the relative value scale assigns numerical values to medical services. These values reflect the amount of skill and time the procedures require of physicians. For example, in an obstetrics practice, a hysterectomy has a higher RVS number than does a dilation and curettage (D&C), because the hysterectomy is a more complicated surgical procedure and is considered to require more skill. To calculate the fee, the value assigned by the RVS is multiplied by a dollar conversion factor.

THINKING IT THROUGH 12.5

If a participating provider has two different fees for a particular CPT code for Medicare and a private payer, which should be lower?

> **TIP**
>
> **Setting Fees**
>
> Most practices set their fees slightly above those paid by the highest reimbursing plan in which they participate. Medicare rules state that the amount billed Medicare must not be higher than the lowest fee billed any payer for the same service.

Resource-Based Relative Value Scale

The payment system used by Medicare is called the **resource-based relative value scale (RBRVS).** The RBRVS establishes relative value units for services. It replaces providers' consensus on fees–the historical charges–with a relative value that is based on resources– what each service really costs to provide.

There are three parts to an RBRVS fee:

1. **The nationally uniform relative value unit** The relative value is based on three cost elements: the physician's work, the practice cost (overhead), and the cost of malpractice insurance.
2. **A geographic adjustment factor** A geographic adjustment factor called the geographic practice cost index (GPCI) is a number that is used to multiply each relative value element so that it better reflects a geographic area's relative costs. For example, the cost of the provider's work is affected by average physician salaries in an area. The cost of the practice depends on things such as office rental prices and local taxes. Malpractice expense is also affected by where the work is done.
3. **A nationally uniform conversion factor** A uniform conversion factor is a dollar amount used to multiply the relative values to produce a payment amount. It is used by Medicare to make adjustments according to changes in the cost of living index.

TIP

Updating Fee Schedules

Fee schedules must be updated when new CPT codes are released. For example, if the definition of a surgical package changes, a surgeon's fees need to be altered to tie exactly to the revised elements of the package, or a new procedure may need to be included. Providers may refer to the national databases or, more likely, review those databases and the Medicare rate of pay to establish the new fees.

Medicare Physician Fee Schedule

Medicare Physician Fee Schedule (MPFS) RBRVS-based allowed fees that are the basis for Medicare reimbursements

Each part of the RBRVS–the relative values, the GPCI, and the conversion factor–is updated each year by CMS. The year's RBRVS is published by CMS in the *Federal Register* and is available through the CMS website. Many private payers use the **Medicare Physician Fee Schedule (MPFS)** as the basis for the fees they pay as well.

chapter 12 summary

KEY TERMS

allowed charge
balance billing
Blue Cross Blue Shield Association (BCBS)
capitation
capitation rate
Civilian Health and Medical Program of the Department of Veterans Affairs (CHAMPVA)
disability compensation program
discounted fee-for-service
dual-eligible
Employee Retirement Income Security Act of 1974 (ERISA)
Federal Employees Health Benefits (FEHB)
fee schedule
fee-for-service
group health plan (GHP)
health maintenance organizations (HMO)
individual health plan (IHP)
Medi-Medi beneficiary
Medicaid
Medicare
Medicare Part A
Medicare Part B
Medicare Part C (Medicare Advantage)
Medicare Part D
Medicare Physician Fee Schedule (MPFS)
Medigap
Original Medicare Plan
point-of-service (POS) plan
preferred provider organization (PPO)
primary care physician (PCP)
relative value scale (RVS)
resource-based relative value scale (RBRVS)
self-insured health plans
Supplementary Medical Insurance (SMI)
third-party payer
TRICARE
usual fees
usual, customary and reasonable (UCR)
workers' compensation insurance

LEARNING OUTCOME	KEY CONCEPTS/EXAMPLES
12.1 Compare the major features of health plans.	• PPO • HMO • Independent practice association model • POS • Indemnity plans
12.2 Discuss third-party payment methods.	Table 12.1 reviews the payment methods of the types of health plans. Payers use one of three main methods of paying providers: allowed charges, contracted fee schedules, and capitation.
12.3 Discuss the organization and regulation of employer-sponsored group health plans and self-insured plans.	The major payers of medical insurance are either private payers or government-sponsored programs. Private payers are: • Employer-sponsored medical insurance • The Federal Employees Health Benefits Program • Self-insured health plans • Individual health plans • The Blue Cross Blue Shield Association

LEARNING OUTCOME	KEY CONCEPTS/EXAMPLES
12.4 Explain the purpose of government-sponsored insurance programs, workers' compensation, and disability plans.	Many patients are insured under one of the four major government-sponsored insurance programs: • Medicare • Medicaid • TRICARE • CHAMPVA When someone is injured accidentally in the course of performing work or a work-related duty or becomes ill as a result of the employment environment, the cost of medical care for the injury or illness is covered by a federal or state plan known as workers' compensation insurance. Disability compensation programs pay benefits for lost income when an illness or injury prevents a person from working. Unlike workers' compensation programs, which also include compensation for lost income, the illness or injury does not have to be work-related.
12.5 Identify the three methods most payers use to pay providers.	1. usual, customary, and reasonable; 2. relative value scale; and 3. resource-based relative value scale.

chapter 12 review

MATCHING QUESTIONS

Match the key terms with their definitions.

_____ 1. *[LO 12.2]* allowed charge

_____ 2. *[LO 12.1]* third-party payer

_____ 3. *[LO 12.5]* relative value scale (RVS)

_____ 4. *[LO 12.4]* Medicare

_____ 5. *[LO 12.5]* fee schedule

_____ 6. *[LO 12.1]* point-of-service (POS) plan

_____ 7. *[LO 12.4]* Medicaid

_____ 8. *[LO 12.3]* preferred provider organization (PPO)

_____ 9. *[LO 12.1]* group health plan (GHP)

_____ 10. *[LO 12.1]* health maintenance organization (HMO)

a. Managed health care system in which providers offer health care to members for fixed periodic payments.

b. Managed care network of health care providers who agree to perform services for plan members at discounted fees.

c. Maximum charge a plan pays for a service or procedure.

d. Federal and state assistance program that pays for health care services for people who cannot afford them.

e. Federal health insurance program for people sixty-five or older and some people with disabilities.

f. Managed care plan that permits patients to receive medical services from non-network providers.

g. Plan of an employer or employee organization to provide health care to employees, former employees, and/or their families.

h. System of assigning unit values to medical services based on their required skill and time.

i. Document that specifies the amount the provider bills for services.

j. Private or government organization that insures or pays for health care on behalf of beneficiaries.

MULTIPLE-CHOICE QUESTIONS

Select the letter that best completes the statement or answers the question.

1. *[LO 12.4]* _____ helps beneficiaries pay for physician services, outpatient hospital services, medical equipment, and other supplies and services.
   a. Medicare Part A
   b. Medicare Part B
   c. Medicare Part C
   d. Medicare Part D

2. *[LO 12.1]* ______ have the most stringent guidelines and the narrowest choice of providers.
   a. Health maintenance organizations (HMOs)
   b. Preferred provider organizations (PPOs)
   c. Point-of-service (POS) plans
   d. Indemnity plans

3. *[LO 12.2]* What is it called when the difference between the insurance payment and the provider's usual charge is subtracted from the patient's bill and never collected?
   a. capitation
   b. allowed charge
   c. write-off
   d. fee schedule

4. *[LO 12.2]* This amount is the most the payer will pay any provider for that CPT code.
   a. usual fee
   b. usual charge
   c. allowed charge
   d. capitation (cap) rate

5. *[LO 12.4]* The Medicare program is managed by the ______ under the Department of Health and Human Services (HHS).
   a. Centers for Medicare and Medicaid Services (CMS)
   b. Blue Cross Blue Shield Association (BCBS)
   c. Federal Employees Health Benefits (FEHB) program
   d. Civilian Health and Medical Program of the Department of Veterans Affairs (CHAMPVA)

6. *[LO 12.5]* The payment system used by Medicare is called the ______.
   a. relative value scale (RVS)
   b. usual, customary, and reasonable (UCR) approach
   c. resource-based relative value scale (RBRVS)
   d. all of the above

7. *[LO 12.1]* The most popular type of health plan is the ______, which contracts with physicians, hospitals, clinics, and pharmacies to provide a network of care providers for its beneficiaries.
   a. health maintenance organization (HMO)
   b. preferred provider organization (PPO)
   c. point-of-service (POS) plan
   d. indemnity plan

8. *[LO 12.1]* ______ or fee-for-service plans require premium, deductible, and coinsurance payments.
   a. Health maintenance organizations (HMOs)
   b. Preferred provider organizations (PPOs)
   c. Point-of-service (POS) plans
   d. Indemnity plans

9. *[LO 12.4]* Workers' compensation covers what kinds of situations that require medical care?
   a. traumatic injury
   b. occupational disease or illness
   c. veterans with service-related disabilities
   d. both (a) and (b)

10. *[LO 12.3]* The largest employer-sponsored health program in the United States is the ______.
    a. Blue Cross Blue Shield Association (BCBS)
    b. Medicare program
    c. Federal Employees Health Benefits (FEHB) program
    d. Medicaid program

SHORT-ANSWER QUESTIONS

Define the following abbreviations.

1. *[LO 12.4]* CMS ____________________
2. *[LO 12.3]* ERISA ____________________
3. *[LO 12.4]* CHAMPVA ____________________
4. *[LO 12.1]* PCP ____________________
5. *[LO 12.3]* BCBS ____________________
6. *[LO 12.3]* FEHB ____________________
7. *[LO 12.5]* UCR ____________________

APPLYING YOUR KNOWLEDGE

12.1 *[LO 12.1, 12.3]* Read this information from a medical insurance policy and answer the questions that follow.

Policy Number: 054351278
Insured: Jane Hellman Brandeis
Premium Due Quarterly: $1,414.98

AMOUNT PAYABLE

Maximum Benefit Limit, per *covered person*	$2,000,000
Stated Deductible per *covered person,* per *calendar year*	$ 2,500

EMERGENCY ROOM DEDUCTIBLE (for each visit for *illness* to an emergency room when not directly admitted to the hospital)	$ 50

Note: After satisfaction of the emergency room deductible, *covered expenses* are subject to any applicable *deductible amounts* and coinsurance provisions.

PREFERRED PROVIDER BENEFITS, per *calendar year*

For *covered expenses* in excess of the applicable stated deductible.	100%

NON-PREFERRED PROVIDER BENEFITS
If *covered expenses* are incurred at a non-Preferred Provider, benefits will be reduced to 80% of Preferred Provider plan benefits. This reduction is limited to a *calendar year* maximum amount of $5,000 per *covered person.*

a. What type of health plan is described, an HMO, a PPO, or an indemnity plan?

b. What is the premium?

c. What is the annual deductible?

d. What percentage of preferred provider charges does the patient owe after meeting the deductible each year?

e. After the annual deductible has been met, the insured incurs a $6,000 out-of-network medical bill. How much will the health plan pay?

12.2 *[LO 12.4]* A physician's usual fee for a routine eye examination is $80. Under the discounted fee-for-service arrangement the doctor has with Plan A, the fee is discounted 15 percent for Plan A members. This month, the doctor has seen five Plan A members for routine eye exams.

a. What is the physician's usual fee for five patients?

b. What will the physician be paid for one Plan A member's exam?

c. What will the physician be paid for the five Plan A eye exams?

chapter **13**

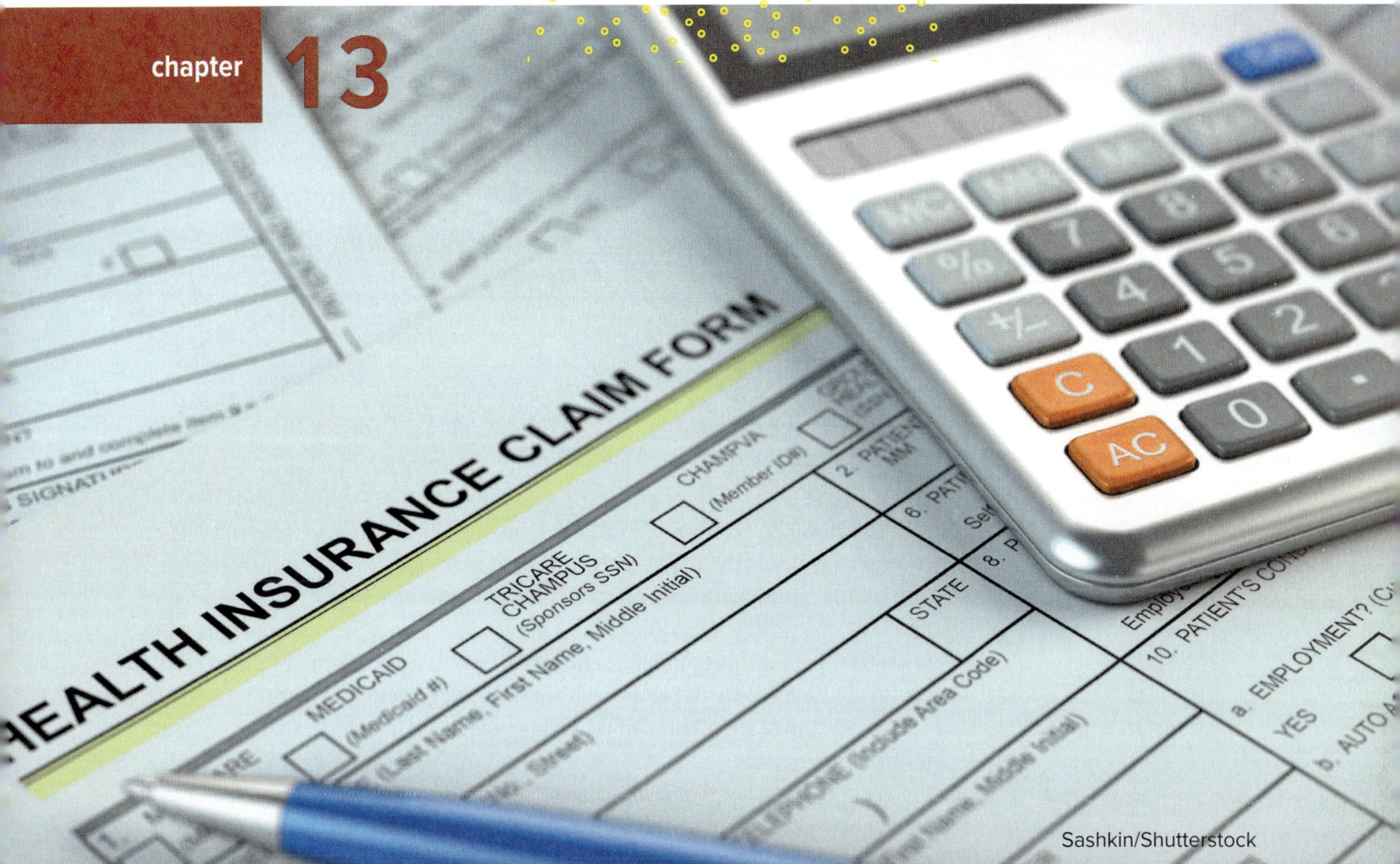

Sashkin/Shutterstock

Claim Management

LEARNING OUTCOMES

When you finish this chapter, you will be able to:

13.1 Describe health care claims.

13.2 Discuss how to create a claim.

13.3 Describe the different methods to submit claims.

13.4 Identify primary, secondary, and tertiary claims.

13.5 Explain how to send an electronic claim attachment.

13.6 Explain claim adjudication.

13.7 Discuss how to monitor claim status.

Claim Accuracy

Trilogy Family Care Center's revenue cycle manager, Elrene Harrison, has been auditing claim submissions. She finds that many claims were rejected due to inaccurate data entry, such as misspelled patient names, wrong dates of birth, and missing information. She decides to contract with a clearinghouse to improve the claim approval rate.

As you read this chapter, consider this scenario and the importance of claim accuracy. How will using a clearinghouse help Trilogy Family Care Center to improve their claim approval rates?

13.1 Introduction to Health Care Claims

Health insurance claims are created for patients with insurance coverage. The insurance claim is the most important document for obtaining correct reimbursement from health care plans. Claims communicate information about a patient's diagnosis, procedures, and charges to a payer. Technology makes it possible for practices to create, send, and track a large volume of claims efficiently and effectively to ensure that they receive prompt payment.

The administrative team must submit clean claims with all the correct information necessary for payer processing. An error on a claim may cause the claim to be delayed or denied. Rejected claims can cost the practice twice as much as clean claims and can result in reduced cash flow. Claims that are not paid in full also have a negative effect on the practice's bottom line.

Claims must also be submitted within the **timely filing** requirements of each health plan. These rules specify the number of days after the date of service that the practice has to file the claim. If it is sent later, it is not eligible for payment. For example, under the Patient Protection and Affordable Care Act (PPACA), the timely filing requirement for Medicare claims is one calendar year after the date of service.

timely filing health plan's rules specifying the number of days after the date of service that the practice has to file the claim

HIPAA X12 837 Health Care Claim HIPAA standard format for electronic transmission of the claim to a health plan

CMS-1500 (08/05) claim the mandated paper insurance claim form

National Uniform Claim Committee (NUCC) organization responsible for claim content

Claim Formats

For many years, the CMS-1500 was the universal health claim form accepted by most payers. The familiar red and black printed form was completed and mailed to payers. Sending paper claims has become rare with the increased use of information technology (IT) in physician practices. HIPAA/HITECH, with its emphasis on electronic transactions, has made the use of IT mandatory except in the case of very small practices and those that never send any kind of electronic health care transactions.

Today, almost all claims are sent electronically. The HIPAA standard transaction for electronic claims is the **HIPAA X12 837 Health Care Claim,** usually called the "837 claim" or the "HIPAA claim." The paper format is known as the **CMS-1500 (08/05) claim** form. Both types of insurance claims are prepared in the PM/EHR.

Claim Content

The **National Uniform Claim Committee (NUCC),** led by the American Medical Association, determines the content of both the HIPAA 837 and the CMS-1500.

CMS-1500

The concept of the health care claim is easier to understand by studying the CMS-1500, since it is a paper-based document. In this section, we provide a listing of the data elements on the CMS-1500 and the corresponding location of those data in Medisoft Network Professional (see Table 13.1). Of course, claims are not filled out by transferring information from other office documents and completing a paper form. Instead, claims are created when the PM/EHR is used to capture and organize databases of claim information. The program automates the formerly laborious task of creating correct claims, making it easy to update, correct, and manage the claim process.

TABLE 13.1 CMS-1500 Fields and Corresponding Data Locations in Medisoft Network Professional (MNP)

Box	CMS-1500 Field Name	Data Source in MNP	Dialog Box/Tab/Field Name in MNP
Top 1	Insurance Name/Address	Insurance	***Insurance Carrier,*** Address, *Name, etc.*
Top 2	Primary, Secondary, Tertiary	Insurance	Determined by claim form selected
1	Insurance Type	Insurance	***Insurance Carrier,*** EDI/Eligibility, *Type*
1a	Insured's ID No.	Case	***Case,*** Policy 1, 2, 3, *Policy No.*
2	Patient's Name	Patient	***Patient/Guarantor,*** Name, Address, *Last Name, First Name, Middle Initial*
3	Patient's Birth Date, Sex	Patient	***Patient/Guarantor,*** Name, Address, *Birth Date, Sex*
4	Insured's Name	Case	***Case,*** Policy 1, 2, 3, *Insured*
5	Patient's Address	Patient	***Patient/Guarantor,*** Name, Address, *Street, City, State, Zip Code*
6	Patient Relation to Insured	Case	***Case,*** Policy 1, 2, 3, *Relationship to Insured*
7	Insured's Address	Patient	***Patient/Guarantor,*** Name, Address, *Street, City, State, Zip Code*
8	Patient Status	Case	***Case,*** Personal, *Marital Status, Student Status, Employment Status*
9	Other Insured's Name	Case	***Case,*** Policy 1, 2, 3, *Insured*
9a	Other Insured's Policy/Group No.	Case	***Case,*** Policy 1, 2, 3, *Policy Number, Group Number*
9b	Other Insured's Date of Birth, Sex	Patient	***Patient/Guarantor,*** Name, Address, *Birth Date, Sex*
9c	Employer/School	Patient	***Patient/Guarantor,*** Other Information, *Employer*
9d	Insurance Plan Name, Program	Insurance	***Insurance Carrier,*** Address, *Plan Name;* if empty, prints carrier name
10a	Condition Related to Employment	Case	***Case,*** Condition, *Employment Related* checkbox
10b	Condition Related to Auto Accident	Case	***Case,*** Condition, *Accident, Related To*
10c	Condition Related to Other Accident	Case	***Case,*** Condition, *Accident, Related To*
10d	Local Use	Case	***Case,*** Miscellaneous, *Local Use A*

(continued)

TABLE 13.1	**(continued)**		
Box	**CMS-1500 Field Name**	**Data Source in MNP**	**Dialog Box/Tab/Field Name in MNP**
11	Insured's Policy Group/FECA #	Case	***Case,*** Policy 1, *Policy Number, Group Number*
11a	Insured's Date of Birth, Sex	Patient	***Patient/Guarantor,*** Name, Address, *Birth Date, Sex*
11b	Employer/School	Patient	***Patient/Guarantor,*** Other Information, *Employer*
11c	Insurance Plan Name/ Program	Insurance	***Insurance Carrier,*** Address, *Plan Name;* if empty, prints carrier name
11d	Another Health Benefit Plan?	Case	***Case,*** Policy 2, 3, *Insurance 2* or *Insurance 3*
12	Patient Signature or Authorized Signature	Patient	***Patient/Guarantor,*** Other Information, *Signature on File;* ***Insurance Carrier,*** Options and Codes, *Patient Signature on File*
13	Insured's Signature or Authorized Signature	Patient	***Patient/Guarantor,*** Other Information, *Signature on File;* ***Insurance Carrier,*** Options and Codes, *Insured Signature on File*
14	Date Current Ill/Inj/LMP	Case	***Case,*** Condition, *Injury/Illness/LMP Date*
15	Same/Similar Date	Case	***Case,*** Condition, *Date Similar Symptoms*
16	Dates Unable to Work	Case	***Case,*** Condition, *Dates—Unable to Work*
17	Referring Provider	Case	***Case,*** Account, *Referring Provider*
17a	Referring Provider, Other Identifier, Qualifier	Referring Provider	***Referring Provider,*** Referring Provider IDs, *NPI*
17b	Referring Provider NPI	Referring Provider	***Referring Provider,*** Referring Provider IDs, *NPI*
18	Hospitalization Dates	Case	***Case,*** Condition, *Dates—Hospitalization*
19	Local Use	Case	***Case,*** Miscellaneous, *Local Use B*
20	Outside Lab? $ Charges	Case	***Case,*** Miscellaneous, *Outside Lab Work*
21	Diagnosis	Case	***Case,*** Diagnosis, Principal Diagnosis, *Default Diagnosis 1, 2, 3, 4*
22	Medicaid Resubmission	Case	***Case,*** Medicaid and Tricare, *Resubmission No., Original Reference*
23	Prior Authorization #	Case	***Case,*** Miscellaneous, *Prior Authorization Number*
24A	Dates of Service	Transaction	***Transaction Entry,*** *Date From, Date To*
24B	Place of Service	Transaction	***Transaction Entry,*** *Place of Service*
24C	EMG	Case	***Case,*** *Condition, Emergency*
24D	Procedures, Services, or Supplies	Transaction	***Transaction Entry,*** *Procedure, M1, M2, M3, M4*
24E	Diagnosis Pointer	Transaction	***Transaction Entry,*** *Diag 1, Diag 2, Diag 3, Diag 4*
24F	$ Charges	Transaction	***Transaction Entry,*** *Amount*
24G	Days or Units	Transaction	***Transaction Entry,*** *Units*
24H	EPSDT	Case	***Case,*** Medicaid and Tricare, *EPSDT*
24I	Rendering Provider, Other ID, Qualifier	Provider	***Provider,*** Provider IDs
24J	Rendering Provider ID #	Provider	***Provider,*** Provider IDs

TABLE 13.1 (continued)

Box	CMS-1500 Field Name	Data Source in MNP	Dialog Box/Tab/Field Name in MNP
25	Federal Tax ID	Practice	***Provider,*** Provider IDs, *Tax ID/SSN*
26	Patient's Account No.	Patient	***Patient/Guarantor,*** Name, Address, *Chart No.*
27	Accept Assignment?	Case	***Case,*** Policy 1, 2, 3, *Assignment of Benefits/Accept Assignment*
28	Total Charge	Transaction	Calculated field
29	Amount Paid	Transaction	***Transaction Entry,*** *Payment*
30	Balance Due	Transaction	Calculated field
31	Physician's Signature	Provider	***Provider,*** Address, *Signature on File;* Insurance Carrier, Address, *Signature on File*
32	Facility Address	Practice	***Facility,*** Address
32A	Facility NPI	Address	***Facility,*** Facility IDs, *NPI*
33	Billing Provider Information	Provider	***Provider,*** Address, *First Name, Middle Initial, Last Name, Street, City, State, Zip*
33A	Billing Provider NPI	Provider	***Provider:*** Provider IDs, *NPI*

TIP

Health Plans Comply

Health plans cannot require providers to make changes or additions to the content of the HIPAA claim, and they cannot refuse to accept the standard transaction or delay payment of any correctly transmitted HIPAA transaction, claims included.

The CMS-1500 claim has thirty-three numbered boxes representing about 150 discrete data elements. **Data elements** are the smallest units of information in a transaction. The CMS-1500 is pictured in Figure 13.1.

data element smallest unit of information in a HIPAA transaction

The HIPAA 837 Transaction

In contrast to the CMS-1500, the HIPAA 837 has a maximum of 244 segments representing about 1,054 elements. However, many of these data elements are conditional and apply to particular specialties only. Some different terms are in use with the HIPAA 837 claim, though, and a few additional information items must be relayed to the payer. For example, the HIPAA 837 uses the term *subscriber* for the insurance policyholder or guarantor, meaning the same as *insured* on the CMS-1500 claim. The HIPAA claim also requires a claim filing indicator code, which is an administrative code that identifies the type of health plan, such as Medicare Part B, Medicaid, HMO, PPO, and so on.

Examples of HIPAA claims data elements are a patient's first name, middle name or initial, and last name. Although these are essentially the same as the data elements used to complete a CMS-1500, they are organized in a manner that is efficient for electronic transmission, rather than for use on a paper form. For example, since computers interpret blank spaces as characters, the efficient transfer of data requires removal of such spaces. As a result, the messages are not easy to read, since there is no space or line break at the end of a line.

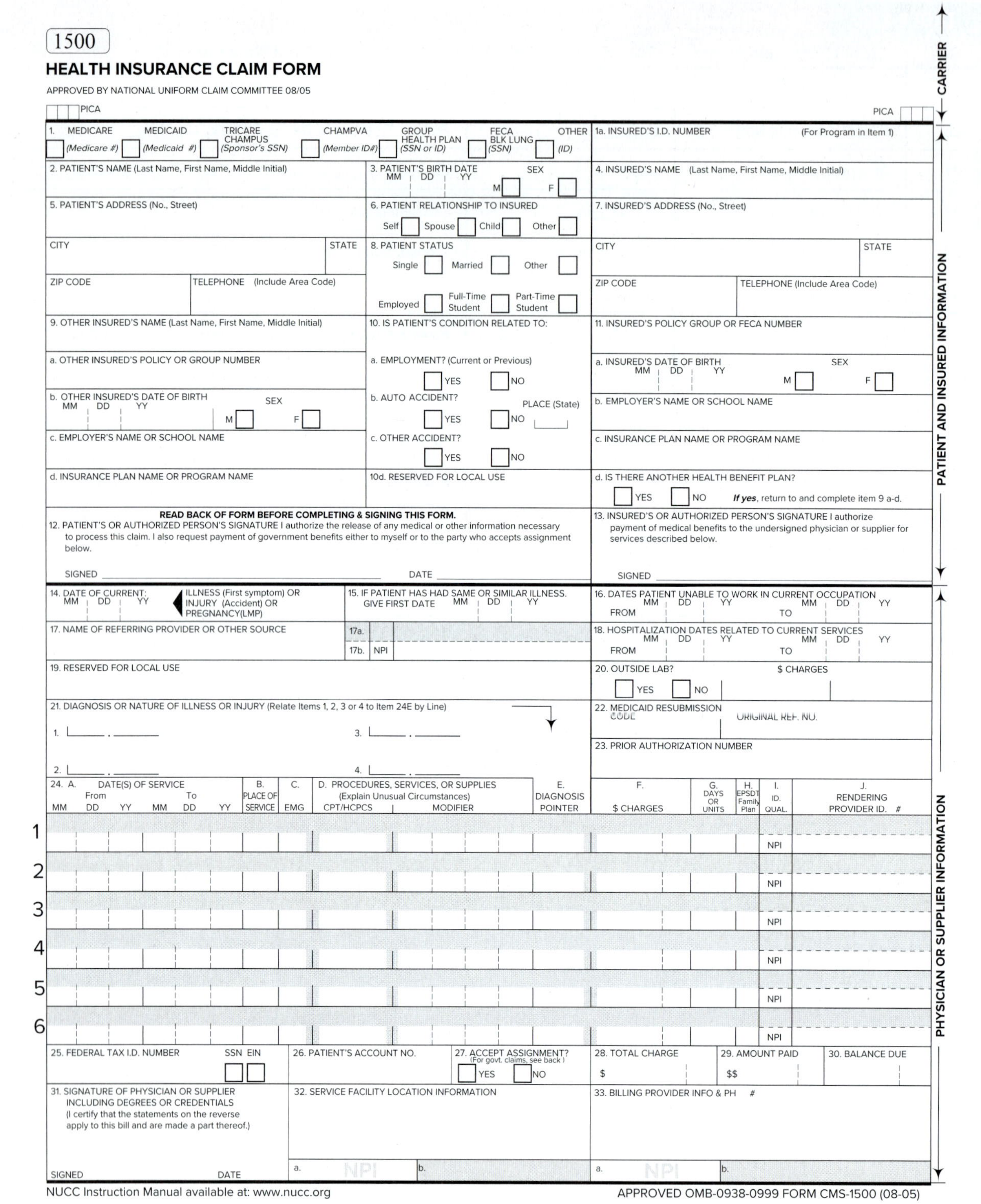
1500

HEALTH INSURANCE CLAIM FORM

APPROVED BY NATIONAL UNIFORM CLAIM COMMITTEE 08/05

PICA | PICA

CARRIER

1. MEDICARE (Medicare #) | MEDICAID (Medicaid #) | TRICARE CHAMPUS (Sponsor's SSN) | CHAMPVA (Member ID#) | GROUP HEALTH PLAN (SSN or ID) | FECA BLK LUNG (SSN) | OTHER (ID)

1a. INSURED'S I.D. NUMBER (For Program in Item 1)

2. PATIENT'S NAME (Last Name, First Name, Middle Initial)

3. PATIENT'S BIRTH DATE MM DD YY SEX M F

4. INSURED'S NAME (Last Name, First Name, Middle Initial)

5. PATIENT'S ADDRESS (No., Street)

6. PATIENT RELATIONSHIP TO INSURED Self Spouse Child Other

7. INSURED'S ADDRESS (No., Street)

CITY | STATE

8. PATIENT STATUS Single Married Other

CITY | STATE

ZIP CODE | TELEPHONE (Include Area Code)

Employed | Full-Time Student | Part-Time Student

ZIP CODE | TELEPHONE (Include Area Code)

9. OTHER INSURED'S NAME (Last Name, First Name, Middle Initial)

10. IS PATIENT'S CONDITION RELATED TO:

11. INSURED'S POLICY GROUP OR FECA NUMBER

a. OTHER INSURED'S POLICY OR GROUP NUMBER

a. EMPLOYMENT? (Current or Previous) YES NO

a. INSURED'S DATE OF BIRTH MM DD YY SEX M F

b. OTHER INSURED'S DATE OF BIRTH MM DD YY SEX M F

b. AUTO ACCIDENT? YES NO PLACE (State)

b. EMPLOYER'S NAME OR SCHOOL NAME

c. EMPLOYER'S NAME OR SCHOOL NAME

c. OTHER ACCIDENT? YES NO

c. INSURANCE PLAN NAME OR PROGRAM NAME

d. INSURANCE PLAN NAME OR PROGRAM NAME

10d. RESERVED FOR LOCAL USE

d. IS THERE ANOTHER HEALTH BENEFIT PLAN? YES NO *If yes*, return to and complete item 9 a-d.

READ BACK OF FORM BEFORE COMPLETING & SIGNING THIS FORM.

12. PATIENT'S OR AUTHORIZED PERSON'S SIGNATURE I authorize the release of any medical or other information necessary to process this claim. I also request payment of government benefits either to myself or to the party who accepts assignment below.

SIGNED ______ DATE ______

13. INSURED'S OR AUTHORIZED PERSON'S SIGNATURE I authorize payment of medical benefits to the undersigned physician or supplier for services described below.

SIGNED ______

PATIENT AND INSURED INFORMATION

14. DATE OF CURRENT: MM DD YY ILLNESS (First symptom) OR INJURY (Accident) OR PREGNANCY(LMP)

15. IF PATIENT HAS HAD SAME OR SIMILAR ILLNESS. GIVE FIRST DATE MM DD YY

16. DATES PATIENT UNABLE TO WORK IN CURRENT OCCUPATION FROM MM DD YY TO MM DD YY

17. NAME OF REFERRING PROVIDER OR OTHER SOURCE | 17a. | 17b. NPI

18. HOSPITALIZATION DATES RELATED TO CURRENT SERVICES FROM MM DD YY TO MM DD YY

19. RESERVED FOR LOCAL USE

20. OUTSIDE LAB? YES NO $ CHARGES

21. DIAGNOSIS OR NATURE OF ILLNESS OR INJURY (Relate Items 1, 2, 3 or 4 to Item 24E by Line)

1. ___ . ___ 3. ___ . ___

2. ___ . ___ 4. ___ . ___

22. MEDICAID RESUBMISSION CODE | ORIGINAL REF. NO.

23. PRIOR AUTHORIZATION NUMBER

24. A. DATE(S) OF SERVICE From MM DD YY To MM DD YY	B. PLACE OF SERVICE	C. EMG	D. PROCEDURES, SERVICES, OR SUPPLIES (Explain Unusual Circumstances) CPT/HCPCS MODIFIER	E. DIAGNOSIS POINTER	F. $ CHARGES	G. DAYS OR UNITS	H. EPSDT Family Plan	I. ID. QUAL.	J. RENDERING PROVIDER ID. #
1								NPI	
2								NPI	
3								NPI	
4								NPI	
5								NPI	
6								NPI	

25. FEDERAL TAX I.D. NUMBER SSN EIN

26. PATIENT'S ACCOUNT NO.

27. ACCEPT ASSIGNMENT? (For govt. claims, see back) YES NO

28. TOTAL CHARGE $

29. AMOUNT PAID $$

30. BALANCE DUE

31. SIGNATURE OF PHYSICIAN OR SUPPLIER INCLUDING DEGREES OR CREDENTIALS (I certify that the statements on the reverse apply to this bill and are made a part thereof.)

SIGNED DATE

32. SERVICE FACILITY LOCATION INFORMATION a. NPI b.

33. BILLING PROVIDER INFO & PH # a. NPI b.

PHYSICIAN OR SUPPLIER INFORMATION

NUCC Instruction Manual available at: www.nucc.org

APPROVED OMB-0938-0999 FORM CMS-1500 (08-05)

Figure 13.1 The CMS-1500 Claim Form

The elements in the 837 claim are transmitted in the five major sections, or levels, of the claim:

1. Provider
2. Subscriber (guarantor/insured/policyholder) and patient (the subscriber or another person)

3. Payer
4. Claim details
5. Services

These levels are set up as a hierarchy, with the provider at the top, so that when the claim is sent electronically, data elements have to be sent only when they do not repeat previous data. For example, when the provider is sending a batch of claims, provider information is sent once for the entire batch. When the subscriber and the patient are the same, the patient information is not needed. But if the subscriber and the patient are different people, information about both is transmitted.

Figure 13.2 shows a claim in CMS-1500 format, and Figure 13.3 shows the same claim in 837 format.

> **TIP**
>
> **Physician Claims: The 837P**
>
> The HIPAA transaction for electronic claims generated by physicians is called the HIPAA 837P, for professional services. The hospital version of the claim is called the 837I (institutional services), and dentists use a version called the 837D (dental services).

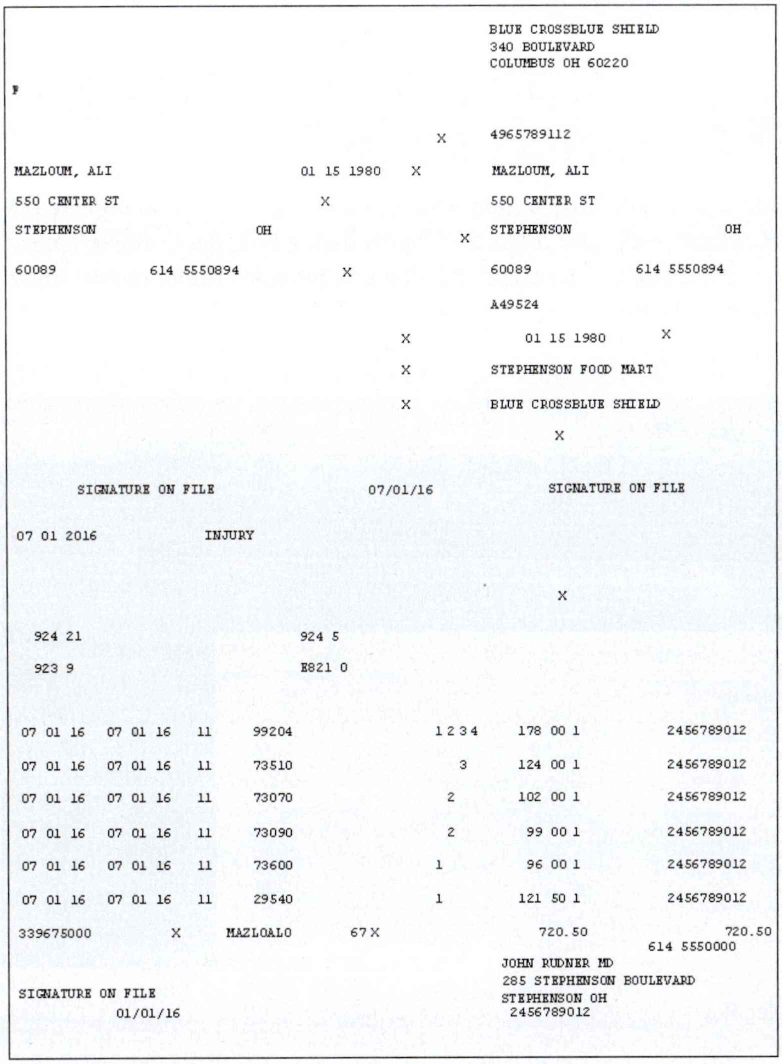

BLUE CROSSBLUE SHIELD
340 BOULEVARD
COLUMBUS OH 60220

X 4965789112

MAZLOUM, ALI 01 15 1980 X MAZLOUM, ALI
550 CENTER ST X 550 CENTER ST
STEPHENSON OH X STEPHENSON OH
60089 614 5550894 X 60089 614 5550894
A49524
X 01 15 1980 X
X STEPHENSON FOOD MART
X BLUE CROSSBLUE SHIELD
X

SIGNATURE ON FILE 07/01/16 SIGNATURE ON FILE

07 01 2016 INJURY

X

924 21 924 5
923 9 E821 0

07 01 16 07 01 16 11 99204 1234 178 00 1 2456789012
07 01 16 07 01 16 11 73510 3 124 00 1 2456789012
07 01 16 07 01 16 11 73070 2 102 00 1 2456789012
07 01 16 07 01 16 11 73090 2 99 00 1 2456789012
07 01 16 07 01 16 11 73600 1 96 00 1 2456789012
07 01 16 07 01 16 11 29540 1 121 50 1 2456789012

339675000 X MAZLOALO 67X 720.50 720.50
614 5550000
JOHN RUDNER MD
285 STEPHENSON BOULEVARD
SIGNATURE ON FILE STEPHENSON OH
01/01/16 2456789012

Figure 13.2 Sample Claim in CMS-1500 Format

```
ISA*00*    *01*CYCTRANS*ZZ*P123456*ZZ*CLAIMSCH*101108*0300*U*00401*000000001*1*P*:~
GS*HC*P123456*ECGCLAIMS*20101108*0300*1*X*004010X098A1~ST*837*0001~BHT*0019*00*11A
AAA*20101108*0300*CH~REF*87*004010X098A1~NM1*41*2*FAMILY CARE
CLINIC*****46*123456123456~PER*IC*JOHN SMITH*TE*5555555555~NM1*40*2*RELAY
HEALTH*****46*4300~HL*1*1*20*1~NM1*85*2*FAMILY CARE CLINIC*****24*033987562~N3*285
STEPHENSON BOULEVARD~N4*STEPHENSON*OH*60089~HL*1*1*22*1~SBR*P*18*A49524*BLUE
CROSS/BLUE SHIELD*****BL~NM1*IL*1*MAZLOUM*ALI****MI*4965789112~N3*550 CENTER ST.*APT
1B~N4*STEPHENSON*OH*60089~DMG*D8*19800115*M~NM1*PR*2*BLUE CROSS/BLUE
SHIELD*****PI*45678~N3*340
BOULEVARD~N4*COLUMBUS*OH*60220~CLM*67*720.5***11::1*Y*A*Y*Y*B~DTP*454*D8*20160701
~DTP*304*D8*20160701~DTP*431*D8*20160701~HI*BK:92421*BF:9239*BF:9245*BF:E8210~LX*1~SV
1*HC:99204*178*UN*1***1:2:3:4**Y~DTP*472*D8*20160701~REF*6R*600~LX*1~SV1*HC:73510*124
*UN*1***3**Y~DTP*472*D8*20160701~REF*6R*601~LX*1~SV1*HC:73070*102*UN*1***2**Y~DTP*4
72*D8*20160701~REF*6R*602~LX*1~SV1*HC:73090*99*UN*1***2**Y~DTP*472*D8*20160701~REF*
6R*603~LX*1~SV1*HC:73600*96*UN*1***1**Y~DTP*472*D8*20160701~REF*6R*604~LX*1~SV1*HC:
29540*121.5*UN*1***1**Y~DTP*472*D8*20160701~REF*6R*605~SE*9999*0001~GE*9999*1~
IEA*9999*000000001~
```


Figure 13.3 Sample Claim in 837 Format

THINKING IT THROUGH 13.1

What are the advantages of transmitting electronic claims? Are there any potential disadvantages?

13.2 Creating Claims

Claims are created after coding and billing compliance are completed. Most EHR systems will have a Create Claims dialog box. An example appears in Figure 13.4. The Create Claims dialog box provides filters to customize the creation of claims.

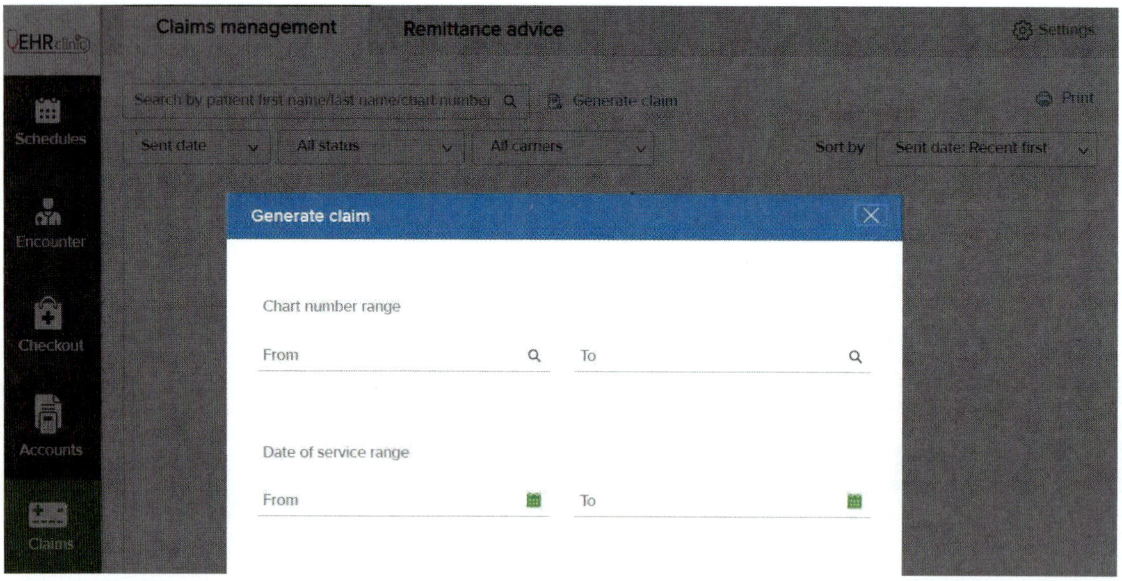

Figure 13.4 Create Claims Dialog Box

Claim Filters

A **filter** is a condition that data must meet to be selected. For example, claims can be created for services performed between the first and the fifteenth of the month. In this case, the filter is the condition that services must have been performed between the first and fifteenth of the month. Transactions that meet this criterion are included in the selection; transactions that do not fall within the date range are not included. Filters can be used to create claims for a specific patient, for a specific insurance carrier, and for transactions that exceed a certain dollar amount, among others. The following filters can be applied within the Create Claims dialog box.

filter a condition that data must meet to be selected

Transaction Dates The Transaction Dates boxes are used to specify the starting and ending dates for which claims will be created. If the boxes are left blank, transactions for all dates will be included.

Chart Numbers The Chart Number boxes are used to enter the starting and ending chart numbers for which claims will be created. If the boxes are left blank, all chart numbers will be included.

Primary Insurance The carrier code for the insurance company is entered in the Primary Insurance box. If claims are being sent to a clearinghouse, more than one insurance carrier code can be entered. When more than one code is entered, commas must be placed between the codes. If claims are being sent directly to the carrier, only that carrier's code is entered.

Billing Codes The billing code is entered in the Billing Codes box. If more than one code is entered, commas must be placed between the codes.

Case Indicator If case indicators are used to classify patients (such as by type of illness for workers' compensation cases), the case indicator can be listed in the Case Indicator box. If more than one indicator is entered, commas must be placed between them.

Location Sometimes a sort is needed by location, such as all procedures done at a hospital. The location code is entered in the Location box. If more than one code is entered, commas must be placed between the codes.

Assigned The radio buttons in the Provider box indicate whether the provider is the assigned or attending provider. The assigned provider is the patient's regular physician. In the box to the right of the radio button, the provider code is entered. If more than one code is entered, commas must be placed between the codes.

Attending The attending provider is someone other than the patient's regular physician who provides treatment to the patient. In the box to the right of the radio button, the provider code is entered.

Enter amount The dollar amount entered in this box is the minimum total amount required for a case before a claim can be created.

Any box that is not filled in will default to include all data, and all claims will be included. When all necessary information has been entered, clicking the Create button creates the claims. These will process through the claim scrubber for edits before submission to the payer.

EXERCISE 13.1

Create an Insurance Claim EHRclinic

Create an insurance claim for a patient, and generate a batch of claims using filters.

Your instructor may assign this exercise to you in Connect. Exercise steps and EHRclinic Help Guides can be downloaded at www.mhhe.com/pmehr2.

13.3 Methods of Claim Submission

clearinghouse company that processes electronic health information and executes electronic transactions such as insurance verification and claim submission for providers

Once claims have been created and checked through the claim scrubber, they are ready to be transmitted. Practices handle the transmission of electronic claims in a variety of ways. The three most common methods of transmitting claims are direct transmission to the payer, direct data entry, and transmission through a clearinghouse. **Clearinghouses** accept claim data from providers in nonstandard formats and translate them into the standard format required by the payer. A practice may choose to use a clearinghouse to transmit all claims, or it may use a combination of methods. For example, it may send claims directly to Medicare, Medicaid, and a few major commercial payers and use a clearinghouse to send claims to other payers.

Direct to the Payer

In the direct transmission approach, providers and payers exchange transactions directly without using a clearinghouse. Claims are created in the PM/EHR, and a connection is made to the payer's database. Once connected, the claims are transmitted. In this approach, the medical practice must supply all the HIPAA data elements and follow specific EDI formatting rules. The practice may also have to purchase special software that can communicate with the payer's system.

Direct Data Entry

Direct data entry (DDE) is a method of claim transmission in which a member of the provider's billing staff manually enters claims into an application on the payer's website. Using DDE, the medical practice logs into a secure website hosted by the payer. Once connected, a staff member from the medical practice enters the claim information into an electronic form on the payer's site. Most practices that use a PM/EHR or a PM do not use DDE, since it is inefficient and susceptible to keyboarding errors.

Clearinghouse

Most providers send their electronic claims to a clearinghouse for a number of reasons. While all health care claims must use HIPAA transactions and code sets, each payer has its own set of claim edits and formatting conventions. These are published in what is known as a **companion guide.** Since payers publish their own guides, it would be difficult for a billing specialist to know the rules of each payer. Instead, clearinghouses perform this function. In practices with a large volume of claims, it is not practical to send electronic claims to each payer; when a clearinghouse is used, claims can be sent in one batch to one location.

companion guide guide published by a payer that lists its own set of claim edits and formatting conventions

clean claim a claim that has no edits and can go directly to the payer

> **TIP**
>
> Disclosing Information for Payment Purposes
>
> Under HIPAA, covered entities such as physician practices may disclose patients' PHI for payment purposes. For example, a provider may disclose a patient's name to a financial institution in order to cash a check or to a clearinghouse to initiate electronic transactions.

At the clearinghouse, claims go through a series of edits. Then, a report indicating which claims have passed and/or failed these edits is sent to the provider. Claims that fail must be corrected and resubmitted to the clearinghouse before they can be sent to the payer. Claims that have not failed edits are called **clean claims.**

Once the claims have cleared the clearinghouse's edits, they are sent to the payer. Rather than receive claims directly, some payers also use a clearinghouse. In these instances, the provider's clearinghouse transmits to the payer's clearinghouse. The payer's clearinghouse processes the claims before it sends them to the payer.

When the claim reaches the payer, additional editing is performed, and a status report is generated indicating which claims were accepted and which were rejected. This report is then sent to the clearinghouse, which forwards the information to the provider. Accepted claims are sent to the payer's adjudication system for payment or denial determination. Rejected claims must be corrected and resubmitted before they can be processed.

> **TIP**
>
> Clearinghouses
>
> There are many electronic claim and transaction processing firms in the health care industry. Some of the largest are RelayHealth, Emdeon, Navicure, Availity, and Gateway.

Most clearinghouses charge fees for their services. Some charge a flat fee per month regardless of the number of claims processed, while others charge on a per-claim basis.

The typical flow of a claim that is ready for transmission from a medical practice to a payer is shown in Figure 13.5.

Primary Versus Secondary and Tertiary Claims

When a patient is covered by more than one health plan, the initial claim is transmitted to the patient's primary health plan. For example, if patients are covered by Medicare and Medicaid, their claims are first submitted to

Figure 13.5 Claim Flow Using a Clearinghouse

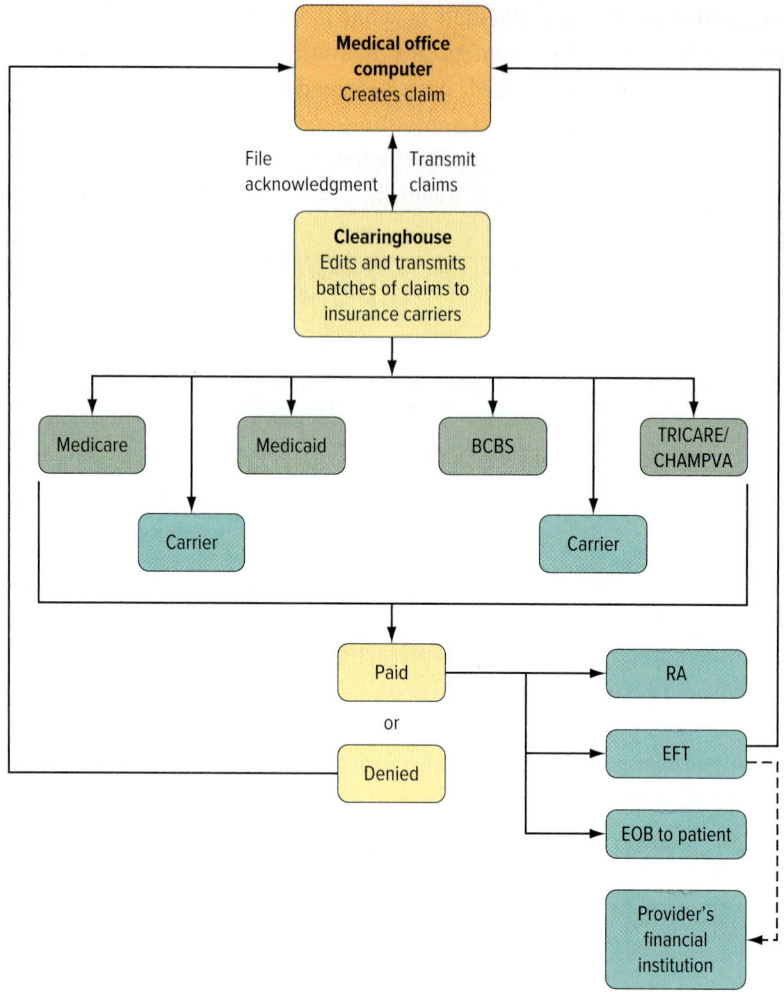

crossover claim claim billed to Medicare and then submitted to Medicaid

Medicare and then to Medicaid. Claims billed to Medicare and then submitted to Medicaid are called **crossover claims.** The majority of Medicare carriers automatically forward crossover claims to the state Medicaid payer. Medicaid is referred to as the "payer of last resort," meaning that under federal policy all other avenues for payment must be followed first before Medicaid will pay a claim.

Some insurance carriers that are secondary to Medicare are classified as complementary crossover carriers. When these carriers are involved, Medicare information about the secondary insurance carrier is already in the Medicare system.

THINKING IT THROUGH 13.2

Why would a medical practice pay to use a clearinghouse for sending electronic claims when the practice could send claims directly to the payer for free?

13.4 Primary, Secondary, and Tertiary Claims

An important step comes before the claims are actually transmitted: checking the claim. Most EHRs provide a way for the billing specialist to review claims for accuracy. This is usually accomplished by using the claim edit feature, which allows claims to be reviewed and edited before they are submitted for payment. The more problems that can be spotted and solved before claims are sent to insurance carriers, the sooner the practice will receive payment.

When a claim is selected, it can be edited by clicking an Edit button, or the claim itself can be double-clicked. Usually this is found in a claim dialog box (see an example in Figure 13.6). In this area you will see the claim number, the date the claim was created, the chart number, the patient's name, and the case number. This information sometimes cannot be edited, per each EHR.

This area is where you will see the payers the claim will be submitted to. Patients will have a primary insurance carrier. Some patients will have a secondary insurance carrier, and some may even have a tertiary payer.

Primary Insurance Carrier

In the EHR you will be able to see the primary insurance carrier. Figure 13.6 shows an example of the Carrier 1 view. This displays information about claims being submitted to the patient's primary insurance carrier. The following boxes are usually listed in this area:

Claim Status The Claim Status box indicates the status of a particular claim: Hold, Ready to send, Sent, Rejected, Challenge, Alert, Done, and Pending.

Billing Method The Billing Method box displays two choices: Paper and Electronic. The button that describes the billing method should be clicked.

Initial Billing Date If the claim was sent more than once, this box automatically displays the initial billing date.

Batch If the claim has been assigned to a batch, the batch number is displayed.

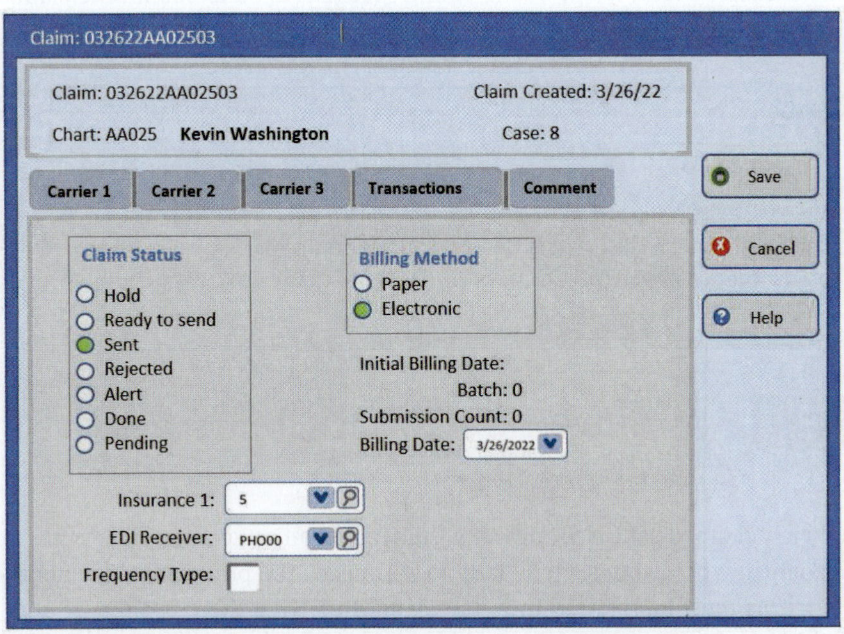

Figure 13.6 Example of a Claim Dialog Box

Submission Count The Submission Count area lists the number of claims submitted.

Billing Date The Billing Date box lists the most recent date the bill was sent (if the claim was submitted more than once).

Insurance 1 The Insurance 1 box lists a patient's primary insurance carrier. This is the patient's main insurance, and the claim must be submitted to this carrier or the claim may be rejected.

Frequency Type This field is used with some insurance carriers when sending claims electronically. Allowed entries in this field are:

1–Original (admission through discharge claim)
6–Corrected (adjustment of prior claim)
10–Replacement (replacement of prior claim)
8–Void (voiding/cancellation of prior claim)

Secondary and Tertiary Carriers

The Carrier 2 and Carrier 3 tabs display information about claims being submitted to a patient's secondary (Carrier 2) and tertiary (Carrier 3) insurance carriers. A secondary insurance carrier is a second insurance plan under which the patient may have coverage. Once the primary has processed the claim, the secondary insurance will cover the balance or another portion of the services. The tertiary insurance carrier is a third insurance plan the patient may have. This is rare, but occasionally it can occur.

The tabs will include the same as the boxes in the Carrier 1 tab, with the exception of the Claim Status box and the Frequency Type box. In the Carrier 2 and Carrier 3 tabs, there is usually no Pending button in the Claim Status box, and there is no Frequency Type box. Otherwise the three tabs are the same in the EHR.

Once the primary insurance carrier has made a decision on the claim, some insurance carriers will send to the secondary and tertiary carriers. If this does not occur, it will be the billing specialist's job to submit the claims to the secondary, then the tertiary insurance carriers.

> **TIP**
>
> **Dropping to Paper**
>
> The phrase "dropping to paper" describes a situation in which a CMS-1500 paper claim needs to be printed and sent to a payer. Some practices, for instance, have a policy of doing this when a claim has been transmitted electronically twice but receipt of the claim is not acknowledged.

13.5 Sending Electronic Claim Attachments

When a claim is sent electronically, sometimes an attachment is needed to accompany the claim, such as radiology films or the provider's documentation. This must be referred to in the claim. In EHRs, there is a report area.

This is called the EDI Report area; it is found within the Diagnosis area. This is used to indicate to the payer that an attachment will accompany the claim and how the attachment will be transmitted.

> **TIP**
>
> **997 Functional Acknowledgment**
>
> When a payer receives a claim transmission, whether from a practice or from a clearinghouse, it sends an electronic acknowledgment of the file transmission, known as the 997 Functional Acknowledgment. This is not a standard HIPAA transaction, but it is used to report that a transaction has been received by the payer. The 997 also lists any additional errors found as a result of edits.

EDI Notes

The EDI Note area can be used for entering extra information for procedures and diagnoses that might be required by the patient's insurance carriers to process the electronic claim.

EDI Report

The EDI Report section can contain three boxes:

Report Type Code This box is used to record the report type code–a two-digit code that indicates the type of report being attached. For example, DG is the code for a diagnostic report. Other codes include:

107	Support data for verification
REFERRAL	To indicate a completed referral form
AS	Admission summary
B2	Prescription
B3	Physician order
B4	Referral form
CT	Certification
DA	Dental models
DG	Diagnostic report
DS	Discharge summary
EB	Explanation of benefits (coordination of benefits or Medicare secondary payer)
MT	Models
NN	Nursing notes
OB	Operative note
OZ	Support data for claim
PN	Physician therapy notes
PO	Prosthetics or orthotic certification
PZ	Physical therapy certification
RB	Radiology films

RR Radiology reports

RT Report of tests and analysis report

Report Transmission Code This area is used to record the report transmission code, a two-character code that indicates the means by which the report will be transmitted to the payer (for example, via mail, email, or fax). Possible codes include:

AA Available on request at provider site. This means that the paperwork is not being sent with the claim at this time. Instead, it is available to the payer (or appropriate entity) at its request.

BM By mail.

EL Electronically only. Indicates that the attachment is being transmitted in a separate X12 functional group.

EM Email.

FX By fax.

Attachment Control Number This box contains the attachment's reference number (up to seven digits, assigned by the practice). This number is required if the transmission code is anything other than AA.

THINKING IT THROUGH 13.3

What is the purpose of the information entered in the EDI Notes and EDI Reports fields? If these fields were not completed, what might happen to a claim with an attachment?

EXERCISE 13.2

Submit Insurance Claims

EHRclinic

A batch of insurance claims has been generated in EHRclinic. Submit the claims to the insurance carrier.

Your instructor may assign this exercise to you in Connect. Exercise steps and EHRclinic Help Guides can be downloaded at www.mhhe.com/pmehr2.

13.6 Claim Adjudication

adjudication series of steps that determine whether a claim should be paid

When the health plan receives claims from the practice, it issues an electronic response to the sender showing that the transmission has been successful. Each claim then undergoes a checking process known as **adjudication,** in which the health plan follows these steps to judge how the claim should be paid:

1. Initial processing
2. Automated review
3. Manual review
4. Determination
5. Payment

Initial Processing

Each claim's data elements are checked by the payer's front-end claims processing system. Paper claims and any paper attachments are date-stamped and entered into the payer's computer system, either by data-entry personnel or by the use of a scanning system. Initial processing might find problems such as the following:

- The patient's name, plan identification number, or place of service code is wrong.
- The diagnosis code is missing or is not valid for the date of service.
- The patient is not the correct sex for a reported gender-specific procedure code.

Claims with errors or simple mistakes are rejected, and the payer transmits instructions to the sender to fix and resubmit them. Such requests from the payer must be answered as quickly as possible by supplying the correct information and, if necessary, submitting another claim. The actual adjudication process begins when a clean claim is accepted by the payer for processing.

Automated Review

Payers' computer systems then apply edits that reflect their payment policies. For example, a Medicare claim is subject to the Correct Coding Initiative (CCI) edits (see Chapter 11). The automated review checks for the following:

Patient eligibility for benefits Is the patient eligible for the services that are billed?

Time limits for filing claims Is the claim sent within the payer's time limits for filing claims?

Preauthorization and referral Are valid preauthorization or referral numbers present as required under the payer's policies?

Duplicate dates of service Is this claim billing for a service on this date that has already been adjudicated?

Noncovered services Are the billed services covered under the patient's policy?

Valid code linkages Are the diagnosis and procedure codes properly linked for medical necessity?

Bundled codes Have surgical code bundling rules and global periods been followed?

Medical review Are the charges for services not medically necessary or over the frequency limits of the plan? The payer's medical director and other professional medical staff have a medical review program to ensure that providers give patients the most appropriate care in the most cost-effective manner. Medical review edits are based on the guidelines of the medical review program.

Utilization review Are the hospital-based health care services delivered to a member of a plan appropriate?

Concurrent care If two or more providers' work is being billed, was it medically necessary to have both treat the patient?

THINKING IT THROUGH 13.4

What effect does performing an edit to check claims before transmission to a health plan have on the speed of claim adjudication?

Manual Review

suspended claim status when the payer is developing the claim

development process of gathering information to adjudicate a claim

determination payer's decision about the benefits due for a claim

medical necessity denial refusal by a plan to pay for a procedure that does not meet its medical necessity criteria

If the automated review finds problems, the claim is **suspended** and set aside for **development**–the term used by payers to indicate that more information is needed for claim processing. Such claims are sent to the medical review department, where a claim examiner reviews them. The examiner may ask the provider for clinical documentation to check:

- Where the service took place
- Whether the treatments were appropriate and a logical outcome of the facts and conditions shown in the medical record
- That the services provided were accurately reported

Determination

For each service line on a claim, the payer makes a payment **determination**–a decision whether to (1) pay it, (2) deny it, (3) hold it for further processing, or (4) pay it at a reduced level. If the service falls within normal guidelines, it will be paid. If it is not reimbursable, the item on the claim is denied. A **medical necessity denial** may result from a lack of a clear, correct linkage between the diagnosis and the procedure.

Payment

If payment is due, the payer sends it to the provider or to the provider's financial institution along with an electronic or paper document explaining the items that were paid. This remittance process is discussed in Chapter 14.

13.7 Monitoring Claims Status

Practices closely track their accounts receivable (A/R)–the money that is owed for services rendered–using the PM/EHR. The accounts receivable is made up of payments due from payers and from patients. For this reason, after claims have been accepted for processing by payers, their status is monitored.

Claim Status

Monitoring claims during adjudication requires two types of information. The first is the amount of time the payer is allowed to take to respond to the claim, and the second is how long the claim has been in process.

Timely Payment of Insurance Claims

Sometimes insurance carriers dispute claims. When a carrier contests a claim or delays payment because more information is needed, providers often are not given notice in a timely manner. When further documentation is requested and the physician provides the information, a health plan can further delay payment by asking for additional information or clarification. Resubmitting rejected claims is a time-consuming process, resulting in increased practice expenses and more delay in payment.

Most states have enacted prompt payment laws to ensure that claims are paid in a timely manner. State **prompt payment laws** mandate a time period known as **claim turnaround time** within which clean claims must be paid, and they call for financial penalties to be levied against late payers.

If a clean claim is not paid within the allotted time frame, the payer should be notified in writing that payment has not been received according to applicable prompt payment laws. Practices should also request written explanations of all claim delays, partial payments, and denials. If satisfaction is not achieved, the appropriate state or federal regulatory agency can be notified of the violation.

prompt payment laws state laws that mandate a time period within which clean claims must be paid; if they are not, financial penalties are levied against the payer

claim turnaround time time period in which a health plan must process a claim

aging classification of accounts receivable by length of time

insurance aging report a report that lists how long a payer has taken to respond to insurance claims

Aging

The other factor in claim follow-up is **aging**—how long a payer has had the claim. The EHR is used to generate an **insurance aging report** that lists the claims transmitted on each day and how long they have been in process with the payer. A typical report, shown in Figure 13.7, shows claims that were sent fewer than thirty days ago, between thirty and sixty days ago, and so on. With the report, it is easy to determine which claims require follow-up. Most practices follow up on claims that are aged less than thirty days in seven to fourteen days.

Primary Insurance Aging Summary

October 31, 2022

Date of Service	Procedure	-Past- 0 to 30	-Past- 31 to 60	-Past- 61 to 90	-Past- 91 to 120	-Past- 121+	Total Balance
McGraw-Hill MedMark							555-620-1975
Claim 69721	Initial Billing Date: 9/23/2022		Last Billing Date: 10/14/2022				
	Insurance Totals:	$0.00	$160.00	$0.00	$0.00	$0.00	$160.00
Ameri-Access							555-315-6607
Claim 63317	Initial Billing Date: 6/30/2022		Last Billing Date: 10/14/2022				
Claim 69721	Initial Billing Date: 8/12/2022		Last Billing Date: 10/14/2022				
	Insurance Totals:	$0.00	$0.00	$465.00	$0.00	$655.00	$1,120.00

Figure 13.7 Primary Insurance Aging Report

> **TIP**
>
> **ANSI ASC X12 5010 Format**
>
> On January 1, 2012, a new version of the standards required to submit electronic transactions took effect. The ASC X12 Version 4010A standards, which had been in place since 2002, were replaced by the ASC X12 Version 5010 standards. The new standards were required to accommodate ICD-10-CM and also provide improvements to a number of electronic transactions.

HIPAA Health Care Claim Status Inquiry/Response

HIPAA X12 276/277 Health Care Claim Status Inquiry/Response electronic format used to ask payers about claims

claim status category codes used to report the status group for a claim

pending claim status in which the payer is waiting for information before making a payment decision

claim status codes used to provide a detailed answer to a claim status inquiry

The status of a claim can also be determined at any time by sending an electronic inquiry to the payer. The **HIPAA X12 276/277 Health Care Claim Status Inquiry/Response** is the standard electronic transaction to obtain the current status of a claim during the adjudication process. The inquiry is the 276, and the response returned by the payer is the 277. Some EHRs track how many days claims have been unpaid and automatically send a claim status inquiry after a certain number of days. For example, if a particular payer pays claims on the twentieth day, the program transmits a 276 for any unpaid claims aged twenty-one days.

The HIPAA 277 transaction from the payer uses **claim status category codes** for the main types of responses:

- *A* codes are an acknowledgment that the claim has been received.
- *P* codes indicate that a claim is **pending,** that is, that the payer is waiting for information before making a payment decision.
- *F* codes indicate that a claim has been finalized.
- *R* codes indicate that a request for more information has been sent.
- *E* codes indicate that an error has occurred in transmission; usually these claims need to be resent.

These codes are further detailed by **claim status codes**, as shown in Table 13.2.

Working with Health Plans

Ensuring that claims are processed as quickly as possible requires being familiar with payers' claim-processing procedures, including:

- The timetable for submitting corrected claims, as well as for filing secondary claims (usually a period of time from the date of payment by the primary payer)
- How to resubmit corrected claims that are denied for missing or incorrect data (some payers have an online or automated telephone procedure that can be used to resubmit a claim after missing information has been supplied)
- How to handle requests for additional documentation required by the payer

Requests for information should be answered as quickly as possible and should be courteous and complete.

TABLE 13.2	Selected Claim Status Codes
1	For more detailed information, see remittance advice.
2	More detailed information in letter.
3	Claim has been adjudicated and is awaiting payment cycle.
4	This is a subsequent request for information from the original request.
5	This is a final request for information.
6	Balance is due from the subscriber.
7	Claim may be reconsidered at a future date.
9	No payment will be made for this claim.
12	One or more originally submitted procedure codes have been combined.
15	One or more originally submitted procedure codes have been modified.
16	Claim/encounter has been forwarded to entity.
29	Subscriber and policy number/contract number mismatched.
30	Subscriber and subscriber ID mismatched.
31	Subscriber and policyholder name mismatched.
32	Subscriber and policy number/contract number not found.
33	Subscriber and subscriber ID not found.

THINKING IT THROUGH 13.5

What action from the health plan would you expect if notified that a claim response is claim status code 3? Code 12?

EXERCISE 13.3

Correct Claim Errors for Resubmission

EHRclinic

An insurance carrier sent a remittance advice (RA) to notify Trilogy Family Care Center that a procedure on a patient's claim was denied due to lack of medical necessity and improper code linkage. Correct the error in EHRclinic and resubmit the claim.

Your instructor may assign this exercise to you in Connect. Exercise steps and EHRclinic Help Guides can be downloaded at www.mhhe.com/pmehr2.

chapter 13 summary

KEY TERMS

adjudication
aging
claim status codes
claim status category codes
claim turnaround time
clean claim
clearinghouse
CMS-1500 (08/05) claim
companion guide
crossover claim
data elements
determination
development
filter
HIPAA X12 276/277 Health Care Claim Status Inquiry/Response
HIPAA X12 837 Health Care Claim
insurance aging report
medical necessity denial
National Uniform Claim Committee (NUCC)
pending
prompt payment laws
suspended
timely filing

LEARNING OUTCOME	KEY CONCEPTS/EXAMPLES
13.1 Describe health care claims.	Health insurance claims are created for patients with insurance coverage. The insurance claim is the most important document for correct reimbursement from health care plans. Claims communicate information about a patient's diagnosis, procedures, and charges to a payer.
13.2 Discuss how to create a claim.	Claims are created after coding is completed and after billing compliance. Filters are used to create the claim. A filter can be used to create claims for a specific patient, for a specific insurance carrier, and for transactions that exceed a certain dollar amount, among others. This is all completed within the PM/EHR.
13.3 Describe the different methods to submit claims.	The three most common methods of transmitting claims are direct transmission to the payer, direct data entry, and transmission through a clearinghouse.
13.4 Identify primary, secondary, and tertiary claims.	Patients can have primary insurance, secondary insurance, and sometimes tertiary insurance. This can be identified in the claim dialog box. There will be tabs for Carrier 1, 2, or 3. Here you can identify the claim and what insurance it should be submitted to.
13.5 Explain how to send an electronic claim attachment.	Sometimes additional information is needed for adjudication. When an attachment is added to the claim, it is noted on the claim. The area is called the EDI Report area, which is found within the Diagnosis area. This is used to indicate to the payer that an attachment will accompany the claim and how the attachment will be transmitted. There are code sets used to indicate how and what will be sent in addition to the claim.

LEARNING OUTCOME	KEY CONCEPTS/EXAMPLES
13.6 Explain claim adjudication.	Each claim undergoes a checking process known as adjudication. The health plan follows these steps to judge how the claim should be paid: 1. Initial processing 2. Automated review 3. Manual review 4. Determination 5. Payment
13.7 Discuss how to monitor claim status.	Monitoring claims during adjudication requires two types of information. The first is the amount of time the payer is allowed to take to respond to the claim, and the second is how long the claim has been in process.

chapter 13 review

MATCHING QUESTIONS

Match the key terms with their definitions.

______ 1. *[LO 13.7]* claim turnaround time
______ 2. *[LO 13.3]* crossover claims
______ 3. *[LO 13.6, 13.7]* adjudication
______ 4. *[LO 13.2]* filter
______ 5. *[LO 13.1]* timely filing
______ 6. *[LO 13.6]* determination
______ 7. *[LO 13.7]* pending
______ 8. *[LO 13.1]* data elements
______ 9. *[LO 13.7]* aging
______ 10. *[LO 13.6]* development

a. Claim status during adjudication when the payer is waiting for information from the submitter.

b. A condition that data must meet to be selected.

c. A payer's decision about the benefits due for a claim.

d. The smallest units of information in a HIPAA transaction, such as a person's name.

e. The time period in which a health plan is obligated to process a claim.

f. The term used by payers to indicate that more information is needed for claim processing.

g. The rules that specify the number of days after the date of service that the practice has to file the claim.

h. Classification of accounts receivable by the length of time an account is due.

i. Claims that are billed to Medicare and then submitted to Medicaid.

j. The process followed by health plans to examine claims and determine benefits.

MULTIPLE CHOICE QUESTIONS

Select the letter that best completes the statement or answers the question.

1. *[LO 13.1]* The HIPAA standard transaction for paper claims is known as the ________.
   a. HIPAA X12 837 Health Care Claim
   b. HIPAA claim
   c. CMS-1500 (08/05) claim
   d. HIPAA X12 276/277 Health Care Claim Status Inquiry/Response

2. *[LO 13.2]* Filters can be used to create claims to meet multiple criteria; which of the following is NOT a filter criterion to generate a claim?
   a. by patient
   b. by insurance
   c. by date range
   d. by diagnosis

3. *[LO 13.2]* A ________ is a condition that data must meet to be selected.
   a. transaction standard
   b. filter
   c. data element
   d. crossover claim
4. *[LO 13.3]* The ________ method of submitting electronic claims requires manual entry of data on the payer's website.
   a. clearinghouse
   b. direct to the payer
   c. direct data entry
   d. all of the above
5. *[LO 13.5]* The EDI Note area can be used for entering extra information for procedures and diagnoses. What box is used to record a two-digit code that indicates the type of report being attached?
   a. Claim Management box
   b. Claim Edit Code box
   c. Report Type Code box
   d. Report Transmission Code box
6. *[LO 13.4]* The ________ box indicates the status of a particular claim: Hold, Ready to send, Sent, Rejected, Challenge, Alert, Done, and Pending.
   a. Batch
   b. Submission count
   c. Billing method
   d. Claim Status
7. *[LO 13.3]* Claims billed to Medicare and then submitted to Medicaid are called ________.
   a. HIPAA claims
   b. CMS-1500 (08/05) claims
   c. crossover claims
   d. all of the above
8. *[LO 13.6, 13.7]* Each claim undergoes a checking process known as ________, made up of the steps the health plan follows to judge how it should be paid.
   a. adjudication
   b. aging
   c. development
   d. pending
9. *[LO 13.6]* A ________ may result from the lack of a clear, correct linkage between the diagnosis and the procedure.
   a. determination
   b. medical necessity denial
   c. filter
   d. crossover claim
10. *[LO 13.7]* The ________ is the standard electronic transaction to obtain the current status of a claim during the adjudication process.
    a. HIPAA X12 837 Health Care Claim
    b. HIPAA claim
    c. CMS-1500 (08/05) claim
    d. HIPAA X12 276/277 Health Care Claim Status Inquiry/Response

SHORT ANSWER QUESTIONS

Define the following abbreviations.

1. *[LO 13.1]* NUCC ________________________
2. *[LO 13.1]* HIPAA X12 276/277 ________________________
3. *[LO 13.1]* HIPAA X12 837 ________________________

APPLYING YOUR KNOWLEDGE

Answer the questions below in the space provided.

13.1 *[LO 13.1]* Why do you think health plans have timely filing requirements?

____

____

13.2 *[LO 13.7]* Why do medical practices monitor the status of the claims they submit?

____

____

13.3 *[LO 13.1]* Why are there timely response limits on health plans to respond to claims?

____

____

13.4 *[LO 13.3]* What are the advantages of submitting claims via each of the following methods?

a. direct data entry

____

b. directly to the payer

____

c. clearinghouse

____

13.5 *[LO 13.4]* What would a reason be for a patient to have a tertiary claim?

____

____

chapter 14

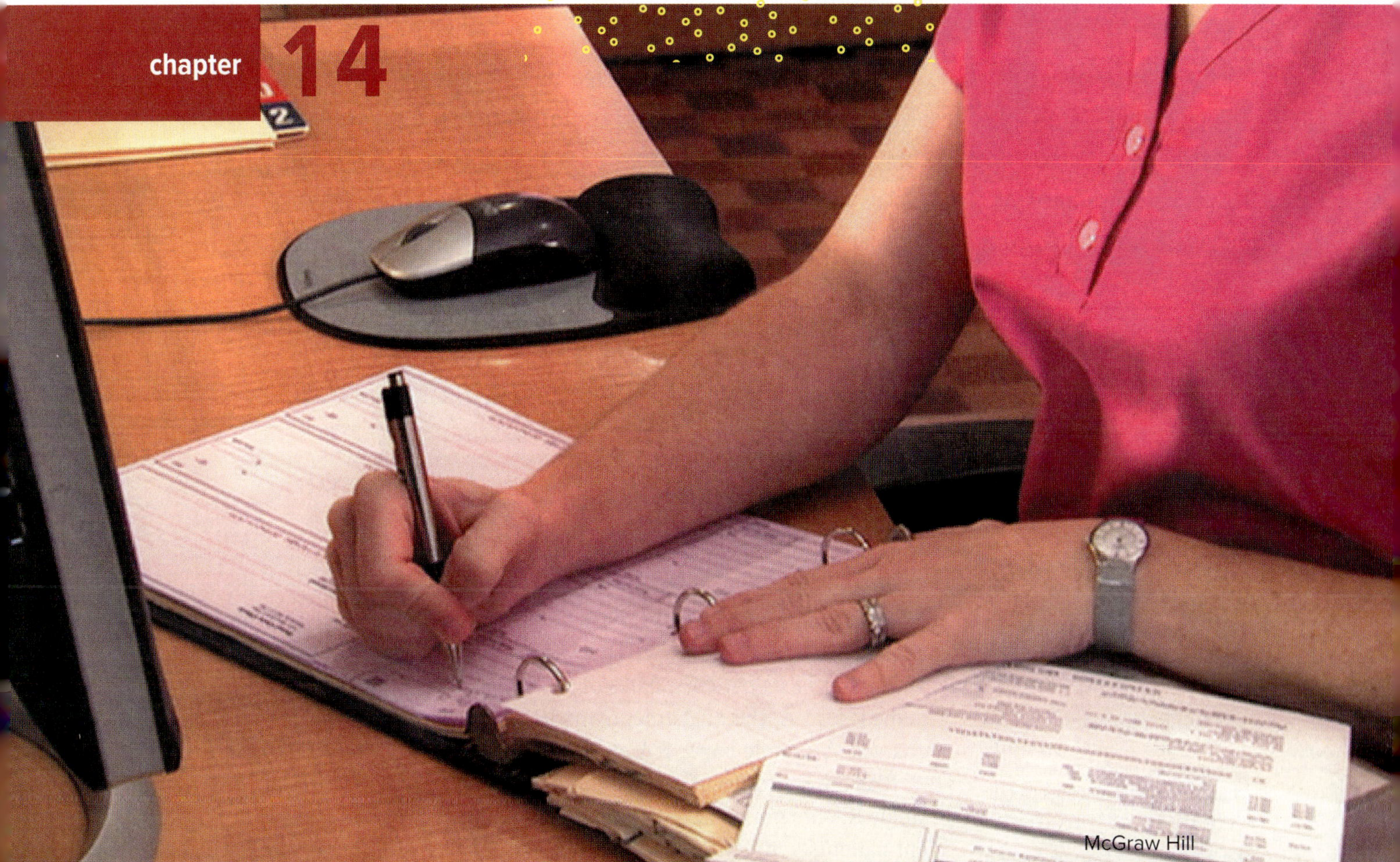
McGraw Hill

Posting Payments and Creating Statements

LEARNING OUTCOMES

When you finish this chapter, you will be able to:

14.1 Describe working with the electronic remittance advice (ERA).

14.2 Discuss posting insurance payments for fee-for-service and capitation plans.

14.3 Describe appeals, postpayment audits, overpayments, and billing secondary payers.

14.4 Describe how to create statements.

14.5 Explain how to record patient payments.

Claim Adjudication

Trilogy Family Care Center received an electronic remittance advice (ERA) from McGraw-Hill Healthmark insurance. All of the claims listed on the ERA were paid in full, except for Dominic Rizzo's.

Upon reviewing the EHR, the coder determines that Dominic's claim for a lipid profile was denied with a reason code indicating that the service is not covered for patients under age 35. Dominic, however, is 43 years old.

Considering this scenario, what do you think probably happened to cause the claim to be denied with that reason code? What are the coder's next steps? How could denial of this claim have been prevented?

14.1 Working with the Electronic Remittance Advice (ERA)

remittance advice (RA) document describing a payment resulting from a claim adjudication

electronic remittance advice (ERA) electronic document that lists patients, dates of service, charges, and the amounts paid or denied by the insurance carrier

X12 835 Remittance Advice Transaction electronic transaction for payment explanation

claim control number unique number assigned to a claim by the sender

autoposting software feature enabling automatic entry of payments from a remittance advice

Once a claim has been received and accepted for adjudication, the health plan determines the payment it will make for each charge. The payer then generates a remittance advice (RA) and sends it to the provider. A **remittance advice (RA)** lists patients, dates of service, charges, and the amounts paid or denied—that is, the adjustments made by the insurance carrier to the billed charges. A sample paper RA appears in Figure 14.1.

RAs cover groups of claims, not just a single claim. The claims paid on a single RA are not consecutive or logically grouped; they are usually for different patients and various dates of service. RAs list the claims that have been adjudicated within the payment cycle in different orders; they may be sorted alphanumerically by the patient account number assigned by provider, alphabetically by client name, or numerically by internal control number. A corresponding EOB sent to the patient, on the other hand, lists just the information for the recipient.

The RA may be sent in electronic format, called an **electronic remittance advice (ERA),** or in paper format. Although similar information is contained on an ERA and a paper RA, the ERA may offer additional data. The ERA that is mandated for use by HIPAA is called the **X12 835 Remittance Advice Transaction,** or simply the 835. In addition to physicians, other health care providers receiving the 835 include hospitals, nursing homes, laboratories, and dentists.

Claim Control Number

When the practice sends a claim, the PM/EHR will assign it a **claim control number,** also known as an ID number. This number, a maximum of twenty characters, is unique to that claim. The claim control number appears on the section of the ERA for that particular claim, and it is used to match the claim with the payment.

Autoposting

In practices that enable certain advanced electronic communication features of PM/EHRs, a capability called **autoposting** is used to automatically post

Figure 14.1 Example of a Payer's Remittance Advice

United Healthcare

PROVIDER REMITTANCE
THIS IS NOT A BILL

Trilogy Family Care Center

PAGE: 1 OF 1
DATE: 04/17/2022
ID NUMBER: NW43915367

PROVIDER: PAUL MCGRATH, M.D.

PATIENT: Dae Kim CLAIM: 03262020025

FROM DATE	THROUGH DATE	PROC CODE	UNIT	AMT BILL	AMT ALLOW	AMT PAID	DED	COPAY	ADJ	COIN	PROV PAID	REASON CODE*
03/26/22	03/26/22	93015	1	205.00	181.15	0.00	181.15	0.00	23.85	0.00	0.00	PR2
03/26/22	03/26/22	93224	1	219.00	194.07	0.00	194.07	0.00	24.93	0.00	0.00	PR2
03/26/22	03/26/22	93225	1	61.00	49.52	0.00	49.52	0.00	11.48	0.00	0.00	PR2
03/26/22	03/26/22	80048	1	68.00	44.11	0.00	44.11	0.00	23.89	0.00	0.00	PR2
03/26/22	03/26/22	80060	1	64.00	43.82	10.10	31.15	0.00	20.18	2.57	10.10	PR2
03/26/22	03/26/22	93000	1	37.00	21.49	17.19	0.00	0.00	15.51	4.30	17.19	PR2
CLAIM TOTALS				654.00	534.16	27.29	500.00	0.00	119.84	6.87	27.29	

PAYMENT SUMMARY		TOTAL ALL CLAIMS		EFT INFORMATION	
TOTAL AMOUNT PAID	27.29	AMOUNT CHARGED	654.00	NUMBER	031110197475
PRIOR CREDIT BALANCE	.00	AMOUNT ALLOWED	534.16	DATE	04/17/22
CURRENT CREDIT DEFERRED	.00	DEDUCTIBLE	500.00	**AMOUNT**	**27.29**
PRIOR CREDIT APPLIED	.00	COPAY	0.00		
NEW CREDIT BALANCE	.00	COINSURANCE	6.87		
NET DISPERSED	27.29				

*REASON CODES

PR1 - Deductible PR2 – Paid PR3 – Co-pay PR4 – Denied V – VOID ADJ – Adjustment

* DENIAL CODES

PR41 – Inconsistent age PR42 – Inconsistent gender PR43 – Duplicate claim/service PR44 – Provider type inconsistency
PR45 – Lack of medical necessity/code linkage PR46 – DOB after DOS PR47 – DOD before DOS PR48 – Precert require

payments listed on an ERA. This capability greatly speeds the process of handling ERAs. The biller in this case performs an audit (review) function rather than a data-entry task. The program lists the posting from the ERA, and the biller accepts or overrides it.

Adjustments

An adjustment means that the payer is paying a claim or a service line in an amount different from what was billed. The adjustment may be that the item is

- Denied
- Zero pay (if accepted as billed but no payment is due)
- Reduced amount paid (most likely paid according to the allowed amount)
- Less because a penalty is subtracted from the payment

To explain the determination to the provider, payers use a combination of codes: (1) a claim adjustment group code, (2) a claim adjustment reason code, and (3) a remittance advice remark code.

TIP

Code Updates

Claim adjustment reason codes and remark codes are updated three times each year; access https://x12.org/codes/claim-adjustment-reason-codes for the updated lists.

claim adjustment group code (CAGC) used on an RA/EOB to indicate the general type of reason code for an adjustment

claim adjustment reason code (CARC) used on an RA/EOB to explain why a payment does not match the amount billed

remittance advice remark code (RARC) code that explains a payer's payment decision

Claim Adjustment Group Codes

Claim adjustment group codes (CAGCs) consist of two alpha characters that assign the responsibility of a claim adjustment on the insurance EOB.

- **PR (patient responsibility)** Appears next to an amount that can be billed to the patient or insured. This group code typically applies to deductible and coinsurance or copayment adjustments.
- **CO (contractual obligations)** Appears when a contract between the payer and the provider resulted in an adjustment. This group code usually applies to allowed charges (also known as allowed amounts). CO adjustments are not billable to the patient under the contract.
- **CR (corrections and reversals)** Appears to correct a previous claim.
- **OA (other adjustments)** Used only when neither PR nor CO applies, as when another insurance is primary.
- **PI (payer-initiated reduction)** Appears when the payer thinks that the patient is not responsible for the charge, but there is no contract between the payer and the provider that states this; it might be used for medical review denials.

TIP

Patient Balance Billing

A group code PR with an associated reason code indicates whether a provider may bill a beneficiary for the nonpaid balance of the furnished services.

Claim Adjustment Reason Codes

Payers use **claim adjustment reason codes (CARCs)** to provide details about an adjustment. They must communicate why a claim or service line was paid in an amount different from what was billed. A few examples of these codes and their meanings are provided in Table 14.1.

Remittance Advice Remark Codes

Payers may also use **remittance advice remark codes (RARCs)** for more explanation. Remark codes are maintained by CMS but can be used by all payers. Codes that start with *M* are from a Medicare code set that was in place before HIPAA but is still used, including Medicare outpatient adjudication (MOA) remark codes. Codes that begin with *N* are new. Table 14.2 shows selected remark codes.

TABLE 14.1	Selected Claim Adjustment Reason Codes
1	Deductible amount.
2	Coinsurance amount.
3	Copayment amount.
4	The procedure code is inconsistent with the modifier used, or a required modifier is missing.
5	The procedure code or bill type is inconsistent with the place of service.
6	The procedure or revenue code is inconsistent with the patient's age.
7	The procedure or revenue code is inconsistent with the patient's gender.
8	The procedure code is inconsistent with the provider type or specialty (taxonomy).
9	The diagnosis is inconsistent with the patient's age.
10	The diagnosis is inconsistent with the patient's gender.
11	The diagnosis is inconsistent with the procedure.
12	The diagnosis is inconsistent with the provider type.

TABLE 14.2	Selected Remark Codes
M11	DME (durable medical equipment), orthotics and prosthetics must be billed to the DME carrier who services the patient's Zip code.
M12	Diagnostic tests performed by a physician must indicate whether purchased services are included on the claim.
M37	Service not covered when the patient is under age 35.
M38	The patient is liable for the charges for this service as you informed the patient in writing before the service was furnished that we would not pay for it, and the patient agreed to pay.
M39	The patient is not liable for payment for this service as the advance notice of non-coverage you provided the patient did not comply with program requirements.
N14	Payment based on a contractual amount or agreement, fee schedule, or maximum allowable amount.
N15	Services for a newborn must be billed separately.
N16	Family or member out-of-pocket maximum has been met. Payment based on a higher percentage.
N210	You may appeal this decision.
N211	You may not appeal this decision.

Steps for Checking an Electronic Remittance Advice

Since an ERA is not easily readable, the PM/EHR will have a feature to translate it to a readable report to view. Once this is translated, these steps must be completed to check the electronic remittance data:

1. Check the patient's name, claim control number, and date of service against the claim.
2. Verify that all billed CPT codes are listed.

3. Check the payment for each CPT code against the expected amount, which may be an allowed charge or a percentage of the usual fee. Many PM/EHRs build records of the amount each payer has paid for each CPT code as these data are entered. When another ERA payment for the same CPT is posted, the program highlights any discrepancy for review.
4. Analyze the payer's adjustment codes to locate all unpaid, downcoded, or denied claims for closer review.
5. Pay special attention to ERAs for claims submitted with modifiers. Some payers' claim processing systems automatically ignore modifiers, and underpayment may need to be appealed.
6. Decide whether there are any items on the ERA that need clarification from the payer, and follow up as necessary.

THINKING IT THROUGH 14.1

Why is it important to double-check the data on the electronic remittance advice?

Denial Management

In most cases, insurance carriers do not fully pay the amount billed by the provider. The provider bills according to the provider's fee schedule, while the payer's rate is determined by a contract with the provider. When the ERA is reviewed, the billing specialist checks to see that the amount paid is the expected amount, per the provider's contract with the payer. If a payment is not as expected, the specialist must determine the reason for the discrepancy.

Typical problems and solutions are:

- **Rejected claims** A claim that is not paid due to incorrect information must be corrected and sent to the payer according to its procedures.
- **Procedures not paid** If a procedure that should have been paid on a claim was overlooked, another claim is sent for that procedure.
- **Partially paid, denied, or downcoded claims** If the payer has denied payment, the first step is to study the adjustment codes to determine why. If a procedure is not a covered benefit or if the patient was not eligible for that benefit, typically the next step will be to bill the patient for the noncovered amount. If the claim is denied or downcoded for lack of medical necessity, a decision about the next action must be made. The options are to bill the patient, write off the amount, or challenge the determination with an appeal, as discussed later in this chapter. Some provider contracts prohibit billing the patient if an appeal or necessary documentation has not been submitted to the payer.

EXERCISE 14.1

Post a Noncovered Service from an RA

EHRclinic

A new patient was seen for a complete physical examination, including a Pap smear. The remittance advice (RA) sent by her insurance carrier indicated that the Pap smear was a noncovered service because she already had one done within the year with her previous provider. Post the denied service and bill the patient for the balance of the noncovered service.

Your instructor may assign this exercise to you in Connect. Exercise steps and EHRclinic Help Guides can be downloaded at http://www.mhhe.com/pmehr2.

14.2 Posting Insurance Payments (Fee-for-Service and Capitation)

Many practices that receive ERAs authorize the health plan to provide payment with an **electronic funds transfer (EFT)** from the health plan's bank to the provider's bank. In this case, payments are deposited directly into the provider's bank account. Otherwise, the payer sends a check to the practice, and the check is taken to the practice's bank for deposit. In either case, insurance payments must be processed so that patients' accounts are brought up to date, reflecting payments on their behalf that reduce their financial responsibility.

electronic funds transfer (EFT) electronic routing of funds between banks

In contrast to patient payments, which are usually entered in a Transaction Entry screen of the PM/EHR, insurance payments are usually entered into a Deposit Entry screen (see Figure 14.2). The name of the area where deposits are entered for insurance payments may vary in different PM/EHRs, but the action of documentation is the same. This area of the PM/EHR is efficient for entering large insurance payments that must be split up and applied to a number of different patients.

The Deposit Entry Screen

Regardless of the PM/EHR system used, deposit entry screens are typically consistent with the following information:

Deposit Date Some PM/EHR systems display the current date. The date should be changed by keying over the default date and entering the deposit date.

Show All Deposits If this box is checked, all payments are displayed, regardless of the date entered.

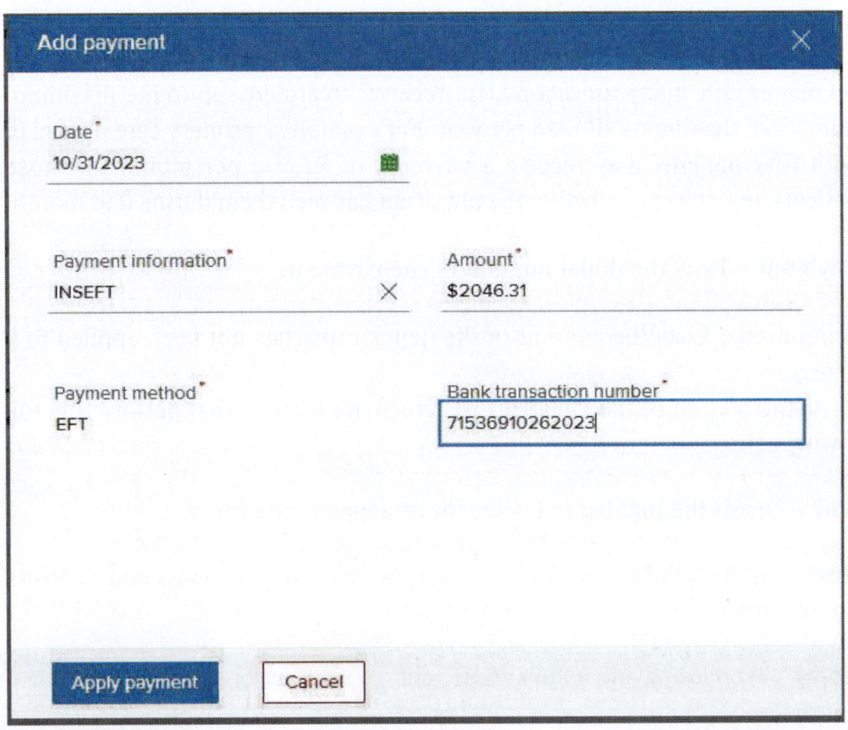

Figure 14.2 Deposit Entry Screen

Show Unapplied Only If the Show Unapplied Only box is checked, only payments that have not been fully applied to charge transactions are displayed. If the box is not checked, all payments—both applied and unapplied—are listed.

Sort By The Sort By drop-down list offers several choices for how payment information is listed. Usually the default for sorting payments is by date and description. Payments can also be sorted by other data fields.

Locate buttons The Locate and Locate Next buttons are usually indicated by magnifying glass icons. These are used to search for a deposit.

Detail To view a specific deposit in more detail, highlight the deposit, and click the Detail button. Another dialog box opens with more information about the selected deposit.

In the Deposit List window, information is listed for each deposit and payment, including the following:

Deposit Date Lists the date of the deposit or payment.

Description Displays whatever was entered in the Description or Check Number box in the Deposit Entry screen. The Deposit Entry screen is where new payments and deposits are recorded.

Payer Name Lists the name of the insurance carrier or individual who made the payment.

Payer Type A classification column that lists whether the payment is an insurance payment, a patient payment, or a capitation payment. Capitation payments are made to physicians on a regular basis (such as monthly) for providing services to patients in a managed care insurance plan (discussed more later in the chapter). In traditional insurance plans, physicians are paid for the specific procedures they perform and the number of times the procedures are performed. Under a capitated plan, a flat fee is paid to the physician no matter how many times a patient receives treatment, up to the maximum number of treatments allowed per year. For example, a primary care physician with fifty patients may receive a payment of $2,500 per month for those patients, regardless of whether the physician has seen them during that month.

Payment Lists the dollar amount of the payment.

Unapplied Lists the amount of the deposit that has not been applied to a charge.

At the bottom of the Deposit List screen are buttons that perform the following actions:

Edit Opens the highlighted payment or deposit for editing.

New Opens the Deposit Entry screen, where new payments and deposits are recorded.

Apply Applies payments to specific charge transactions.

Print Sends a command to print the deposit list.

Delete Deletes the highlighted transaction.

Export Exports the data in a spreadsheet program, per the medical practice preference.

Close Exits the Deposit List screen.

New Deposit Entry Screen

The New Deposit Entry screen should contain the following fields:

Deposit Date The PM/EHR's current date is displayed by default and must be changed if it is not the date of the deposit.

Payer Type The drop-down options in this box indicate whether the payer is an insurance carrier, a capitation plan, or a patient. If Insurance is selected, the dialog box is as illustrated in Figure 14.3. If Capitation is selected, all the boxes below Insurance disappear. If Patient is chosen, the boxes listed below Deposit Code become Chart Number, Payment Code, Adjustment Code, and Copayment Code.

Payment Method This box lists whether the payment is check, cash, credit card, or electronic.

Check Number If payment is made by check, the number of the check is entered in this box.

Description/Bank No. This box can be used to enter a description of the payment, if desired.

Payment Amount The total amount of the payment is entered in this box.

Deposit Code This field can be used by practices to sort deposits according to user-defined categories.

Insurance The insurance carrier that is making the payment is selected.

Payment Code, Adjustment Code, Withhold Code, Deductible Code, and Take Back Code The appropriate codes for the insurance carrier are selected.

Once all the information has been entered and checked for accuracy, the deposit is saved.

Posting a Capitation Payment

Capitation payments are entered in the Deposit List screen as well as a fee-for-service payment. To indicate a capitation payment, Capitation is selected from the Payer Type drop-down list in the New Deposit Entry screen (see Figure 14.3). As you can see, the boxes below Insurance are gone.

When a capitation payment is entered in a PM/EHR, the payment is not applied to the charges of individual patients. Under **capitated plans,** the

capitation payments payments made to physicians on a regular basis for providing services to patients in a managed care plan

capitated plan insurance plan in which prepayments made to a physician cover the physician's services to a plan member for a specified period of time

Figure 14.3 New Deposit Entry Screen for a Capitation Payment

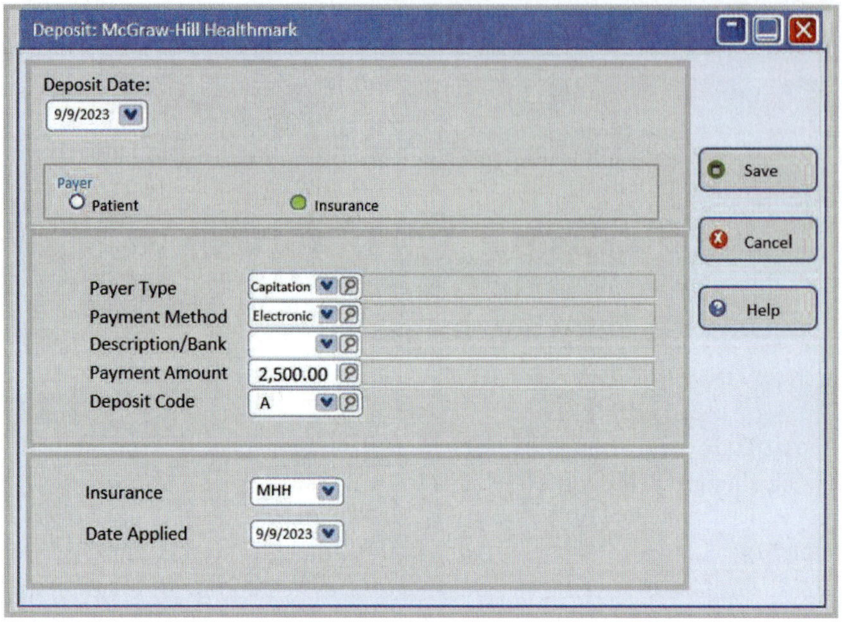

health plan pays the practice a set fee to cover all the insured patients who elect to use the practice. This designated payment is made regardless of whether any of the patients visit the practice or how often they visit. However, the charges in the account of each patient who has used the practice during the month covered by the capitation payment still must be adjusted to a zero balance to indicate that the plan has met its obligation (through the capitation payment) and that the patient has also done so (by paying a copayment at the time of the office visit).

In order to adjust the patient accounts of those covered by the capitated plan, a second deposit is entered as an insurance payment with a zero amount.

Once the zero amount deposit is saved, the deposit appears in the Deposit List. The Payment column lists EOB Only, since there is no payment associated with the zero amount deposit.

The next step is to locate patients who have claims during the month covered by the capitation payment. This can be accomplished by sorting services provided during the month and insurance in the PM/EHR.

Once patients have been identified, the search area will be closed, and the Deposit List is opened. The identified patient accounts must be adjusted to a zero balance in the Apply Payment/Adjustments to Charges screen of the PM/EHR.

EXERCISE 14.2 Post Insurance Payments Using an RA

EHRclinic

Trilogy Family Care Center received a remittance advice (RA) from an insurance carrier with an electronic payment for multiple patients. Post the insurance deposit to the patient accounts in EHRclinic.

Your instructor may assign this exercise to you in Connect. Exercise steps and EHRclinic Help Guides can be downloaded at http://www.mhhe.com/pmehr2.

Post a Deductible from an RA EHRclinic

EXERCISE 14.3

A remittance advice (RA) was received from an insurance carrier, indicating that a patient has not yet met his deductible for a portion of the charges. Apply the insurance deposit and post the payment to the patient's account. Bill the patient for the balance of the allowed charges.

Upon receipt of the statement, the patient comes in to pay his balance. Record the patient's deductible and coinsurance payments.

Your instructor may assign this exercise to you in Connect. Exercise steps and EHRclinic Help Guides can be downloaded at http://www.mhhe.com/pmehr2.

14.3 Appeals, Postpayment Audits, Overpayments, and Billing Secondary Payers

After ERAs are reviewed and processed by the practice, events that may follow can alter the amount of payment. When a claim has been denied or a payment reduced by the health plan, an appeal may be filed with the payer for reconsideration, possibly reversing the nonpayment. Postpayment audits by payers may change the initial determination. Under certain conditions, refunds may be due to either the payer or the patient. Similarly, in some situations, additional claims need to be created in order to generate full payments on behalf of insured patients.

The General Appeal Process

An **appeal** is a process that can be used to challenge a payer's decision to deny, reduce, or otherwise downcode a claim. A provider may begin the appeal process by asking for a review of the payer's decision. Patients, too, have the right to request appeals. The person filing the appeal is the **claimant** or the **appellant,** whether that individual is a provider or a patient.

appeal request for reconsideration of a claim adjudication

claimant person or entity exercising the right to receive benefits

appellant person who appeals a claim decision

Basic Steps

Each payer has consistent procedures for handling appeals. These procedures are based on the nature of the appeal. The practice staff reviews the appropriate procedure before starting an appeal and plans its actions according to these rules.

Appeals must be filed within a specified time after the claim determination. Most payers have an escalating structure of appeals, such as (1) a complaint, (2) an appeal, and (3) a grievance. The claimant must move through the three levels in pursuing an appeal, starting at the lowest and continuing to the highest, final level. Some payers also set a minimum amount that must be involved in an appeal process, so that a lot of time is not spent on a small dispute.

Options after Appeal Rejection

A claimant can take another step if the payer has rejected all the appeal levels on a claim. Because they license most types of payers, state insurance commissions have the authority to review appeals that payers reject. If a claimant decides to pursue an appeal with the state insurance commission, copies of the complete case file—all documents that relate to the initial claim determination and the appeal process—are sent, along with a letter of explanation.

> **TIP**
>
> **Late Claims Not Appealable**
>
> A claim that is denied because it was not filed on time is not subject to appeal.

Postpayment Audits

audit formal examination or review, such as a review to determine whether an entity is complying with regulations

postpayment audit review conducted after a claim is adjudicated

Recovery Audit Contractor (RAC) entity that audits Medicare claims to determine where there are opportunities to recover incorrect payments from previously paid but noncovered services, erroneous coding, and duplicate services

An **audit** is a systematic examination of a representative sample of documents intended to show whether particular situations exist. There are tax audits that seek underpayment, coding audits that look for upcoding, and compliance audits that seek to uncover fraudulent activities. Some audits are internal—that is, they are done in the practice by staff members or consultants to review claims and coding—and others are external, done by an outside entity such as a health plan or a government agency like the HHS Office of the Inspector General.

Health plans often conduct **postpayment audits.** Most are reviews that are used to build clinical information. Payers use audits of practices, for example, to study treatments and outcomes for patients with similar diagnoses. The patterns that are determined are used to confirm or alter best practice guidelines.

At times, however, a payer does a postpayment audit to verify the medical necessity of reported services or to uncover fraud and abuse. The audit may be based on detailed records about each provider's services that are kept by payers' medical review departments. Some payers keep records that go back for many months or years. The payer analyzes these records to assess patterns of care from individual providers and to flag outliers—those that differ from what other providers do. A postpayment audit might be conducted to check the documentation of the provider's cases or, in some cases, to check for fraudulent activities.

A good example of a postpayment audit payer program is the **Recovery Audit Contractor (RAC)** initiative of the Medicare program. The purpose of an RAC is to audit Medicare claims and determine where there are opportunities to recover incorrect payments from previously paid but noncovered services (including services that were not medically necessary), erroneous coding, and duplicate services.

RACs use a software program to analyze claims based on a practice's claim history, looking for:

- Obvious "black-and-white" coding errors (such as a well-woman exam billed for a male patient)
- Medically unnecessary treatment or wrong setting of care where information in the medical record does not support the claim
- Multiple or excessive number of units billed

Offices should respond to all RAC inquiries, since requests for information must be answered within forty-five days, or an error is declared and penalties may result.

Refunds of Overpayments

A postpayment audit may show that the health plan has overpaid a claim. From the payer's point of view, **overpayments** (also called credit balances and payer **takebacks**) are improper or excessive payments resulting from billing errors for which the provider owes refunds.

overpayment improper or excessive amount received by provider from payer

takeback balance that a provider owes a payer following a postpayment audit

EXAMPLE

A payer may mistakenly overpay a claim.

A payer's postpayment audit may find that a claim that has been paid should be denied or downcoded because the documentation that was examined later does not support it.

A provider may collect a primary payment from Medicare when another payer is primary.

In such cases, the payer will ask for a refund (with the possible addition of interest for Medicare). If the audit shows that the claim was for a service that was not medically necessary, the provider also must refund any payment collected from the patient.

Often, the procedure is to promptly refund the overpayment. Many states require the provider to make the refund payment unless the overpayment is contested, which it may be if the provider thinks it is erroneous. A refund request may also be challenged because many practices set a time period beyond which they will not automatically issue a refund. State law may also provide for a reasonable time limit during which payers can recoup overpayments.

Billing of Secondary Payers

If a patient has additional insurance coverage, after the primary payer's ERA has been posted, the next step is to bill the second payer. The initial claim gave the primary payer information about the patient's secondary insurance policy. The secondary payer now needs to know what the primary payer paid on the claim in order to coordinate benefits. The primary claim crosses over automatically to the secondary payer in many cases—for Medicare–Medicaid and Medicare–Medigap claims as well as for others—and no additional claim is filed. For noncrossover claims, an additional claim is prepared for the secondary payer and sent with a copy of the primary payer ERA.

Electronic Claims

A claim transmitted to the secondary payer with the primary RA is sent either electronically or on paper according to the payer's procedures. The secondary payer determines whether additional benefits are due under the policy's coordination of benefits (COB) provisions and sends payment with another RA to the practice.

The practice does not send a claim to the secondary payer when the primary payer handles the coordination of benefits transaction. In this case, the primary payer electronically sends the COB transaction, which is the same HIPAA 837 that reports the primary claim, to the secondary payer. When the primary payer forwards the COB transaction, a message appears on the primary payer's ERA. For example, an ERA may contain the phrase "Claim information forwarded to," followed by the name of the secondary payer.

THINKING IT THROUGH 14.2

Discuss the importance of correct billing procedures to avoid problems that can arise during postpayment audits.

Paper Claims

If a paper RA is received, the procedure is to use the CMS-1500 to bill the secondary health plan that covers the beneficiary. The practice completes the claim form and sends it with the primary RA attached.

EXERCISE 14.4

Post Secondary Insurance Payments Using an RA

EHRclinic

After the primary insurance carrier payments were posted to patient accounts, their secondary insurance carriers were billed. A remittance advice (RA) was received with an electronic payment from the secondary insurance carrier. Post the secondary insurance payments to the patient accounts.

Your instructor may assign this exercise to you in Connect. Exercise steps and EHRclinic Help Guides can be downloaded at http://www.mhhe.com/pmehr2.

14.4 Creating Statements

patient statement list of the amount of money a patient owes, the procedures performed, and the dates the procedures were performed

explanation of benefits (EOB) document showing how the amount of a benefit was determined

A **patient statement** lists the amount of money a patient owes, organized by the amount of time the money has been owed, the procedures performed, and the dates the procedures were performed. A patient statement is created after an insurance claim has been filed and a remittance advice received.

A patient statement is sent to collect an account balance that is the patient's responsibility. This may include coinsurance charges and charges for procedures that were not covered by the insurance company. At the same time the practice receives an ERA that covers a particular claim, the patient or guarantor receives a notice, called an **explanation of benefits (EOB),** that provides the same information in language appropriate for general readers. The EOB presents the charges for a date of service, the amount the insurance paid, and the amount the patient is now responsible for. By the time the practice sends a statement to an insured patient, the patient has received prior notice of what the statement will entail.

Statements are created using the PM/EHR. The Claim Management area provides a range of options for billing insurance carriers. The Statement Management area of the PM/EHR offers multiple choices for billing patients.

Statement Management Screen

The Statement Management area will vary depending on the PM/EHR. However the screens will be very similar. Usually the medical billing specialist will access this area by clicking on an Activities menu to select the Statement Management action. The Statement Management screen will then populate. This lists all statements that have already been created. Several actions can be performed in this dialog box: Existing statements can be reviewed and edited, new statements can be created, the status of existing statements can be changed, and statements can be printed.

Statement Management screens should include the following:

Stmt # The Stmt # column lists the statement numbers, which are generated by the program in sequential order.

Guarantor In the Statement Management screen, guarantors rather than patients are listed because statements are created only for the people who are financially responsible for accounts. For example, if a patient's father is the guarantor, a statement is created for the patient's father, not for the patient. In the Statement Management screen, the statement is listed under the father's chart number. If a man is also the guarantor on his wife's account, his chart number will appear twice in the Statement Management section. When statements are printed, however, all transactions for the guarantor's child and wife are billed on one statement.

Phone The Phone columns list the guarantors' phone number.

Status The status assigned to each statement depends on whether the statement has been billed and whether the account has a zero balance:

- **Ready to Send** Transactions that have not been billed
- **Sent** Transactions that have been billed but not fully paid
- **Done** Transactions that have been billed and fully paid

Some PM/EHRs will assign additional sections and activities:

Initial Billing The date the statement was initially sent appears in the Initial Billing column. If a statement has been sent more than once, the most recent date is shown in the Billing Date field located in the General tab of the Statement area, which is used for editing statements.

Batch The batch number assigned by the PM/EHR is displayed. This is the number that identifies when the statements were generated.

Media The format for the statement, either paper or electronic, is designated.

Type The type of statement, either Standard or Remainder, is listed.

Figure 14.4 Create Statements Screen

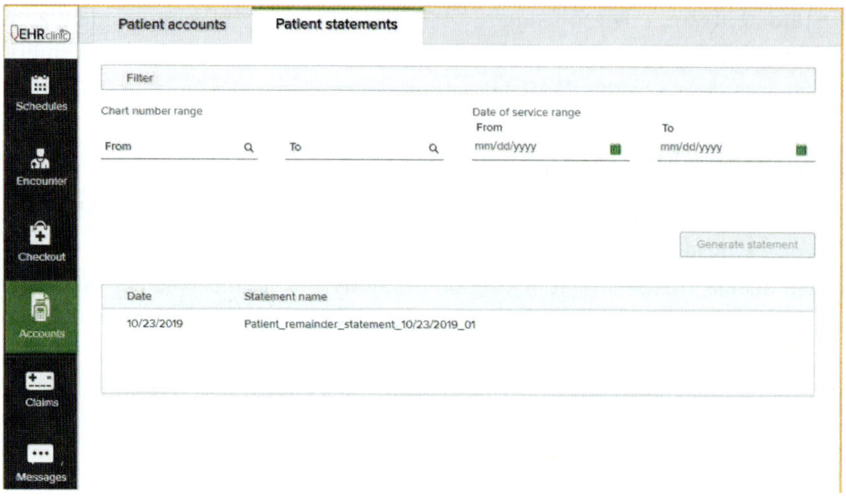

Create Statements Screen

The Create Statements screen is where information is entered that determines which statements are generated (see Figure 14.4).

The following filters can be applied in the Create Statements screen:

Transaction Dates A range of dates is entered to select transactions that occur within those dates. The dates can be entered directly by keying into the boxes, or they can be selected from the calendar that appears when the drop-down arrow is clicked.

Chart Numbers In the Chart Numbers boxes, the starting and ending chart numbers for which statements will be created are entered. If the boxes are left blank, all chart numbers will be included.

Select Transactions that Match The options in this portion of the dialog box provide filters for creating statements for billing codes, case indicators, locations, and provider. In all instances except provider, commas must be placed between entries if more than one code is entered.

Create Statements if the Remainder Total Is Greater Than . . . Enter Amount The dollar amount entered in this box is the minimum outstanding balance required for a statement to be created. For example, if 5.00 is entered in this box, the program will not create statements for accounts with balances below $5.00. If this field is left blank, statements will be created for all accounts, regardless of the balances.

standard statements statements that show all charges regardless of whether the insurance carrier has paid on the transactions

remainder statements statements that list only charges that are not paid in full after all insurance carrier payments have been received

Statement Type **Standard statements** show all available charges regardless of whether the insurance has paid on the transactions. **Remainder statements** list only those charges that are not paid in full after all insurance carrier payments have been received. Once a statement type is selected, the setting remains in effect until the other type of statement is selected.

After all selections are complete in the Create Statements screen, clicking the Generate button instructs the program to create new statements.

Create Patient Statements (Batch Invoicing) EHRclinic

EXERCISE 14.5

Trilogy Family Care Center performs *cycle billing,* in which billing statements are sent out in batches throughout the month. Create patient statements for the first batch in the cycle. Once the statements are printed, they will be mailed to the patients' homes.

Your instructor may assign this exercise to you in Connect. Exercise steps and EHRclinic Help Guides can be downloaded at http://www.mhhe.com/pmehr2.

14.5 Recording Patient Payments

Payments collected from the patient are an important part of cash flow, but not all are collected in the office. Payments can be made at the time of service and made after the encounter. All payments need to be posted on the patient's account and in the medical practice's PM/EHR.

Types of Payments

As discussed in Chapter 11, practices routinely collect payment for the following types of charges:

- Previous balances
- Copayments or coinsurance
- Noncovered or overlimit fees
- Charges of nonparticipating providers
- Charges for self-pay patients
- Deductibles for patients with consumer-driven health plans (CDHPs)

Each practice's financial procedures are different. Some charges may be collected at check-in, at check-out, electronically, or mailed to the office.

THINKING IT THROUGH 14.3

Why is it important to record the payments at the time the office receives the payment?

Payments Made at the Time of Service

Patient payments made at the time of an office visit are entered into the PM/EHR from the Transaction Entry screen. Payments that are received electronically or by mail, such as insurance payments and mailed patient payments, are entered in the Deposit List screen, which was discussed earlier in the chapter. The Deposit List feature is very efficient for entering large insurance payments that must be split up and applied to a number of different patients.

The first step when entering a patient payment is to select a patient's chart number and case number in the Transaction Entry screen. After the chart and case numbers have been selected, a payment transaction can be entered. Payments are entered in the Payments, Adjustments, and Comments section of the Transaction Entry screen (see Figure 14.5).

Figure 14.5 Payments, Adjustments, and Comments Area of the Transaction Entry Screen

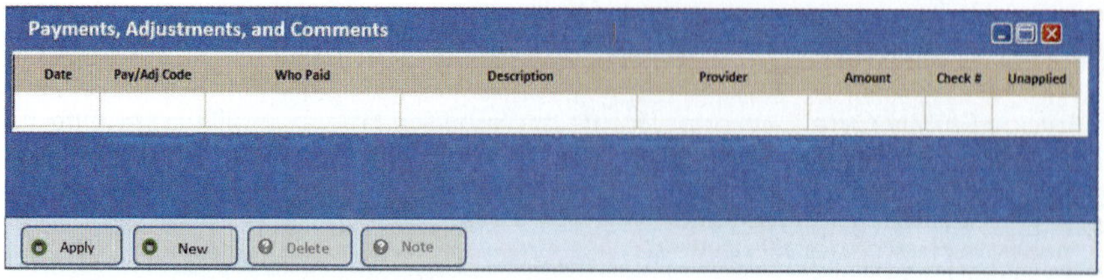

The process of creating a payment transaction begins with clicking the New button. When the New button is clicked, the PM/EHR will automatically enter the current date in the Date box. If this is not the date on which the payment was received, the date must be changed. To change the default date for these boxes, either of these two methods can be used:

- The Set Program Date calendar can be clicked to enter the appropriate date.
- The date that is already in the Date box can be keyed over.

Pay/Adj Code Once the correct date is entered, pressing the Tab key moves the cursor to the Payment/Adjustment Code box. Or you may use your mouse to click into the Payment/Adjustment Code box. The code for a payment is selected from the drop-down list of payment codes already entered in the system (see Figure 14.6).

Who Paid After the code is selected and you move to the next field either by the Tab key or by clicking into the Who Paid box, the PM/EHR will automatically complete the field based on information stored in the database. The Who Paid field displays a drop-down list of guarantors and carriers that are assigned in the patient case folder.

Description The Description field can be used to enter other information about the payment, if desired.

Provider The Provider column lists the code number of the provider.

Amount The Amount field contains the amount of payment received. If the payment is a copayment from a patient, this box is completed automatically when a payment/adjustment code is selected. PM/EHRs can be programed to auto-populate field information stored in the database.

Check Number The Check Number field is used to record the number of the check used for payment.

Figure 14.6 Payment/Adjustment Code Drop-Down List

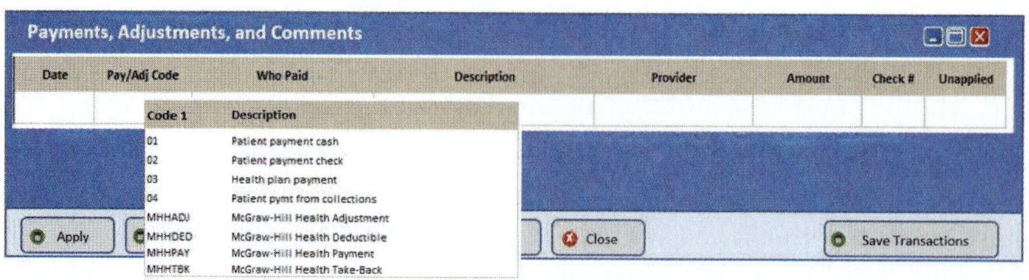

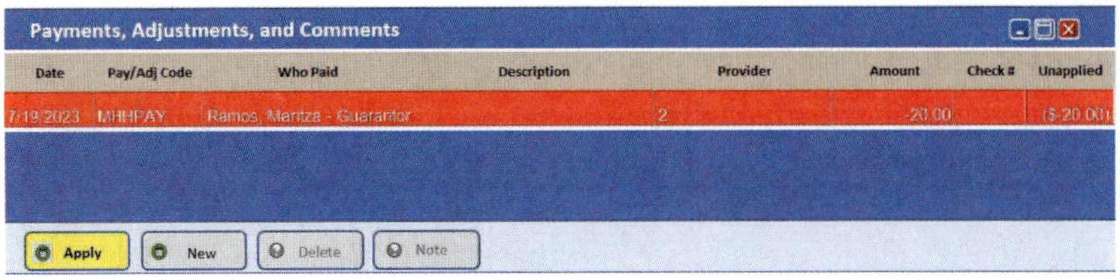

Figure 14.7 Payments, Adjustments, and Comments Area with a Color-Coded Unapplied Payment and with Apply Button Highlighted

Unapplied The dollar value in the Unapplied box is the amount that has not yet been applied to a charge transaction.

Applying Payments to Charges

PM/EHRs should indicate payment status when recording payments. For this model, the payments are color-coded to indicate payment status (see Figure 14.7). Some PM/EHRs will have icons instead of color coding. The payment status color codes that are usually applied are:

1. Partially applied payment (blue)
2. Unapplied payment (red)
3. Overapplied payment (pink)

Payments that have been fully applied are not colored and appear white.

Once all the necessary information is entered, it is time to apply the payment to specific charges. This is accomplished by clicking the Apply button, which causes the Apply Payment to Charges dialog box to be displayed. The Apply Payment to Charges screen lists information about all unpaid charges for a patient, including the date of the procedure, the document number, the procedure code, the charge, the balance, and the total amount paid (see Figure 14.8).

In the upper-right corner of the screen, the amount of the payment that has not yet been applied to charges is listed in the Unapplied box.

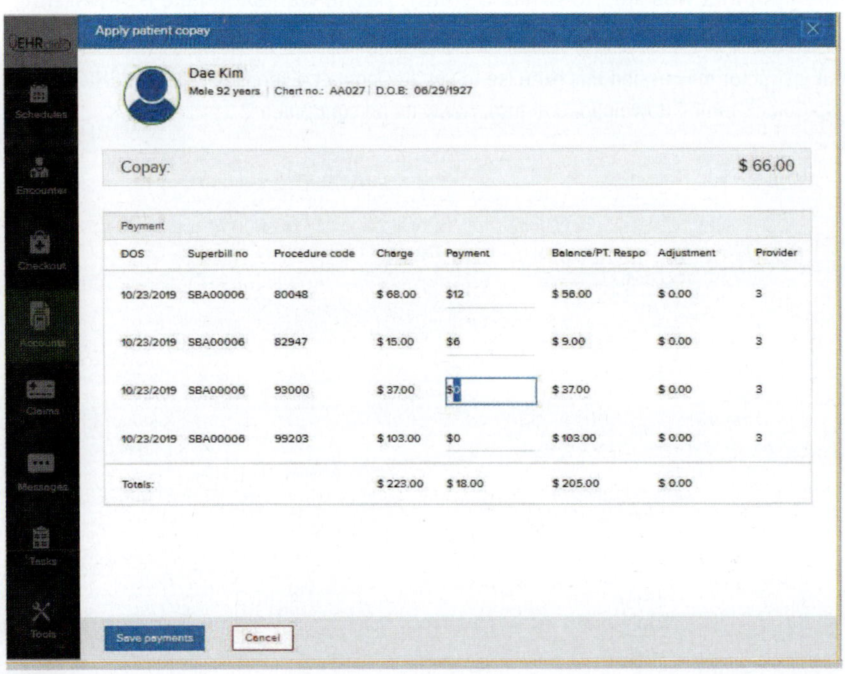

Figure 14.8 Apply Payment to Charges Screen

The first step in applying a payment is to determine the charge(s) to which the payment should be applied. Payments may be applied to charges that require a copayment, charges that are the oldest, or any other charges.

If the payment is a copayment, then the Apply to Copay button is clicked. When the Apply to Copay button is clicked, the program automatically applies the payment to the charge on that date that requires a copayment. Information about whether a procedure code requires a copayment is located in the General tab of the Procedure/Payment/Adjustment box for that code.

If the payment should be applied to the oldest charge, the Apply to Oldest button is clicked. When the Apply to Oldest button is used, the PM/EHR automatically applies the payment to the oldest charge.

Payments may also be manually applied by clicking in the box in the This Payment column on the line that contains the charge. Clicking in the box causes a dotted rectangle to appear around the outside of the box. Then you can enter the amount. The payment is applied, and the Unapplied Amount entry is lowered by the amount of the payment.

A payment can be applied to more than one charge. For example, suppose that the payment is $200.00 and that three charges have not been paid. The $200.00 payment can be applied to one, two, or all three of the charges.

Once the Apply Payment to Charges screen is closed, the payment appears in the Payments, Adjustments, and Comments area of the Transaction Entry screen,

Saving Payment Information

When all the information on a payment has been entered and checked for accuracy, it must be saved. Payment transactions are saved by clicking the Save Transactions button.

EXERCISE 14.6 Apply a Patient Payment

EHRclinic

A patient walks into Trilogy Family Care Center. He brings in the most recent statement that was sent to him and states that he wants to make a payment. Post the patient's payment and apply it to his outstanding charges.

Your instructor may assign this exercise to you in Connect. Exercise steps and EHRclinic Help Guides can be downloaded at http://www.mhhe.com/pmehr2.

chapter 14 summary

KEY TERMS

appeal
appellant
audit
autoposting
capitated plan
capitation payment
claim adjustment group code (CAGC)
claim adjustment reason code (CARC)
claim control number
claimant
electronic funds transfer (EFT)
electronic remittance advice (ERA)
explanation of benefits (EOB)
overpayments
patient statement
postpayment audits
Recovery Audit Contractor (RAC)
remainder statements
remittance advice (RA)
remittance advice remark code (RARC)
standard statements
takeback
X12 835 Remittance Advice Transaction

LEARNING OUTCOME	KEY CONCEPTS/EXAMPLES
14.1 Describe working with the electronic remittance advice (ERA).	Once a claim has been received and accepted for adjudication, the health plan determines the payment it will make for each charge. The payer then generates a remittance advice (RA) and sends it to the provider. A remittance advice (RA) lists patients, dates of service, charges, and the amounts paid or denied—that is, the adjustments made by the insurance carrier to the billed charges.
14.2 Discuss posting insurance payments for fee-for-service and capitation plans.	Insurance payments must be processed so that patients' accounts are brought up to date, reflecting payments on their behalf that reduce their financial responsibility. These payments are sent electronically and need to be applied to the correct patient using the Deposit Entry screen.
14.3 Describe appeals, postpayment audits, overpayments, and billing secondary payers.	When a claim has been denied or a payment reduced by the health plan, an appeal may be filed with the payer for reconsideration, possibly reversing the nonpayment. Postpayment audits by payers may change the initial determination. Under certain conditions, refunds may be due to either the payer or the patient. Similarly, in some situations additional claims need to be created in order to generate full payments on behalf of insured patients.
14.4 Describe how to create statements.	A patient statement is sent to collect an account balance that is the patient's responsibility. To do this, information is entered into the Statement Management screens of the PM/EHR.
14.5 Explain how to record patient payments.	Payments collected from the patient are an important part of cash flow, but they may not occur while in the office. Payments can be made at the time of service or after the encounter. All payments need to be posted on the patient's account and in the medical practice's PM/EHR. Patients' payments are entered in the Transaction screens to be applied to services.

chapter 14 review

MATCHING QUESTIONS

Match the key terms with their definitions.

_____ 1. *[LO 14.3]* appeal

_____ 2. *[LO 14.3]* appellant

_____ 3. *[LO 14.2]* capitated plan

_____ 4. *[LO 14.2]* capitation

_____ 5. *[LO 14.3]* claimant

_____ 6. *[LO 14.3]* overpayment

_____ 7. *[LO 14.3]* audit

_____ 8. *[LO 14.3]* Recovery Audit Contractor (RAC)

_____ 9. *[LO 14.3]* takebacks

_____ 10. *[LO 14.4]* standard statements

a. A prepayment covering a provider's services for a plan member for a specified period.

b. A person who appeals a claim decision.

c. An entity that audits Medicare claims to determine where there are opportunities to recover incorrect payments from previously paid but noncovered services, erroneous coding, and duplicate services.

d. An improper or excessive amount received by the provider from the payer.

e. An insurance plan in which prepayments made to a physician cover the physician's services to a plan member for a specified period of time.

f. A balance that a provider owes a payer following a postpayment audit.

g. Statements that show all charges regardless of whether the insurance carrier has paid on the transactions.

h. A person or entity exercising the right to receive benefits.

i. A formal examination or review.

j. A request for reconsideration of a claim adjudication.

MULTIPLE CHOICE QUESTIONS

Select the letter that best completes the statement or answers the question.

1. *[LO 14.1]* What is the mandated ERA called?
   a. X12 835 Remittance Advice Transaction
   b. CAGCs
   c. remittance advice (RA)
   d. EFT

2. *[LO 14.1]* Which of the following are claim adjustment group codes (CAGCs)?
   a. patient responsibility
   b. corrections and reversals

c. payer-initiated reduction
d. all of the above

3. *[LO 14.2]* What should the Data Entry screen include?
   a. show all deposits
   b. deposit date
   c. both (a) and (b)
   d. none of the above

4. *[LO 14.3]* A(n) ______ is a systematic examination of a representative sample of documents intended to show whether particular situations exist.
   a. autoposting
   b. capitation
   c. audit
   d. X 835

5. *[LO 14.3]* Which of the following is an example of a postpayment audit program?
   a. Recovery Audit Contractor (RAC)
   b. Claim Adjustment Group Codes (CAGCs)
   c. Remittance Advice Remark Codes (RARCs)
   d. Explanation of Benefits (EOB)

6. *[LO 14.3]* Who sends a secondary claim when the primary payer handles the coordination of benefits transaction?
   a. secondary payer
   b. primary payer
   c. EOB
   d. RAC

7. *[LO 14.4]* A(n) ______ lists the amount of money a patient owes, organized by the amount of time the money has been owed, the procedures performed, and the dates the procedures were performed.
   a. overpayment
   b. standard statement
   c. remainder statement
   d. patient statement

8. *[LO 14.4]* The ______ screen is where information is entered that determines which statements are generated.
   a. Deposit Entry
   b. Transaction Entry
   c. Create Statement
   d. Deposit List

9. *[LO 14.5]* Which of the following are NOT types of charges to collect at the time of service?
   a. previous balances
   b. copayments
   c. deductibles
   d. secondary nonpayments

10. *[LO 14.5]* What is displayed in the Who Paid box in the Payments, Adjustments, and Comments area screen?
    a. guarantors and payers
    b. patients and dates
    c. guarantors and providers
    d. guarantors and dates

SHORT ANSWER QUESTIONS

Define the following abbreviations.

1. *[LO 14.1]* RA ______________________
2. *[LO 14.1]* ERA ______________________
3. *[LO 14.1]* CAGCs ______________________
4. *[LO 14.1]* CARCs ______________________
5. *[LO 14.1]* RARCs ______________________
6. *[LO 14.2]* EFT ______________________
7. *[LO 14.3]* RAC ______________________
8. *[LO 14.4]* EOB ______________________

APPLYING YOUR KNOWLEDGE

Answer the questions below in the space provided.

14.1 *[LO 14.3]* What are the three levels of appeals?

____

____

14.2 *[LO 14.5]* What is the difference between PAR and nonPAR providers?

____

____

14.3 *[LO 14.1]* What is the difference between an RA and an ERA?

____

____

14.4 *[LO 14.2]* Where in the PM/EHR are insurance payments entered?

____

____

part four

Producing Reports and Following Up

chapter 15

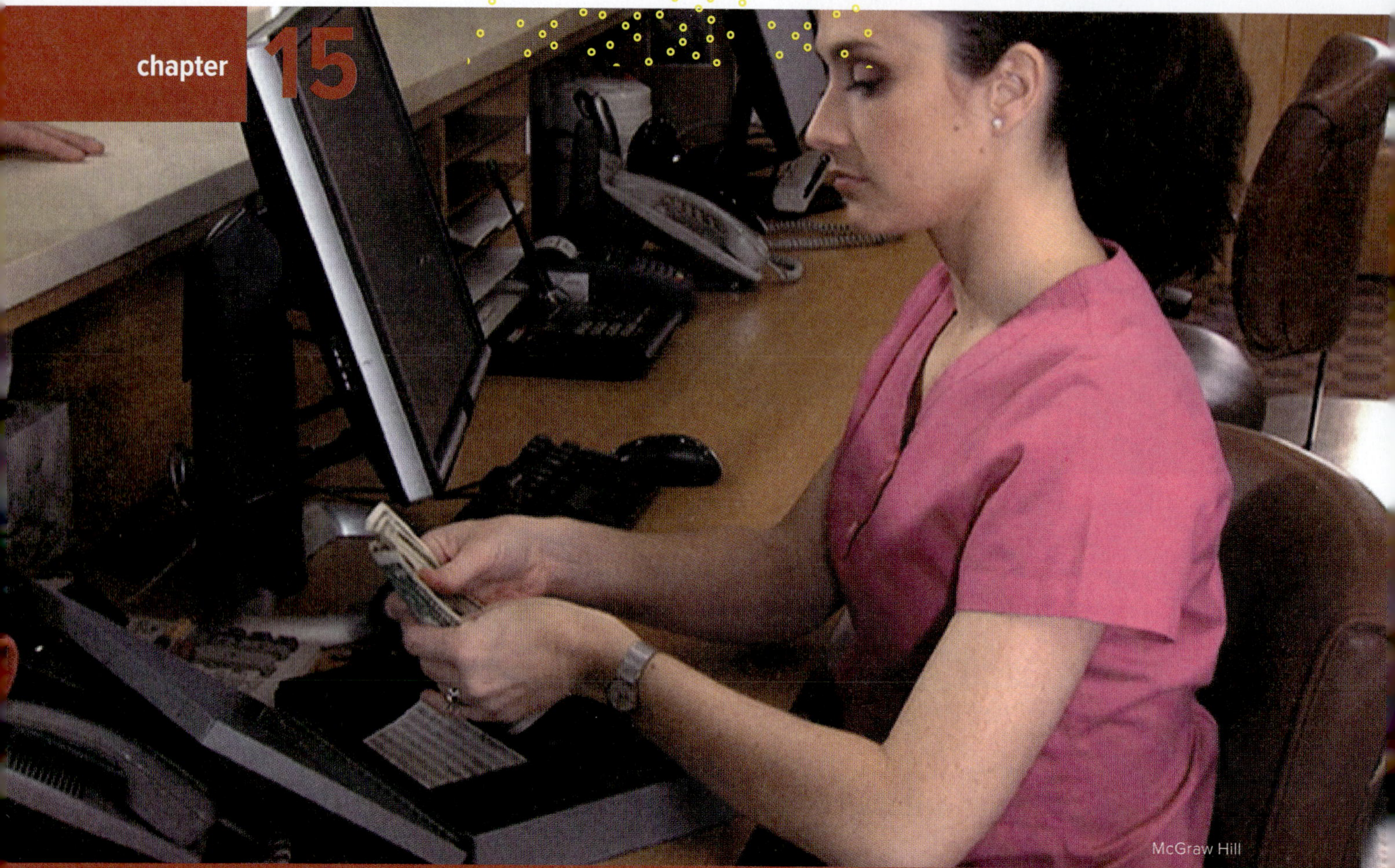

McGraw Hill

Accounts Receivable Follow-Up and Collections

LEARNING OUTCOMES

When you finish this chapter, you will be able to:

15.1 Discuss the importance of patient collections.

15.2 Explain the financial policy and payment expectations.

15.3 Describe collection procedures.

15.4 Discuss laws governing patient collections.

15.5 Explain what is included in collection letters.

15.6 Explain regulations of payment plans.

15.7 Describe collection agencies.

15.8 Explain the difference between write-offs and refunds.

Accounts Receivable and Collections

Elrene Harrison, Trilogy Family Care Center's revenue cycle manager, is reviewing the practice's accounts receivable. She performs a patient aging analysis and asks the billers to initiate collection efforts for several past-due accounts.

Elrene assigns batches to the following billers to resolve:

- Mariel Brown, 31–60 days past-due accounts
- Rodney Calhoun, 61–90 days past-due accounts
- Ginger Amato, 91–120 days past-due accounts
- Lashelle Williams, 120+ days past-due accounts

As you read this chapter, consider the collection strategies each biller should use for his or her batch of past-due accounts. Why are there different collection strategies for various stages of past-due balances? What are some options for debt resolution?

15.1 The Importance of Patient Collections

Receiving full payment for services is a critical factor in determining the financial success of a medical practice. Out-of-pocket spending for patients grew 4.6 percent to $406.5 billion in 2019, or 11 percent of the total national health expenditure (NHE), according to the Centers for Medicare and Medicaid Services (CMS). Sums that are not collected must be subtracted from the practice's income, reducing working capital, meaning that the practice might have to borrow funds and pay interest on those amounts just to pay bills. The physician and clinical services expenditures grew 4.6 percent to $772.1 billion in 2019. Collecting payments from the patient is vital for the medical practice to succeed. The practice cannot rely only on insurance payments.

Patients' payments are collected both at the time of service (TOS) and, for insured patients, after claim adjudication by payers. At TOS, practices routinely collect copayments and overdue balances, and they may also collect either partial or full payment for visits. The majority of payments, however, are collected from patients after the payer's remittance advice and payment are transmitted to the office. A statement is then mailed to the patient indicating the balance due. The collection process begins with sending these statements to patients promptly. It continues until the bill is collected or the amount due is determined to be uncollectible.

While most patients pay their bills on time, every practice has some patients who do not. Patients' reasons for not paying may include:

- Lack of insurance coverage
- Lack of financial resources
- Significant medical costs
- Consumer-directed health plans with high out-of-pocket costs
- Lack of understanding that payment is their responsibility

Members of the billing staff may be asked to work with patients to follow up on overdue accounts. The goal of the follow-up is to resolve problems and collect payments.

15.2 The Financial Policy and Payment Expectations

The patient collection process begins with a clear financial policy and effective communications with patients about their financial responsibilities. When patients understand the charges and the practice's financial policy in advance, collecting payments is not usually problematic. As a result, as detailed in Chapter 5 and reviewed here, it is important to have a written financial policy that spells out patients' responsibilities.

The financial policy of a medical practice explains how the practice handles financial matters. When new patients register, they should be given copies of the financial policy along with the practice's HIPAA privacy policies and patient registration material. The policy should tell patients how the practice handles:

- Collecting copayments and past-due balances
- Setting up financial arrangements for unpaid balances
- Providing charity care or using a sliding scale for patients with low incomes
- Collecting payments for services not covered by insurance
- Collecting prepayment for services
- Accepting cash, checks, money orders, and credit and debit cards
- Process for handling **nonsufficient funds (NSF)** payments

nonsufficient funds (NSF) check or debit that is not honored by the bank because the account lacks funds to cover it

THINKING IT THROUGH 15.1

After receiving a statement in the mail, a patient calls the practice and asks to speak to the billing department. The patient believes that she has been overcharged. In your opinion, what first steps should the biller take to respond to the call? What tone should the biller use?

THINKING IT THROUGH 15.2

Based on the financial policy shown in Figure 15.1:

- Who is responsible for charges?
- What fee is charged if a copay is not paid at TOS?

If the practice's printed or displayed payment policy covers adding finance charges on late accounts, it is acceptable to do so. The amount of the finance charge must comply with federal and state law.

Additionally, most practices handle nonsufficient funds in a similar manner. A patient who submits a payment by check or an electronic payment will typically incur an NSF fee if there is insufficient money in the account to cover the charge. When this occurs, the original charges must be applied back to the patient's account (because the practice wasn't paid for them), and then the NSF fee will be added.

Trilogy Family Care Center

Financial Policy

Thank you for choosing Trilogy Family Care Center for your health care needs. The following information is being provided to assist you in understanding our financial policies and to address the questions most frequently asked by our patients.

Account Responsibility
You are responsible for all charges incurred on your account. It is also your responsibility to make sure all information on your account is current and accurate. Incorrect information can cause payment delays, which may result in late fees being applied to your account. Many people are under the impression that it is up to the physician and staff to make sure that all charges are paid or covered by insurance. This is not the case. Please remember that the insurance contract is between you and the insurance company, not the physician. It is your responsibility to know what your contract covers and pays and to communicate this to physicians and staff. Therefore, you are responsible for charges incurred regardless of insurance coverage.

Insurance Billing
If you have medical insurance, we will be happy to bill your insurance carrier for you. As a courtesy, we will also bill the carrier of any secondary insurance coverage that you may have. Trilogy Family Care Center contracts with many insurance companies, but due to the fact that these companies have a variety of plans available, it is impossible for us to know if your specific plan is included. It is your responsibility to check with your insurance company in advance. Please remember that your insurance may not cover or pay all charges incurred. Any unpaid balance after insurance payments are posted is your responsibility.

Copays
All copays are due at time of service. A $5.00 billing fee is assessed if your copay is not paid at time of service. This fee will not be waived. It is your responsibility to know whether your insurance plan requires you to pay a copay.

No Insurance
If you have no insurance, payment in full is expected at time of service, unless payment arrangements have been made prior to your visit.

Late Fees
All patient balances are to be paid in full within 60 days. This refers to balances after your insurance has paid. If you are unable to pay your balance in full within 60 days, please contact the business office to set up a payment plan. A late fee of $20.00 per month will be assessed on patient balances over 60 days.

Cash Only
If your account has been turned over to collection, it will also be changed to a cash-only account. This means that all services will need to be paid in full at time of service. A letter will be sent to inform you if your account has been changed to a cash-only

Dishonored Checks (Non-Sufficient Funds)
A $25.00 service charge will be assessed with all dishonored checks or checks that are returned for insufficient funds.

Payment Methods
Express, and Discover. Payments can be made at any reception area. For your convenience, an ATM is located in the lobby of the building.

Figure 15.1 A Sample Medical Practice Financial Policy

Figure 15.1 shows a sample financial policy of a medical practice.

EXERCISE 15.1

Handle a Returned NSF Check

EHRclinic

When reviewing deposits, you notice that a patient's check was returned for nonsufficient funds (NSF). Post the original charges back to the patient's account and then apply the $35 NSF fee, per Trilogy Family Care Center's financial policy.

Your instructor may assign this exercise to you in Connect. Exercise steps and EHRclinic Help Guides can be downloaded at http://www.mhhe.com/pmehr2.

15.3 Collection Procedures

Despite the practice's efforts to communicate the financial policy to all patients, some people still do not pay in full and on time. Nonpayment of patient statements initiates the collection process, which involves identifying the overdue accounts and organizing them for effective follow-up.

Working with Patient Aging Reports

The medical office tracks overdue bills by reviewing the patient aging report. Like the insurance aging report, it is analyzed to determine which patients are overdue on their bills and to group them into categories for efficient

Trilogy Family Care Center

Patient Aging by Date of Service

Show all data where Charges/Payments/Adj is on or before 10/31/2022

Chart	Name	-Past- 0 to 30	-Past- 31 to 60	-Past- 61 to 90	-Past- 91 to 120	-Past- 121+	Total
AA004	Jack Kyser	50.00					50.00
AA007	Anthony Battistuta	21.17	7.47				28.64
AA008	Pauline Battistuta				720.50		720.50
AA011	Jonathan Bell	49.18		15.52			64.70
AA024	Randall Klein		18.91				18.91
AA026	Raj Patel	-10.00					-10.00
AA031	James Smolowski				93.64		93.64
Report Totals:		110.35	26.38	15.52	814.14		966.39

Figure 15.2 Example of a Patient Aging Report

collection efforts (see Figure 15.2). The patient aging report includes the patient's chart number, name, aging amounts, and total balance. The aging period begins on the date of the bill. The report is divided into the following categories based on each statement's beginning date:

- Current or up-to-date: 30 days
- Past due: 31–60 days
- Past due: 61–90 days
- Past due: 91+ days

Each practice sets its own procedures for the collection process. Large bills have priority over smaller ones. Usually, an automatic reminder notice and a second statement are mailed when a bill has not been paid thirty days after it was issued. Some practices phone a patient with a thirty-day overdue account. If the bill is not then paid, a series of collection letters is generated at intervals, each more stringent in its tone and more direct in its approach.

Table 15.1 provides an example of one practice's collection timeline; different approaches are used in other practices. Some practices send all accounts that are past thirty days to an outside agency.

THINKING IT THROUGH 15.3

What are the benefits of reviewing the patient aging report monthly?

TABLE 15.1 Patient Collection Timeline

Amount Past Due	Action
30 days	Bill patient
45 days	Call patient regarding bill
60 days	Letter 1
75 days	Letter 2 and call
80 days	Letter 3
90 days	Turn over to collections

Adding an Account to the Collection List

Once overdue accounts have been identified, the next step is to add collection items to a collection list. The **collection list** is designed to track activities that need to be completed as part of the collection process. Ticklers or collection reminders are displayed as collection list items. A **tickler** is a reminder to follow up on an account that is entered on the collection list.

collection list tool for tracking activities that need to be completed as part of the collection process

tickler reminder to follow up on an account

Using the Collection List Window

In some PM/EHR systems, Collection List displays ticklers that have already been entered into the database (see Figure 15.3). The information displayed on the screen depends on the dates entered in the Date boxes. For example, if 10/13/2022 is entered in both boxes, only ticklers marked for follow-up on October 13, 2022, will be listed.

Options for controlling what appears in the Collection List window vary per PM/EHR but may include the following:

Date Items can be displayed for the current date, for a range of dates, or for all dates. By default, the current date is usually used as the range of dates, and only those tickler items that are due on that date are displayed.

Show All Ticklers Selecting this box results in the listing of all tickler items.

Show Deleted Only Selecting this box displays only ticklers that have been deleted.

Exclude Deleted Selecting this box indicates that deleted ticklers are not displayed.

The Collection List contains the following information about each tickler item:

Item This unique number identifying a tickler item is assigned automatically by the program.

Responsible Party This field contains the chart number (patient/guarantor) or insurance code (insurance carrier) that identifies the responsible party for

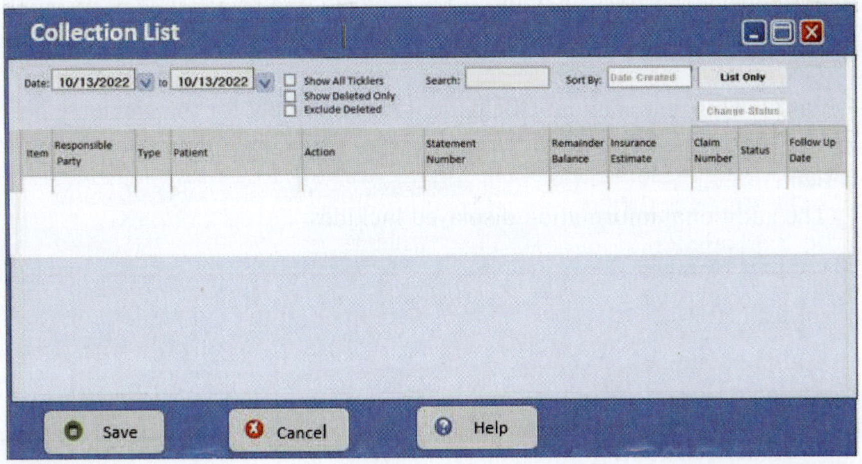

Figure 15.3 Collection List Dialog Box

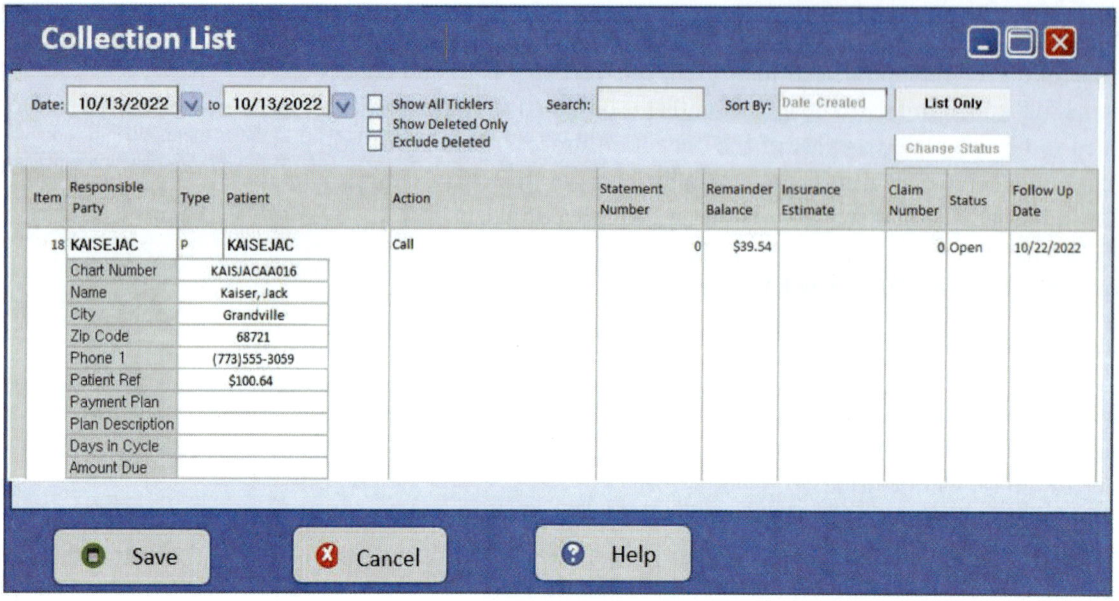

Figure 15.4 Additional Information Displayed When the Responsible Party Is a Patient/Guarantor

this item. Often this field can be expanded to view more information about the responsible party.

The following additional information is displayed (see Figure 15.4):

- Chart Number
- Name
- City
- Zip Code
- Phone/Cell
- Patient Reference Balance
- Payment Plan
- Plan Description
- Days in Cycle
- Amount Due

Type The type is either a *P* for Patient or an *I* for Insurance. If the type is *P*, the responsible party is a patient. If the type is *I*, the responsible party is the insurance carrier.

Patient This field contains the patient chart number for this tickler. Clicking in this field expands the window to show more information on the patient.

The additional information displayed includes:

- Chart Number
- Last Name
- First Name
- Middle Initial
- Phone/Cell

- Zip Code
- Date of Birth
- Sex
- Patient Reference Balance
- Social Security Number

Other information in the Collection List includes the following:

Action This field lists the action required. To see all of the text entered for this field, double-click in the field. This opens a window showing the complete text entry.

Statement Number If the tickler is for a patient, the statement number is listed.

Remainder Balance If the responsible type is Patient, the balance reported is the patient's balance as listed in Transaction Entry. If the responsible type is Insurance, the balance reported is an estimated balance for the patient's specified carrier. This is the balance at the time the tickler is created. This balance does not refresh when payments are made to the patient's account. To manually update the amounts, the tickler must be edited and saved again.

Insurance Estimate This field displays an estimate of the amount of payment expected from the insurance carrier.

Claim Number If the tickler is for an insurance carrier, the claim number is listed in this column.

Claim Total If the tickler is for an insurance carrier, the total amount of charges on the claim is listed here.

Status The entries in the field are Open, Resolved, and Deleted.

Follow-Up Date This is the date the tickler will appear on the collection list.

Date Resolved This is the date that the status of the item was changed to Resolved. Resolution is determined by the user.

User ID The User ID identifies the user who is responsible for following up on the item. In an actual practice, users are assigned log-in names and passwords in the Security Setup area of the program.

Entering a Tickler Item

A new tickler item is created by pressing the New button in the Collection List screen. This action opens the Tickler Item. The Tickler Item is displayed in Figure 15.5.

The Tickler Item contains two areas for information: Tickler and Office Notes.

Tickler Tab

The following information is entered in the Tickler tab:

Figure 15.5 Tickler Item

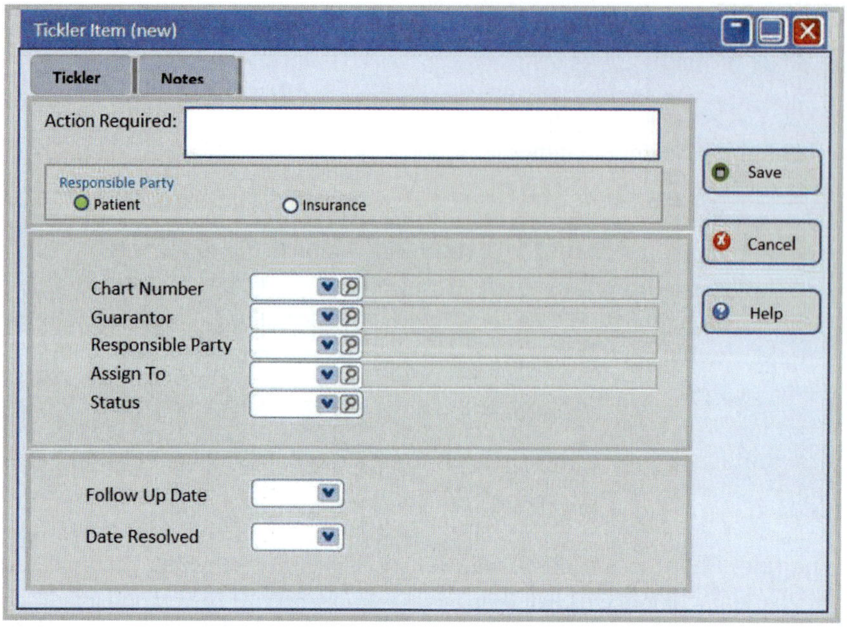

Action Required The Action Required field specifies the action that is to be taken to remedy the problem. Up to eighty characters of text can be entered.

Responsible Party type The button selected in this field indicates whether the patient or the insurance carrier is responsible for the account balance. This entry also controls the contents of the drop-down lists for the Responsible Party field below.

Chart Number The patient's chart number is selected from the list.

Guarantor The Guarantor field lists the account guarantor chart number for this tickler item.

Responsible Party If the responsible party type is Patient, a chart number is selected from the drop-down list. If the responsible party type is Insurance, the code for an insurance carrier is selected.

Assign To The Assign To box lists the name of the person responsible for following up on the tickler item. These names are set up by the practice's management team, who have access to add staff working with the collection process.

Status The status of the tickler item is chosen from a drop-down list. The options are Open, Resolved, or Deleted.

Follow-Up Date This is the date the tickler will appear on the collection list if the Date range in the Collection List window is used. By default, it is usually set as the current date.

Date Resolved This field lists the date on which the status of the item was changed to Resolved. When the status is set to Resolved, the Date Resolved is set to the current date.

Office Notes Tab

The Office Notes tab consists of several buttons and a large area in which to enter notes. Notes that relate to the collection process of the selected tickler are entered in the text box displayed.

Most PM/EHR systems use short phrases or smart phrases to help staff document correspondences quickly with the patient. When the right mouse button is clicked within the typing area, a drop-down box will display where the collection staff can choose the most appropriate phrase. Then the collection staff can personalize the note, such as adding a date. The collection staff can also free-type a note.

Once a new tickler has been saved, the program automatically assigns a unique identifier code to the item.

THINKING IT THROUGH 15.4

A patient account is entered into collections by creating a tickler. One of the fields on the Tickler tab lists the guarantor. Based on what you learned here and in Chapter 5, why is it necessary to list the guarantor in the Tickler tab?

THINKING IT THROUGH 15.5

You are a biller for Trilogy Family Care Center and are asked to call Jennifer Argada about the $40 payment that is overdue for the preschool visit of her child, Jimmy. The amount is overdue thirty days. When you call, you get the answering machine. Write a script for the phone message you would leave in this situation.

TIP

Warning!

When an account is added to the collection list, the current balance for the tickler is determined. Once recorded in the tickler, it is not updated when new transactions are entered in the program.

For patient-responsible ticklers, the balance is the balance shown in the Transaction Entry screen. It could also include insurance balances. For insurance-responsible ticklers, the balance is the estimated amount due from the assigned insurance carrier.

15.4 Laws Governing Patient Collections

Collections from patients are classified as consumer collections and are regulated by federal and state laws. The Federal Trade Commission enforces the **Fair Debt Collection Practices Act of 1977 (FDCPA)** and the **Telephone Consumer Protection Act of 1991** that regulate third-party collections to ensure fair and ethical treatment of debtors. The following guidelines are part of federal regulations and are also best practices in medical offices:

- Contact patients only once daily, and leave no more than three messages per week.
- Do not call a patient before 8:00 A.M. or after 9:00 P.M.

Fair Debt Collection Practices Act of 1977 (FDCPA) federal law regulating collection practices

Telephone Consumer Protection Act of 1991 federal law regulating collection practices

- Do not threaten the patient or use profane language.
- Identify the caller, the practice, and the purpose of the call; do not mislead the patient.
- Do not discuss the patient's debt with another person (called a third party).
- Do not leave a message on an answering machine that indicates the call is about a debt or send an email stating that the topic is debt.
- If a patient requests that all phone calls cease and desist, do not call the patient again, and contact the patient via mail.
- If a patient wants calls to be made to an attorney, do not contact the patient again unless the attorney permits it or the attorney cannot be reached.

15.5 Collection Letters

The practice's collection procedures outline the series of written contacts patients will receive when they have overdue balances.

Collection Letter Series

For most patients, the collection letter is their first notice that their bill is past due. Collection letters are generally brief and to the point while preserving a professional and courteous tone. They remind patients of the practice's payment options and their responsibility to pay the debt. Practices decide what types of letters should be sent to accounts in the various past-due stages. Accounts that are further past due will receive more aggressive letters. For example, Figure 15.6a–c shows the progression in the tone of these letters.

TIP

Collection letters must comply with all debt-collection statutes—federal, state, and local.

Figure 15.6 Samples of Collection Letters

Date:
Patient:
Acct. #:
Balance Due: $

Dear

Your insurance company has paid its portion of your bill. You are now responsible for the remaining balance. Full payment is due, or you must contact this office within 10 days to make suitable payment arrangements. As an added payment option, you may pay by credit card, using the payment form below.

Sincerely,

<Employee signature>
<Employee name and title>

(a) First Letter

Date:
Patient:
Acct. #:
Balance Due: $

Dear

This is a reminder that your account is overdue. If there are any problems we should know about, please telephone or stop in at the office. A statement is attached showing your past account activity.

Your prompt payment is requested.

Sincerely,

<Employee signature>
<Employee name and title>

(b) Second Letter

Date:
Patient:
Acct. #:
Balance Due: $

Dear

Your account is seriously past due and has been placed with our in-house collection department. Immediate payment is needed to keep an unfavorable credit rating from being reported on this account. If you are unable to pay in full, please call to make acceptable arrangements for payment. Failure to respond to this notice within 10 days will precipitate further collection actions.

Sincerely,

<Employee signature>
<Employee name and title>

(c) Third Letter

Creating Collection Letters

A number of actions must be taken within the PM/EHR system before collection letters can be sent. A patient-responsible tickler item for the patient's account must be entered in the collection list. Also, a Collection Letter Report must be created. This report is generated when the Patient Collection Letters option is selected. The Collection Letter Report lists patients with overdue accounts to whom statements have been mailed or need to be mailed. Figure 15.7 shows a printed report. This report can be printed or displayed on the screen. Once this is reviewed, the PM/EHR will provide the option to generate collection letters.

Figure 15.7 Collection Letter Report

Trilogy Family Care Center

Collection Letter Report

10/31/2022

User ID:

Item	Status	Responsible Party	Patient Chart	Date Created	Date Received	Follow Up Date	Balance	# Days Old
19	Open	Kristin Zapata	AA047	10/31/2022		10/31/2022	$247.50	0
18	Open	Elizabeth Jones	AA024	10/31/2022		10/31/2022	$28.64	0
17	Open	Dae Kim	AA027	10/31/2022		10/31/2022	$104.39	0

There will be a button to create these letters, usually named Send Letters. Once this button is clicked, the program generates the collection letters (see Figure 15.8).

Figure 15.8 Patient Collection Letter

Trilogy Family Care Center

Kristin Zapata
109 East Milian Avenue
Stephenson, OH 60089

October 31, 2022

Patient Account: Zapata, Kristin

Dear Kristin Zapata

Our records indicate that your account with us is overdue. The total unpaid balance is $282.50.

If you have already forwarded your payment, please disregard this letter, otherwise please forward your payment immediately.

Please contact us at (586) 555-4100 if you have any questions or concerns about your account.

Sincerely,

Katherine Yan
Office Manager

43514 Bridgewater Ave, Washington, MI 48094 4 (586) 555-4100 4 trilogyfamilycarexy.com

After collection letters are printed, an account alert appears in the Transaction Entry, Quick Ledger, and Appointment Entry windows for staff to see. This alert remains on the account until the patient no longer has an open tickler in the collection list. There are three account alert abbreviations:

1. RB: The patient has a remainder balance greater than the amount specified in the General tab in the Program Options window.
2. DP: The patient is delinquent on his or her payment plan.
3. IC: The patient account is in collections. (For this message to appear, a collection letter must have been printed.)

EXERCISE 15.2

Create a Collection Letter

EHRclinic

Create a collection letter for a patient whose balance is 60 to 90 days past due.

Your instructor may assign this exercise to you in Connect. Exercise steps and EHRclinic Help Guides can be downloaded at http://www.mhhe.com/pmehr2.

Creating a Collection Tracer Report

A **collection tracer report** is used to keep track of collection letters that were sent. The report lists the tickler item number, the responsible party, the chart number, the account balance (as of the date the tickler was created), the date the collection letter was sent, and the reasons the account is in collections (see Figure 15.9).

collection tracer report tool for keeping track of collection letters that were sent

Trilogy Family Care Center

Collection Tracer Report

10/31/2022

Item #	Responsible Party	Patient Chart	Balance	Date Letter Sent	Reasons
Elizabeth Jones					
2	Elizabeth Jones	AA026	28.64	10/31/2022	The outstanding balance is greater than 0.01
					Total Letters Sent: 1
Kristin Zapata					
3	Kristin Zapata	AA047	247.5	10/31/2022	The outstanding balance is greater than 0.01
					Total Letters Sent: 1

Figure 15.9 Collection Tracer Report

payment plan agreement between a patient and a practice in which the patient agrees to make regular monthly payments over a specified period of time

Equal Credit Opportunity Act (ECOA) law that prohibits credit discrimination on the basis of race, color, religion, national origin, sex, marital status, or age, or because a person receives public assistance

Truth in Lending Act part of the federal Consumer Credit Protection Act that regulates collection practices related to finance charges and late fees

15.6 Payment Plans

For large bills or special situations, some practices may offer payment plans to patients. A **payment plan** is an agreement between a patient and a practice in which the patient agrees to make regular monthly payments over a specified period of time.

Equal Credit Opportunity Act

The Federal Trade Commission (FTC) enforces the **Equal Credit Opportunity Act (ECOA),** which prohibits credit discrimination on the basis of race, color, religion, national origin, sex, marital status, age, or because a person receives public assistance. If the practice decides not to extend credit to a particular patient while extending it to others, under the ECOA the patient has a right to know why. Factors like income, expenses, debts, and credit history are among the considerations lenders use to determine creditworthiness. The practice must be specific in answering such questions.

THINKING IT THROUGH 15.6

In the collection tracer report in Figure 15.9, which patient has the greater balance? How much is the patient's balance?

Financial Agreements

If no finance charges are applied to unpaid balances, this type of arrangement is between the practice and the patient, and no additional legal regulations apply. If, however, the practice adds finance charges or late fees and the payments are to be made in more than four installments, the arrangement is subject to the **Truth in Lending Act,** which is part of the Consumer Credit Protection Act. In this case, the practice notifies the patient in writing about the total amount, the finance charges (stated as a percentage), the amount of each payment and when it is due, and the date the last payment is due. The agreement must be signed by the patient.

For example, the following schedule might be followed:

$50 balance or less: Entire balance due the first month

$51-$500 balance: $50 minimum monthly payment

$501-$1,000 balance: $100 minimum monthly payment

$1,001-$2,500 balance: $200 minimum monthly payment

Over $2,500 balance: 10 percent of the balance due each month

Collection specialists work out payment plans using patient information such as the amount of the bill, the patient's payday, the amount of disposable income the patient has, and any other contributing factors.

Assigning a Payment Plan to a Patient's Account

Most practices have a number of different payment plans that can be offered to patients. These plans vary depending on:

- The day of the month the payment is due (for example, 10th, 20th, 30th)
- How often the payment occurs (for example, every thirty days)
- The amount of the payment (for example, $20 or $40 per payment)

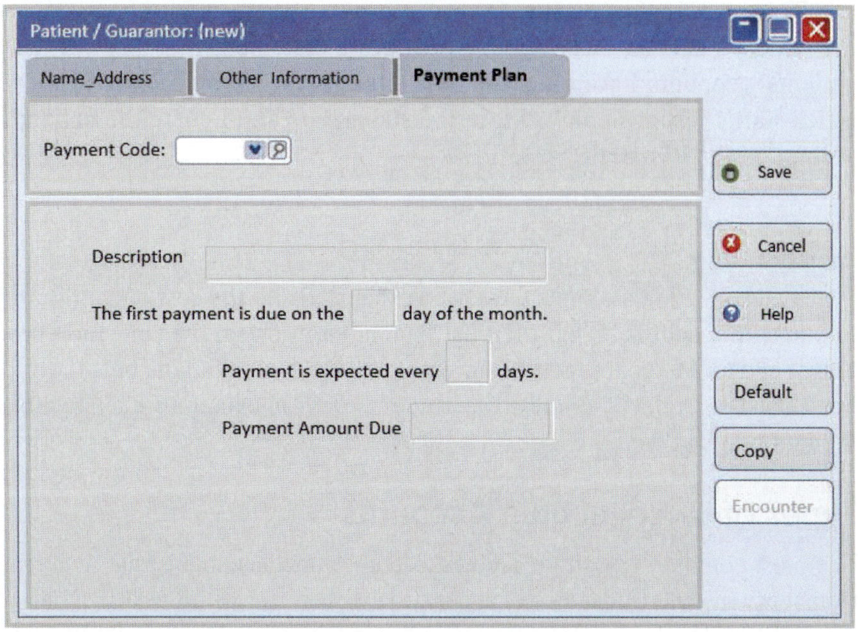

Figure 15.10 Example of Payment Plan Tab

If a payment plan is assigned and the patient follows the plan (that is, pays the required amount by the required date), the patient will not be sent collection letters. However, if the plan is not followed or the patient is in default, letters will be sent.

In a PM/EHR system, payment plans are usually set up in the Patient Payment Plan screen.

Once set up, payment plans are assigned to patient accounts in the Payment Plan tab of the Patient/Guarantor box (see Figure 15.10).

Selecting a plan in the Payment Code field assigns a specific payment amount, due date, and schedule of payments. Once the Payment Code is entered, the program automatically completes the rest of the fields.

15.7 Collection Agencies

Office staff members encounter a number of problems in their collections work. For example, a patient may have moved without leaving a forwarding address. After a number of collection attempts that do not produce results, some practices use collection agencies to pursue large unpaid bills. A **collection agency** is an outside firm hired to collect on delinquent accounts. The agency that is selected should have a reputation for fair and ethical handling of collections.

collection agency outside firm hired to collect on delinquent accounts

When a patient's account is referred to an agency for collection, the office staff members no longer contact the patient or send statements. If a payment is received from a patient while the account is with the agency, the agency is notified. Collection agencies are often paid on the basis of the amount of money they collect. For example, an agency may keep 30 percent of the amount it collects.

THINKING IT THROUGH 15.7

Under HIPAA and HITECH, collection agencies are considered business associates of the practice. Based on the information in Chapter 3, are business associates required to comply with the HIPAA Privacy and Security Rules?

When a payment is received from a collection agency, it must be posted to the patient's account. The agency provides a statement that shows which patients' accounts have paid and the amounts of the payments. It is the office staff's responsibility to take the statements and update the patient's account in the PM/EHR.

15.8 Write-Offs and Refunds

When all collection attempts have been exhausted and the cost of continuing to pursue the debt is higher than the total amount owed, the collection process is ended. Medical practices have policies on how to handle bills they do not expect to collect. Usually, the amount owed is called an **uncollectible account** or a bad debt.

uncollectible account account that does not respond to collection efforts and is written off the practice's expected accounts receivable

means test process of fairly determining a patient's ability to pay

bankruptcy declaration that a person is unable to pay his or her debts

Types of Uncollectible Accounts

The most common reason an account becomes uncollectible is that a patient cannot pay the bill. Under federal and state laws there are **means tests** that help a practice decide whether patients are indigent (categorized as poor). Patients complete a form that is used to evaluate their ability to pay. A combination of factors, such as their income level (verified by recent federal tax returns) compared to the federal poverty level, their other expenses, and the practice's policies, are used to determine what percentage of the bill will be declared uncollectible.

Other reasons for uncollectible accounts include the following:

- A patient cannot be located.
- A patient has died. Large unpaid balances of deceased patients may be pursued, either by filing an estate claim or by working in a considerate manner with the deceased patient's family members.
- A patient has filed for **bankruptcy.** Debtors may choose to file for bankruptcy when they determine that they will not be able to repay the money they owe. When a patient files for bankruptcy, the practice, which is considered to be an unsecured creditor, must file a claim in order to join the group of creditors that may receive some compensation for unpaid bills. Claims must be filed by the date specified by the bankruptcy court, or the right to any money from the bankruptcy case will be forfeited.

> **TIP**
>
> **Warning!**
>
> In the Medicare and Medicaid programs, it is fraudulent to forgive or write off any payments that beneficiaries are responsible for, such as copayments and coinsurance, unless a rigid set of steps has been followed to verify the patient's financial situation. Similarly, it is fraudulent to discount services for other providers or their families, which was formerly a common practice.

Writing Off Uncollectible Accounts

On rare occasions, practices sue individuals to collect the money they are owed. Usually, though, rather than going through the expense of a court case with uncertain results, the practice deems an unpaid balance to be uncollectible and writes it off the expected accounts receivable. A **write-off** is a balance that has been removed from a patient's account.

write-off balance that has been removed from a patient's account

small-balance account overdue patient account in which the amount owed is less than the cost of pursuing payment

patient refund money owed to patient

Small Balances

Practices also have policies that determine when amounts due are not worth pursuing. The cost of dealing with **small-balance accounts** can exceed the amounts eventually collected, making pursuing collection a poor use of the practice's resources.

In PM/EHR systems, small-balance accounts can be written off for a single patient, or in batches for multiple patients. When the program writes off the balances, several other features are updated:

- Write-off entries are created and applied to all patient-responsible charges associated with the patient.
- The Collection List items associated with the account are updated.
- Statements are changed to the status of Done.
- A note is added to the write-off entries.

THINKING IT THROUGH 15.8

Why would a practice write off accounts with small balances? Why not try to collect all monies owed to the practice?

EXERCISE 15.3

Make an Adjustment to a Patient's Account EHRclinic

Trilogy Family Care Center typically writes off small balances for procedures with less than $5 owed. Make an adjustment to a patient's account to write off the balance owed for these procedures.

Your instructor may assign this exercise to you in Connect. Exercise steps and EHRclinic Help Guides can be downloaded at http://www.mhhe.com/pmehr2.

Patient Refunds

The medical office focuses on accounts receivable, but at times the practice may need to issue **patient refunds**. Refunds are made when the practice has overcharged a patient for a service and must return the extra amount, or when a patient has overpaid an account. Note that the balance due must be refunded promptly if the practice has completed the patient's care. However, if the practice is still treating the patient, the credit balance may be carried forward–that is, noted on the patient's statement and account to be applied toward the copayment or other charges for the next visit.

EXERCISE 15.4

Process a Patient Refund EHRclinic

The billing manager at Trilogy Family Care Center identified that a patient overpaid for his coinsurance. Issue a patient refund for the difference in the overpayment.

Your instructor may assign this exercise to you in Connect. Exercise steps and EHRclinic Help Guides can be downloaded at http://www.mhhe.com/pmehr2.

chapter 15 summary

KEY TERMS

bankruptcy
collection agency
collection list
collection tracer report
Equal Credit Opportunity Act (ECOA)
Fair Debt Collection Practices Act of 1977 (FDCPA)
means tests
nonsufficient funds (NSF)
patient refunds
payment plans
small-balance accounts
Telephone Consumer Protection Act of 1991
tickler
Truth in Lending Act
uncollectable account
write-off

LEARNING OUTCOME	KEY CONCEPTS/EXAMPLES
15.1 Discuss the importance of patient collections.	Receiving full payment for services is a critical factor in determining the financial success of a medical practice. Patients' payments are collected both at the time of service (TOS) and, for insured patients, after claim adjudication by payers. At TOS, practices routinely collect copayments and overdue balances, and they may also collect either partial or full payment for visits. The majority of payments, however, are collected from patients after the payer's remittance advice and payment are transmitted to the office.
15.2 Explain the financial policy and payment expectations.	The patient collection process begins with a clear financial policy and effective communications with patients about their financial responsibilities. When patients understand the charges and the practice's financial policy in advance, collecting payments is not usually problematic. The financial policy of a medical practice explains how the practice handles financial matters.
15.3 Describe collection procedures.	Nonpayment of patient statements initiates the collection process, which involves identifying the overdue accounts and organizing them for effective follow-up. The patient aging report will be reviewed for this collection procedure.
15.4 Discuss laws governing patient collections.	Collections from patients are classified as consumer collections and are regulated by federal and state laws. The Federal Trade Commission enforces the Fair Debt Collection Practices Act of 1977 (FDCPA) and the Telephone Consumer Protection Act of 1991.

LEARNING OUTCOME	KEY CONCEPTS/EXAMPLES
15.5 Explain what is included in collection letters.	Collection letters are generally brief and to the point while preserving a professional and courteous tone. They remind the patient of the practice's payment options and their responsibility to pay the debt. Practices decide what types of letters should be sent to accounts in the various past-due stages. Accounts that are further past due will receive more aggressive letters.
15.6 Explain regulations of payment plans.	For large bills or special situations, some practices may offer payment plans to patients. The Federal Trade Commission (FTC) enforces the Equal Credit Opportunity Act (ECOA), which prohibits credit discrimination on the basis of race, color, religion, national origin, sex, marital status, age, or because a person receives public assistance. If the practice decides not to extend credit to a particular patient while extending it to others, under the ECOA the patient has a right to know why.
15.7 Describe collection agencies.	After a number of collection attempts that do not produce results, some practices use collection agencies to pursue large unpaid bills. A collection agency is an outside firm hired to collect on delinquent accounts. The agency that is selected should have a reputation for fair and ethical handling of collections. When a patient's account is referred to an agency for collection, the office staff members no longer contact the patient or send statements.
15.8 Explain the difference between write-offs and refunds.	When all collection attempts have been exhausted and the cost of continuing to pursue the debt is higher than the total amount owed, the collection process is ended. The most common reason an account becomes uncollectible is that a patient cannot pay the bill. The unpaid amount is written off from the patient's account.

chapter 15 review

MATCHING QUESTIONS

Match the key terms with their definitions.

_____ 1. *[LO 15.7]* collection agency

_____ 2. *[LO 15.6]* Equal Credit Opportunity Act (ECOA)

_____ 3. *[LO 15.4]* Fair Debt Collection Practices Act of 1977 (FDCPA)

_____ 4. *[LO 15.4]* Telephone Consumer Protection Act of 1991

_____ 5. *[LO 15.3]* tickler

_____ 6. *[LO 15.8]* means tests

_____ 7. *[LO 15.8]* bankruptcy

_____ 8. *[LO 15.8]* small-balance accounts

_____ 9. *[LO 15.5]* collection tracer report

_____ 10. *[LO 15.6]* payment plans

a. A federal law regulating collection practices.

b. A reminder to follow up on an account.

c. The declaration that a person is unable to pay his or her debts.

d. An outside firm hired to collect on delinquent accounts.

e. The process of fairly determining a patient's ability to pay.

f. Overdue patient account in which the amount owed is less than the cost of pursuing payment.

g. An agreement between a patient and a practice in which the patient agrees to make regular monthly payments over a specified period of time.

h. A tool for keeping track of collection letters that were sent.

i. A federal law regulating collection practices.

j. A law that prohibits credit discrimination on the basis of race, color, religion, national origin, sex, marital status, or age, or because a person receives public assistance.

MULTIPLE CHOICE QUESTIONS

Select the letter that best completes the statement or answers the question.

1. *[LO 15.1]* The medical practice cannot rely only on _________ to survive.
   a. patient payments
   b. insurance payments
   c. collection agency payments
   d. federal grants

2. *[LO 15.1]* What is NOT a reason a patient may not pay their bill?
   a. lack of insurance coverage
   b. lack of understanding their payment responsibility
   c. lack of financial resources
   d. consumer-directed health plans with low out-of-pocket costs

3. *[LO 15.2]* Which of the following should be included in the financial policy?
   a. collecting of copayments
   b. what types of payments the medical practice accepts
   c. both (a) and (b)
   d. none of the above
4. *[LO 15.3]* What report does the practice review to track overdue bills?
   a. collection list
   b. tickler
   c. patient aging report
   d. accounts receivable
5. *[LO 15.4]* Which of the following is a provision of federal debt collection regulations?
   a. You may call the patient at any hour of the day.
   b. Profane language in a collections call is acceptable in some circumstances.
   c. When leaving a message, you must state that it concerns a debt.
   d. You must not discuss the patient's debt with another person.
6. *[LO 15.5]* What is usually the first notice a patient receives about a debt in collections?
   a. collection letter
   b. collection call
   c. refusal of care
   d. personal message on social media
7. *[LO 15.5]* What are the three account alert abbreviations used to flag accounts in collections?
   a. RP, DB, IO
   b. RB, DP, IC
   c. RR, AR, AC
   d. RB, DR. AR
8. *[LO 15.6]* A(n) ________ is an agreement between a patient and a practice in which the patient agrees to make monthly payments.
   a. payment plan
   b. payment installment
   c. audit
   d. equal credit plan
9. *[LO 15.7]* Whose responsibility is it to post payments made through the collection agency?
   a. the collection agency's staff
   b. the medical practice's staff
   c. the provider
   d. the patient
10. *[LO 15.8]* A ________ is a balance that has been adjusted off of the patient's account.
   a. bankruptcy
   b. collections
   c. means test
   d. write-off

SHORT ANSWER QUESTIONS

Define the following abbreviations.

1. *[LO 15.6]* ECOA ______________________

2. *[LO 15.4]* FDCPA ______________________

APPLYING YOUR KNOWLEDGE

Collection Process

15.1 *[LO 15.2]* Why is it important to make patients aware of their financial responsibilities?

____

____

15.2 *[LO 15.1]* Why is it important to collect patient payments?

____

____

15.3 *[LO 15.7]* Why should a collection agency have a reputation for fair and ethical practices?

____

____

15.4 *[LO 15.6]* What are the benefits of offering payment plans?

____

____

15.5 *[LO 15.4]* Why are there laws governing how debts are collected?

____

____

chapter 16

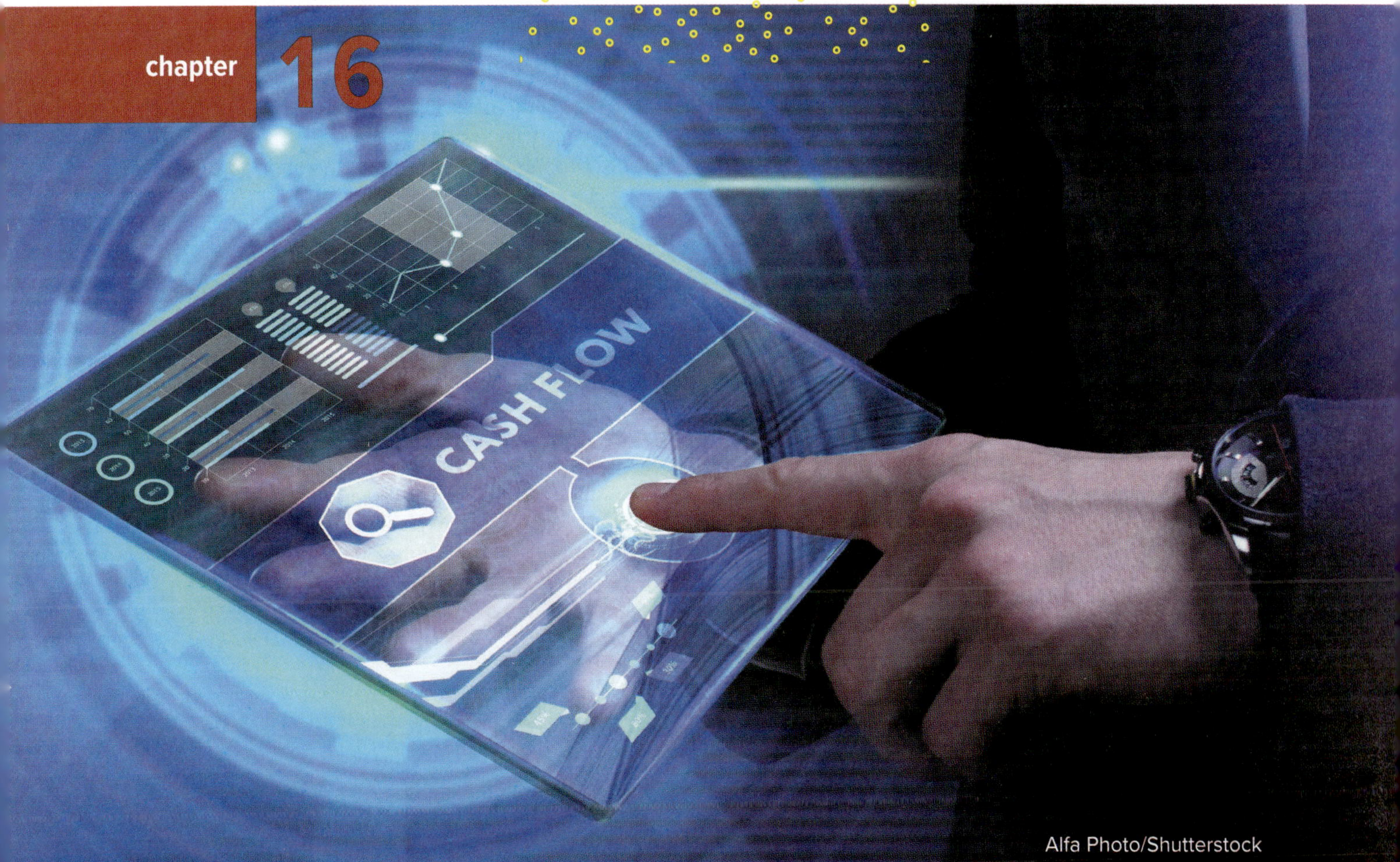

Alfa Photo/Shutterstock

Reports

LEARNING OUTCOMES

When you finish this chapter, you will be able to:

16.1 Describe the use of day sheets.

16.2 Explain the use of practice analysis reports.

16.3 Describe the use of patient ledger reports.

16.4 Explain standard patient lists.

16.5 Explain the importance of aging reports.

16.6 Explain the use of clinical reports.

Practice Reports

Trilogy Family Care Center's new PM/EHR system has the capacity to run a variety of financial and clinical reports.

At the end of each day, the revenue cycle manager, Elrene Harrison, runs the following reports:

- Patient day sheet
- Procedure day sheet

She also runs monthly reports for the following:

- Practice analysis
- Insurance analysis
- Referring providers
- Unapplied deposits

This chapter will describe each report in greater detail. As you review the report types, consider why it is important to run each one daily or monthly. What types of reports should Elrene run and review to determine the length of time a patient bill or insurance claim is outstanding?

16.1 Day Sheets

day sheet a report that provides information on practice activities for a twenty-four-hour period

patient day sheet a summary of patient activity on a given day

procedure day sheet a report that lists all the procedures performed on a particular day, in numerical order

A **day sheet** is a standard report that provides information on practice activities for a twenty-four-hour period. In PM/EHRs, there are usually three types of day sheet reports: patient day sheets, procedure day sheets, and payment day sheets. Options to view or print the three types of day sheets are located on the Reports menu, within the Day Sheets submenu.

Patient Day Sheet

At the end of the day, a medical practice often prints a **patient day sheet,** which is a summary of the patient activity on that day (see Figures 16.1a and 16.1b). It includes:

- Procedures performed for a particular patient or group of patients
- Charges, receipts, adjustments, and balances for a particular patient or group of patients
- A summary of a practice's charges, payments, and adjustments

Procedure Day Sheet

A **procedure day sheet** lists all procedures performed on a particular day and gives the dates, patients, document numbers, places of service, debits, and credits relating to them (see Figure 16.2). Procedures are listed in numerical order. Procedure day sheets are printed by clicking Day Sheets and then Procedure Day Sheet on the Reports menu. The same Search box used for a patient day sheet is displayed, except that a range of procedure codes (CPT/HCPCS codes) rather than patients can be selected. A procedure day sheet will be generated only for data that meet the selection criteria. If any box is left blank, all values are included in the report. The report can be previewed on the screen, printed, or exported to a file.

Trilogy Family Care Center

Patient Day Sheet

Show all data where the Date From is between 9/8/2022 - 9/8/2022

Entry	Date	Document	POS	Description	Provider	Code	Amount
FITZWJO0		Fitzwilliams, John					
380	09/08/2022	100907000	11		2	CHVCPAY	-15.00
471	09/08/2022	506020000	11		2	99211	36.00
472	09/08/2022	506120000	11		2	84478	29.00
				Patient Charges	Patient Receipts	Adjustments	Patient Balance
				$65.00	-$15.00	$0.00	$58.00
FITZWSA0		Fitzwilliams, Sarah					
563	09/08/2022	1010040000	11		1	90471	15.00
565	09/08/2022	1006070000	11		1	90703	29.00
566	09/08/2022	1009070000	11		1	CHVCPAY	-15.00
				Patient Charges	Patient Receipts	Adjustments	Patient Balance
				$44.00	-$15.00	$0.00	$0.00
GARDIJO0		Gardiner, John					
385	09/08/2022	1009070000	11		1	99211	36.00
387	09/08/2022	1009070000	11		1	MCGCPAY	-20.00
				Patient Charges	Patient Receipts	Adjustments	Patient Balance
				$36.00	-$20.00	$0.00	$0.00
KLEINRA0		Klein, Randall					
388	09/08/2022	1109060000	11		2	99211	54.00
389	09/08/2022	1009070000	11		2	MCGCPAY	-20.00
				Patient Charges	Patient Receipts	Adjustments	Patient Balance
				$56.00	-$20.00	$0.00	$0.00

Figure 16.1a Page 1 of a Patient Day Sheet Report

Trilogy Family Care Center

Patient Day Sheet

Show all data where the Date From is between 9/8/2022 - 9/8/2022

Entry	Date	Document	POS	Description	Provider	Code	Amount
				Total # Patients	4		
				Total # Procedures	8		
				Total Procedure Charges	$340.50		
				Total Product Charges	$0.00		
				Total Inside Lab Charges	$0.00		
				Total Outside Lab Charges	$0.00		
				Total Billing Charges	$0.00		
				Total Charges	$340.50		
				Total Insurance Payments	$0.00		
				Total Cash Copayments	$0.00		
				Total Check Copayments	-$50.00		
				Total Credit Card Copayments	$0.00		
				Total Patient Cash Payments	$0.00		
				Total Patient Check Payments	$0.00		
				Total Credit Card Payments	$0.00		
				Total Receipts	-$50.00		
				Total Credit Adjustments	$0.00		
				Total Debit Adjustments	$0.00		
				Total Insurance Debit Adjustments	$0.00		
				Total Insurance Credit Adjustments	$0.00		
				Total Insurance Withholds	$0.00		
				Total Adjustments	$0.00		
				Net Effect on Accounts Receivable	$290.50		

Figure 16.1b Page 2 of a Patient Day Sheet Report

Payment Day Sheet

A **payment day sheet** lists all payments received on a particular day, organized by provider (see Figure 16.3). It is printed by clicking Day Sheets and then Payment Day Sheet on the Reports menu. The same Search box is displayed, but with fewer data fields.

payment day sheet a report that lists all payments received on a particular day, organized by provider

Trilogy Family Care Center

Procedure Day Sheet

Show all data where the Date From is between 9/8/2022 - 9/8/2022

Entry	Date	Chart	Name	Document	POS	Debits	Credits
####							
389	09/08/2022	KLEINRA0	Klein, Randall	1009070000	11	121.50	
		Total of 29540		Quantity:	1	$121.50	0.00
####							
472	09/08/2022	FITZWJO0	Fitzwilliams, John	506020000	11	29.00	
		Total of 84478		Quantity:	1	$29.00	0.00
90471							
563	09/08/2022	FITZWSA0	Fitzwilliams, Sarah	1010040000	11	15.00	
		Total of 90471		Quantity:	1	$15.00	0.00
####							
565	09/08/2022	FITZWSA0	Fitzwilliams, Sarah	1009070000	11	29.00	
		Total of 90703		Quantity:	1	$29.00	0.00
####							
390	09/08/2022	KLEINRA0	Klein, Randall	1009070000	11	20.00	
		Total of 99070		Quantity:	1	$20.00	0.00
99211							
471	09/08/2022	FITZWJO0	Fitzwilliams, John	1506020000	11	36.00	
385	09/08/2022	GARDIJO0	Gardiner, John	1009070000	11	36.00	
		Total of 99211		Quantity:	2	$72.00	0.00
99212							
388	09/08/2022	KLEINRA0	Klein, Randall	1009070000	11	54.00	
		Total of 99212		Quantity:	1	$54.00	0.00
CHVCPAY							
380	09/08/2022	FITZWJO0	Fitzwilliams, John	1009070000	11		-15.00
566	09/08/2022	FITZWSA0	Fitzwilliams, Sarah	1009070000	11		-15.00
		Total of 99211		Quantity:	2	$0.00	-$30.00
MCGPAY							
387	09/08/2022	GARDIJO0	Gardiner, John	1009070000	11		-20.00
		Total of 99211		Quantity:	1	$0.00	-$20.00
					Total of Codes	$340.50	-$50.00
					Balance	$290.50	

Figure 16.2 Procedure Day Sheet

Trilogy Family Care Center

Payment Day Sheet

Show all data where the Date From is between 9/8/2022 - 9/8/2022

Entry	Date	Document	Description	Chart	Code	Amount
1	**Yan, Katherine**					
566	09/08/2022	1009070000		FITZWSA0	CHVCPAY	-15.00
387	09/08/2022	1009070000		GARDIJO0	MCGCPAY	-20.00
			Count 2		Provider Total	-35.00
2	**Rudner, John**					
566	09/08/2022	1009070000		RUDNEJO0	CHVCPAY	-15.00
			Count 2		Provider Total	-35.00
				Report Totals		
				Total # Payments		3
				Total Payments		-50.00

Figure 16.3 Payment Day Sheet

A payment day sheet will be generated only for data that meet the selection criteria. If any box is left blank, all values for that box are included in the report. Again, the report can be previewed on the screen, printed, or exported to a file.

THINKING IT THROUGH 16.1

How do patient day sheets, procedure day sheets, and payment day sheets differ?

Create Day Sheet Reports

EHRclinic

EXERCISE 16.1

At the end of each day, you are responsible for running day sheet reports for Trilogy Family Care Center. Create patient and payment day sheet reports.

Your instructor may assign this exercise to you in Connect. Exercise steps and EHRclinic Help Guides can be downloaded at http://www.mhhe.com/pmehr2.

16.2 Practice Analysis Reports

PM/EHRs can include a number of standard reports that provide information about practice finances. These reports are known as analysis reports. The following paragraphs provide a description of common reports. Not all reports can be created in all PM/EHR software. Reports vary with the system the practice uses along with the needs of the practice.

Billing/Payment Status Report

The billing/payment status report lists the status of all transactions that have responsible insurance carriers, showing who has paid and who has not been billed (see Figure 16.4). The report is in a column format sorted

Family Care Clinic

Billing/Payment Status Report

Show all data where the Patient Reference Balance is between 0.01,999999999999.99
Show all data where the Date From is between 10/1/2016, 10/31/2016

Date	Document	Procedure	Amount	Policy 1	Policy 2	Policy 3	Guarantor	Adjustments	Balance
BARREJO0	**Jorge Barrett (614)509-3637**								
Case 67	1:	Blue Cross/Blue Shield	(614)024-9000						
	2:								
	3:								
10/21/2016	1610210000	99203	120.00	-96.00*	0.00*	0.00*	11/30/2016	0.00	24.00
								SubTotal:	24.00
								Unapplied Payments and Adjustments:	96.00
								Case Balance:	120.00
								Patient Reference Balance:	24.00
BATTIAN0	**Anthony Battistuta (614)500-3619**								
Case 25	1:	Medicare	(215)599-0000						
	2:								
	3:								
10/27/2016	1009280000	82947	25.00	10/31/2016	0.00*	0.00*	Not Billed	0.00	25.00
10/27/2016	1009280000	99212	54.00	10/31/2016	0.00*	0.00*	Not Billed	0.00	54.00
								SubTotal:	79.00
								Unapplied Payments and Adjustments:	0.00
								Case Balance:	79.00
								Patient Reference Balance:	79.00
BROOKLA0	**Lawana Brooks (614)027-4242**								
Case 27	1:	East Ohio PPO	(419)444-1505						
	2:								
	3:								
10/28/2016	1010290000	73600	96.00	10/31/2016	0.00*	0.00*	Not Billed	0.00	96.00
10/28/2016	1010290000	99212	54.00	10/31/2016	0.00*	0.00*	-20.00	0.00	34.00
								SubTotal:	130.00
								Unapplied Payments and Adjustments:	0.00
								Case Balance:	130.00
								Patient Reference Balance:	130.00
FITZWJO0	**John Fitzwilliams (614)002-1111**								
Case 7	1:	ChampVA	(614)024-7000						
	2:								
	3:								
10/3/2016	1006230000	82270	19.00	Not Billed	0.00*	0.00*	Not Billed	0.00	19.00
10/3/2016	1006230000	99212	54.00	Not Billed	0.00*	0.00*	-15.00	0.00	39.00
								SubTotal:	58.00
								Unapplied Payments and Adjustments:	-50.00
								Case Balance:	8.00
								Patient Reference Balance:	58.00

Figure 16.4 Sample First Page of Billing/Payment Status Report

first by chart number and then by case. Every chart number listed shows a patient balance and any unapplied payments or unapplied adjustments. An asterisk (*) next to a number indicates that the payer has made a complete payment for that transaction. Information in this report can be used by a practice to determine whether billing charges can be applied to a patient account.

Insurance Payment Comparison

The insurance payment comparison report isolates a procedure code and shows the payments applied to it from up to five insurance carriers. It is used to determine the average amount different carriers are paying for a given procedure or a range of procedures. In the Insurance Carrier #1 box, the Lookup button is used to select an insurance carrier code. Additional codes are selected using the Add to List button. For each procedure code, the report shows the procedure code and description, the standard charge, the average payment of each insurance carrier selected for the report, and the total current charges for the procedure.

Practice Analysis Report

practice analysis report a report that analyzes the revenue of a practice for a specified period of time

A **practice analysis report** analyzes the revenue of a practice for a specified period of time, usually a month or a year (see Figures 16.5a and 16.5b). The report can be used to generate medical practice financial statements. It can also be used for profit analysis. The summary at the end of the report breaks down the information into total charges, total payments and copayments, and total adjustments.

Family Care Clinic

Practice Analysis

Show all data where the Date From is between 9/1/2016, 9/30/2016

Code	Description	Amount	Units	Average	Cost	Net
02	Patient payment, check	-299.50	2	-149.75	0.00	-299.50
29540	Strapping, ankle	121.50	1	121.50	0.00	121.50
50390	Aspiration of renal cyst by needle	551.00	1	551.00	0.00	551.00
73510	Hip x-ray, complete, two views	124.00	1	124.00	0.00	124.00
84478	Triglycerides test	29.00	1	29.00	0.00	29.00
90471	Immunization administration	15.00	1	15.00	0.00	15.00
90703	Tetanus injection	29.00	1	29.00	0.00	29.00
92516	Facial nerve function studies	210.00	1	210.00	0.00	210.00
93000	Electrocardiogram--ECG with interpr	84.00	1	84.00	0.00	84.00
99070	Supplies and materials provided	20.00	1	20.00	0.00	20.00
99201	OF--new patient, minimal	66.00	1	66.00	0.00	66.00
99211	OF--established patient, minimal	144.00	4	36.00	0.00	144.00
99212	OF--established patient, low	324.00	6	54.00	0.00	324.00
99213	OF--established patient, detailed	216.00	3	72.00	0.00	216.00
99214	OF--established patient, moderate	105.00	1	105.00	0.00	105.00
99394	Preventive est., 12-17 years	222.00	1	222.00	0.00	222.00
AARPAY	AARP Payment	-19.57	3	-6.52	0.00	-19.57
BCBDED	BCBS Deductible	0.00	1	0.00	0.00	0.00
BCBPAY	BCBS Payment	-168.00	2	-84.00	0.00	-168.00
CHVCPAY	ChampVA Copayment	-30.00	2	-15.00	0.00	-30.00
EAPADJ	East Ohio PPO Adjustment	-12.60	2	-6.30	0.00	-12.60
EAPCPAY	East Ohio PPO Copayment	-160.00	8	-20.00	0.00	-160.00
EAPPAY	East Ohio PPO Payment	-73.40	2	-36.70	0.00	-73.40
MCDADJ	Medicaid Adjustment	-479.95	2	-239.97	0.00	-479.95
MCDCPAY	Medicaid Copayment	-10.00	1	-10.00	0.00	-10.00
MCDPAY	Medicaid Payment	-127.05	2	-63.52	0.00	-127.05
MEDADJ	Medicare Adjustment	-212.73	6	-35.46	0.00	-212.73
MEDPAY	Medicare Payment	-209.42	7	-29.92	0.00	-209.42
OHCADJ	OhioCare HMO Adjustment	-50.00	2	-25.00	0.00	-50.00
OHCCPAY	OhioCare HMO Copayment	-40.00	2	-20.00	0.00	-40.00

Figure 16.5a Page 1 of Practice Analysis Report

Family Care Clinic

Practice Analysis

Show all data where the Date From is between 9/1/2016, 9/30/2016

Code	Description	Amount	Units	Average	Cost	Net
	Total Procedure Charges					$2,260.50
	Total Global Surgical Procedures					$0.00
	Total Product Charges					$0.00
	Total Inside Lab Charges					$0.00
	Total Outside Lab Charges					$0.00
	Total Billing Charges					$0.00
	Total Insurance Payments					-$597.44
	Total Cash Copayments					$0.00
	Total Check Copayments					-$240.00
	Total Credit Card Copayments					$0.00
	Total Patient Cash Payments					$0.00
	Total Patient Check Payments					-$299.50
	Total Credit Card Payments					$0.00
	Total Debit Adjustments					$0.00
	Total Credit Adjustments					$0.00
	Total Insurance Debit Adjustments					$0.00
	Total Insurance Credit Adjustments					-$755.28
	Total Insurance Withholds					$0.00
	Net Effect on Accounts Receivable					$368.28
	Practice Totals					
	Total # Procedures					60
	Total Charges					$4,977.50
	Total Payments					-$2,558.64
	Total Adjustments					-$755.86
	Accounts Receivable					$1,712.72

Figure 16.5b Page 2 of Practice Analysis Report

EXERCISE 16.2

Create a Practice Analysis Report

EHRclinic

The revenue cycle manager has asked for a meeting to review the practice's revenue from month to month. Run a practice analysis report to share this month's revenue during the meeting.

Your instructor may assign this exercise to you in Connect. Exercise steps and EHRclinic Help Guides can be downloaded at http://www.mhhe.com/pmehr2.

Insurance Analysis

The insurance analysis report tracks charges, insurance payments received during a specified period, and copayments applied to accounts that include those procedures. It is usually printed at the end of the month. The amount listed as the outstanding balance displays the total charges, subtracting the full amount of the charge if the insurance payment was made.

Referring Provider Report

The referring provider report enables a practice to determine the origins of revenue derived from providers who have referred patients to the practice. The report lists the percentage of total income that was generated by referring providers.

Referral Source Report

The referral source report tracks the source of referrals that are not from other medical offices or providers, such as referrals from established patients.

Facility Report

The facility report tracks the revenue coming in from patients who are treated at different facilities. For the facility report to work properly, facilities must be set up using the Facilities option on the Lists menu within settings. Then the appropriate facility must be entered in the Account tab for each patient's case. The filters include a "case facility" range and a "date from" range.

Unapplied Payment/Adjustment Report

The unapplied payment/adjustment report lists payments or adjustments that have not been fully applied. Information about the payment or adjustment includes the case, document number, posting date, code, code description, transaction amount, and unapplied amount.

Unapplied Deposit Report

The unapplied deposit report lists deposits that have unapplied amounts. The report includes the date, code, payer name, payer type, deposit amount, and unapplied amount.

Copayment Report

This report lists patients who have copayment transactions. It shows the amount paid, how much was applied, and how much, if any, was left unapplied.

Outstanding Copayment Report

This report shows patients who have outstanding copayment transactions. The report shows the copayment amount expected, the actual amount paid, and the amount due.

THINKING IT THROUGH 16.2

What is the importance of the referring provider report?

16.3 Patient Ledger Reports

patient ledger a report that lists the financial activity in each patient's account

A **patient ledger** lists the transaction details of a patient's account, including charges, payments, and adjustments, as shown in Figure 16.6. Like day sheets, analysis reports, and production reports, the patient ledger report is one of the standard reports in a PM/EHR system. The information it provides is especially useful when there is a question about a patient's account.

The patient account ledger report is typically created by clicking Patient Ledger on the Reports menu. After the preview, print, or export selection is made, the Search box is displayed, as it is with the other reports. It provides

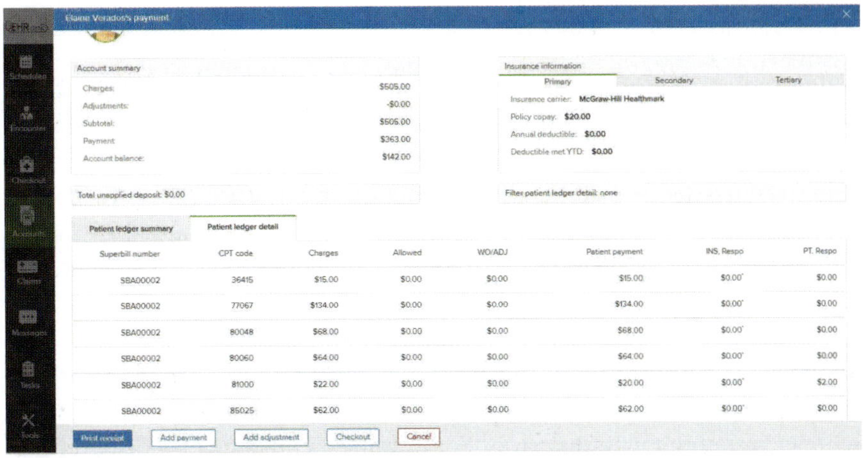

Figure 16.6 Patient Account Ledger Report

options to select by chart numbers, patient reference balances, dates, attending providers, billing codes, and patient indicators. A patient account ledger is generated only for data that meet the selection criteria.

THINKING IT THROUGH 16.3

What are the benefits of a patient ledger report?

16.4 Standard Patient Lists

PM/EHR systems include several convenient reports for identifying patients by diagnosis or insurance carrier. These reports can help track trends within the community and health care coverage.

The patient by diagnosis report lists diagnosis code, chart number, patient name, age, attending provider, facility, and date of last visit. These reports can be used to send to insurance carriers and CMS for tracking measures and reporting of statistics.

THINKING IT THROUGH 16.4

Why would a medical practice review a report based on diagnosis?

The patient by insurance carrier report lists patients sorted by provider or facility, and then by their insurance carrier.

THINKING IT THROUGH 16.5

What types of trends could be found by reviewing an insurance carrier report?

16.5 Aging Reports

aging report a report that lists the amount of money owed to the practice, organized by the amount of time the money has been owed

patient aging report a report that lists a patient's balance by age, date and amount of the last payment, and telephone number, grouping unpaid bills by the length of time they remain due

Aging reports are of particular importance to medical billing specialists. An **aging report** lists the amount of money owed to the practice, organized by the amount of time the money has been owed. Medical practices use aging reports to determine which accounts require follow-up to collect past-due balances. A **patient aging report,** depicted in Figure 16.7, lists a patient's balance by age overdue, date and amount of the last payment, and telephone number.

As shown in Figure 16.8, an insurance aging report shows how long a payer has taken to respond to each claim (also discussed in Chapter 13). This information is used to compare the response time with the terms of the practice's contract with the payer. For example, a practice may discover that a payer is routinely responding to claims ten days later than the claim turn-around time specified in the contract. In that case, the practice manager might review the situation with the payer's customer service manager and ask the payer to adhere to its guidelines.

Trilogy Family Care Center

Patient Aging by Date of Service

Show all data where Charges/Payments/Adj is on or before 10/31/2022

Chart	Name	-Past- 0 to 30	-Past- 31 to 60	-Past- 61 to 90	-Past- 91 to 120	-Past- 121+	Total
AA004	Jack Kyser	50.00					50.00
AA007	Anthony Battistuta	21.17	7.47				28.64
AA008	Pauline Battistuta				720.50		720.50
AA011	Jonathan Bell	49.18		15.52			64.70
AA024	Randall Klein		18.91				18.91
AA026	Raj Patel	-10.00					-10.00
AA031	James Smolowski				93.64		93.64
Report Totals:		110.35	26.38	15.52	814.14		966.39

Figure 16.7 Example of Patient Aging Report

Primary Insurance Aging Summary

October 31, 2022

Date of Service	Procedure	-Past- 0 to 30	-Past- 31 to 60	-Past- 61 to 90	-Past- 91 to 120	-Past- 121+	Total Balance
McGraw-Hill MedMark							555-620-1975
Claim 69721	Initial Billing Date: 9/23/2022		Last Billing Date: 10/14/2022				
	Insurance Totals:	$0.00	$160.00	$0.00	$0.00	$0.00	$160.00
Ameri-Access							555-315-6607
Claim 63317	Initial Billing Date: 6/30/2022		Last Billing Date: 10/14/2022				
Claim 69721	Initial Billing Date: 8/12/2022		Last Billing Date: 10/14/2022				
	Insurance Totals:	$0.00	$0.00	$465.00	$0.00	$655.00	$1,120.00

Figure 16.8 Example of Insurance Aging Report

THINKING IT THROUGH 16.6

What steps should a practice take if they have not received payment from an insurance carrier?

EXERCISE 16.3

Create Aging Reports

EHRclinic

You are responsible for collections and following up outstanding insurance claims for Trilogy Family Care Center. Run a patient aging report and an insurance aging report to ensure that you are using current data to collect overdue payments.

Your instructor may assign this exercise to you in Connect. Exercise steps and EHRclinic Help Guides can be downloaded at http://www.mhhe.com/pmehr2.

16.6 Clinical Reports

PM/EHRs have the potential to substantially improve the delivery of health care. For this reason, the federal government and private payers have established financial incentives to guide EHR implementation.

As discussed in Chapter 3, the HITECH Act requires providers to show that they are going to change the way they practice by using health information technology to improve outcomes and quality and by using EHRs in ways that accomplish the following basic goals:

- Improving quality, safety, and efficiency, while reducing disparities in the care patients receive
- Engaging patients and families in their health care
- Improving care coordination
- Ensuring adequate privacy and security protections for personal health information
- Improving population and public health

Using a PM/EHR system saves countless hours of time and energy by automating the process of sorting through hundreds of records, searching for specific results, and generating lists and reminders for follow-up.

Risk Adjustment Reporting

Each practice's results can be compared to national standards and to the results of other practices. Common areas include the management of diabetes, cardiovascular disease, cancer screening, immunizations, infectious disease, mental health, substance abuse, and obesity. These are tracked by **Hierarchical Condition Category coding (HCC).** ICD-10-CM coding is assigned risk scores to patients. Each HCC is mapped to an ICD-10-CM code. Using algorithms, insurance companies can use a patient's diagnosis to estimate future health care costs and to help paint a full picture of the complexity of patients and the care they are receiving. Practices are given financial incentives yearly when they report HCC coding to payers, including Medicare.

Hierarchical Condition Category Coding (HCC) a risk-adjustment model based on ICD-10-CM coding to assign risk scores to patients to estimate health care cost and give a picture of the complexity of patients

patient registry method of reporting clinical data to payers using an online service rather than claim-based reporting

Reporting Methods

Practices that participate in HCC coding may either report their codes directly to CMS using a claims-based system that is often handled by a clearinghouse or by using a **patient registry.** Patient registries are databases that collect clinical data on all the practice's patients who have specific conditions, such as diabetes or asthma, or that keep track of specific tests, such as mammograms. A registry acts as an online service that coordinates storage and reporting of performance measurement data. The practice can enter the patient data as part of routine clinical activities like documentation using the PM/EHR reports.

THINKING IT THROUGH 16.7

Besides the financial incentives, why would a practice participate in HCC coding?

chapter 16 summary

KEY TERMS

aging report
day sheet
Hierarchical Condition Category coding (HCC)
patient aging report
patient day sheet
patient ledger
patient registry
payment day sheet
practice analysis report
procedure day sheet

LEARNING OUTCOME	KEY CONCEPTS/EXAMPLES
16.1 Describe the use of day sheets.	A day sheet is a standard report that provides information on practice activities for a twenty-four-hour period. In PM/EHRs, there are usually three types of day sheet reports: Patient day sheets Procedure day sheets Payment day sheets
16.2 Explain the use of practice analysis reports.	Reports that provide information about practice finances are known as analysis reports. The various types are: • Billing/Payment Status Report • Insurance Payment Comparison • Practice Analysis Report • Insurance Analysis Report • Referring Provider Report • Referral Source Report • Facility Report • Unapplied Payment/Adjustment Report • Unapplied Deposit Report • Copayment Report • Outstanding Copayment Report
16.3 Describe the use of patient ledger reports.	A patient ledger lists the transaction details of a patient's account, including charges, payments, and adjustments. It is a summary of all transactions of the patient's account.
16.4 Explain standard patient lists.	Standard patient lists are reports for identifying patients by diagnosis or insurance carrier. These reports can help track trends within the community and health care coverage.

LEARNING OUTCOME	KEY CONCEPTS/EXAMPLES
16.5 Explain the importance of aging reports.	An aging report lists the amount of money owed to the practice, organized by the amount of time the money has been owed. Medical practices use aging reports to determine which accounts require follow-up to collect past-due balances. • Patient Aging Report • Insurance Aging Report
16.6 Explain the use of clinical reports.	Each practice can pull data based on clinical results. These can be compared to national standards and to the results of other practices. Hierarchical Condition Category coding (HCC) is used to paint a picture of the complexity of patients for statistical reasons and for additional reimbursement when reported.

chapter 16 review

MATCHING QUESTIONS

Match the key terms with their definitions.

_____ 1. *[LO 16.1]* day sheet

_____ 2. *[LO 16.1]* patient day sheet

_____ 3. *[LO 16.1]* payment day sheet

_____ 4. *[LO 16.2]* practice analysis report

_____ 5. *[LO 16.3]* patient ledger

_____ 6. *[LO 16.5]* patient aging report

_____ 7. *[LO 16.5]* insurance aging report

_____ 8. *[LO 16.6]* patient registry

_____ 9. *[LO 16.1]* procedure day sheet

_____ 10. *[LO 16.5]* aging report

a. A report that analyzes the revenue of a practice for a specified period of time.

b. A summary of patient activity on a given day.

c. A report that lists how long a payer has taken to respond to insurance claims.

d. A report that lists the financial activity in each patient's account.

e. A report that lists all payments received on a particular day, organized by provider.

f. A report that lists a patient's balance by age, date and amount of the last payment, and telephone number, grouping unpaid bills by the length of time they remain due.

g. A report that lists all the procedures performed on a particular day, in numerical order.

h. A report that lists the amount of money owed to the practice, organized by the amount of time the money has been owed.

i. Method of reporting clinical data to payers using an online service rather than claim-based reporting.

j. A report that provides information on practice activities for a twenty-four-hour period.

MULTIPLE CHOICE QUESTIONS

Select the letter that best completes the statement or answers the question.

1. *[LO 16.1]* At the end of the day, a medical practice often prints a _____, which is a summary of the patient activity on that day.
   a. patient day sheet
   b. day sheet
   c. payment day sheet
   d. patient aging report

2. *[LO 16.1]* What is included on a patient day sheet?
   a. amounts owed and charges of the practice
   b. procedures, diagnosis, and charges for the patient
   c. amounts owed by insurance and patient
   d. procedures, charges for patient and practice

3. *[LO 16.2]* The ______ status report lists the status of all transactions that have responsible insurance carriers.
   a. insurance payment
   b. patient payment
   c. billing/payment
   d. practice analysis

4. *[LO 16.2]* A ______ analyzes the revenue of a practice for a specified period of time.
   a. practice analysis report
   b. insurance payment report
   c. practice billing report
   d. patient payment report

5. *[LO 16.2]* What report can be used to track the source of referrals that are not from medical offices?
   a. referring provider report
   b. referral source report
   c. practice billing report
   d. none of the above

6. *[LO 16.3]* A ______ lists the transaction details of a patient's account, including charges, payments, and adjustments.
   a. patient day sheet
   b. patient payment report
   c. patient ledger
   d. insurance report

7. *[LO 16.4]* The ______ report lists patients sorted by provider and then by their insurance carrier.
   a. insurance report
   b. patient by insurance carrier
   c. insurance payment
   d. facility

8. *[LO 16.5]* What type of report lists the amount of money owed to the practice, organized by the amount of time the money has been owed?
   a. analysis report
   b. patient day sheet
   c. patient ledger
   d. aging report

9. *[LO 16.6]* What type of tracking is used to compare data to national standards, also known as risk adjustment reporting?
   a. HCC coding
   b. ICD-10-CM
   c. patient analysis report
   d. Medicare statistic report

10. *[LO 16.6]* Databases that collect clinical data on all of the practice's patients who have specific conditions are called

   a. insurance registry
   b. patient registration
   c. patient registry
   d. none of the above

SHORT ANSWER QUESTIONS

Define the following abbreviations.

1. *[LO 16.6]* HCC ________________________

APPLYING YOUR KNOWLEDGE

Answer the questions below in the space provided.

16.1. *[LO 16.1]* Why does a practice print and review the patient day sheet?

____

____

16.2. *[LO 16.2]* List the different practice analysis reports a PM/EHR may have.

____

____

16.3. *[LO 16.6]* The HITECH Act requires providers to show that they are going to change the way they practice by using health information technology to improve outcomes and quality of care. How do reports factor into the quality of care and outcomes?

____

____

16.4. *[LO 16.1]* List the three day sheets used in a medical practice, and define the use of each.

____

____

chapter 17

Messaging and Administrative Tasks

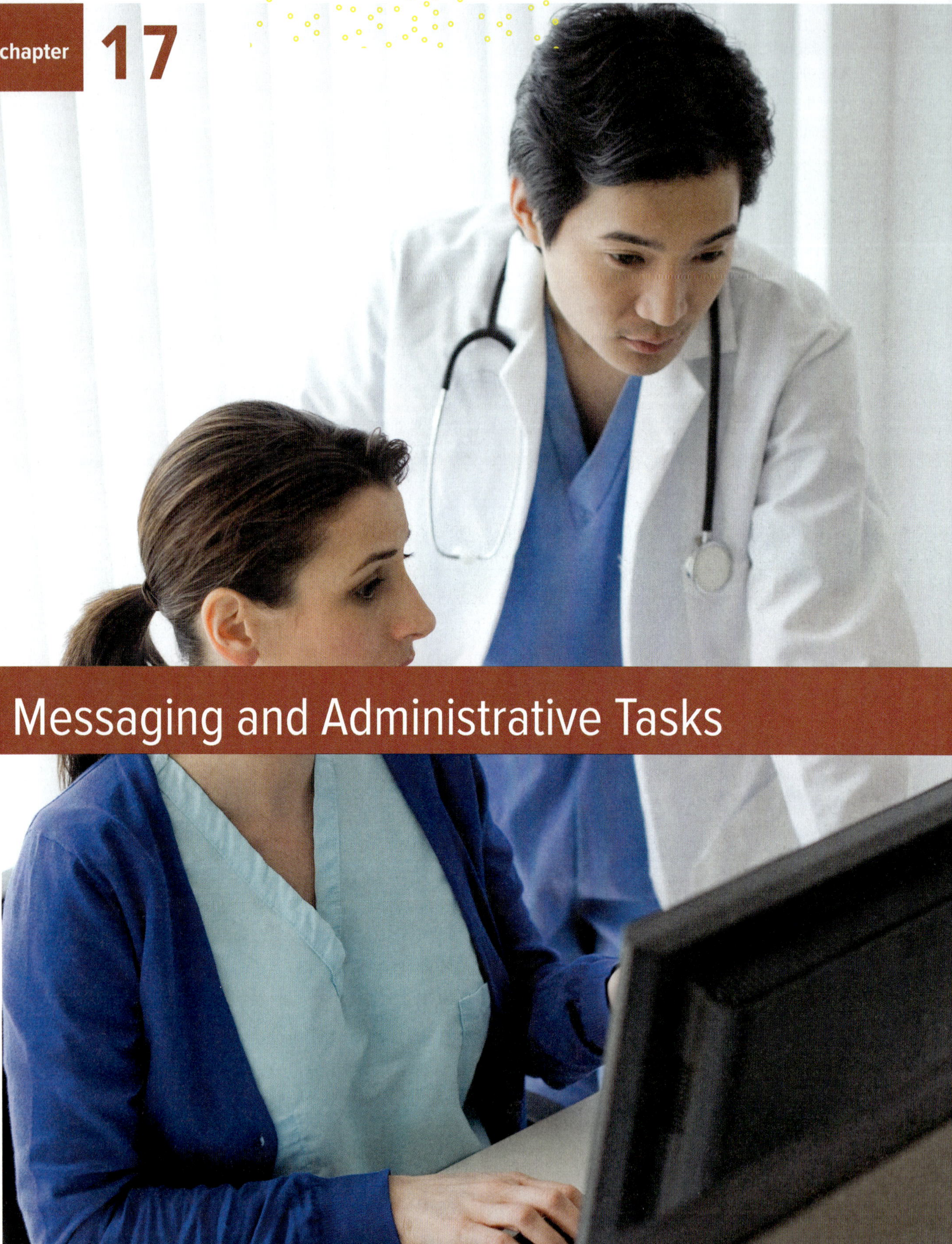

Tetra Images/Getty Images

LEARNING OUTCOMES

When you finish this chapter, you will be able to:

17.1 Describe how emails and telephone encounters are used in electronic health records.

17.2 Demonstrate the professional use of written communications in an electronic health record.

17.3 Explain how tasks and recall lists are used to communicate in a medical practice.

Communication Is Key

Anthony Davis calls the Trilogy Family Care Center and asks to leave a message for Dr. Williams because he is out of town and has lost his medications. He needs his asthma and hypertension medications called into a local pharmacy so he can pick them up.

As you read this chapter, consider the type of message that Anthony Davis would leave. Is this an urgent message? Why or why not? What kind of information would you need to obtain from Mr. Davis to ensure that the message can be handled efficiently?

17.1 Electronic Messaging

Messages are an important part of communication in any medical practice. They are used to communicate internally among staff or externally with patients, vendors, and other outside providers or health systems. Most messaging systems provide two-way communication in which two or more individuals or entities can initiate or receive messages as well as respond to them. This is typically done in email or telephone message formats.

Communication Through Messages

As previously mentioned, messages are used as a form of **two-way communication**. The **sender** initiates a message by calling, at which point the message is recorded, or the message is sent through an email. The message is then forwarded to the **recipient,** who will review it and return a response, usually in the form of a returned call or another email.

Message Types

In a medical practice, messages from phone calls are typically recorded as **electronic telephone messages.** An electronic telephone message is initiated when a caller wishes to leave a message for the provider or another member of the health care team. If the call is related to a patient, the message is entered directly into the patient's electronic health record, at which point each response is documented and becomes a part of the patient's legal medical record.

Similarly, **emails** are commonly used to communicate to health care providers or the health care team. These are messages that are delivered

two-way communication when one person is the sender of a message that is transmitted to another person (the receiver)

sender an individual who initiates a message to another person or entity

recipient a person, persons, or entity who receives a message

electronic telephone message communication that is transmitted by telephone and entered into an electronic health record for response and resolution

email messages delivered electronically through a network to one or more recipients

electronically through a network to one or more recipients. Most patient portals have email capability in which patients can communicate directly with the medical practice through the portal. Responses are also provided through the portal, and then email notifications are sent to the patient. Like electronic telephone messages, patient-related emails are automatically documented within the patient's EHR.

Internal and External Messages Messages are identified as being either internal or external. Internal messages are communications within a medical practice or health care system. External messages are those that come from outside of the practice, such as from a patient or another health care system, provider, lab, or outside source.

Patient and Nonpatient Messages There are also two main types of messages; those related to patients and those that are not related to patients or patient care. When taking messages, it is important to first identify if the caller is a patient or calling about a patient.

EXAMPLES

Here are some examples of internal, external, patient, and nonpatient messages:

Internal nonpatient message Dr. Williams sends the office manager, Elrene, an email asking her to order lunch for the office.

Internal patient message Dr. Cheng sends an email to the lab requesting that a patient's urinalysis be processed STAT (immediately).

External nonpatient message Dr. Mancini's son calls and leaves a telephone message to let her know that he does not need to be picked up from soccer practice.

External patient message Janice Washington calls and leaves a message with this week's at-home blood pressure readings for Dr. McGrath. The message is recorded in an electronic telephone message and linked to the patient's EHR.

Effective Message Documentation

In a medical practice, there is no room for misunderstanding of messages. Unclear messages can be dangerous for patients and a liability for providers. The following strategies can help to ensure that messages are delivered clearly and with the least opportunity for error.

The C's of Communication

Whether they are by phone or email, messages–sending and receiving–are an important part of communication in a medical practice, so it is essential to understand the "C's of communication." These guidelines that should be followed to ensure that messages are effective and accurate.

The C's of communication should be applied to messages so they will be:

Clear Be clear about the purpose of a message, and ensure that the content is understandable. When documenting a telephone message, be sure to clarify information from the caller.

Correct Accuracy is essential when taking messages. Make sure that the information documented is error-free (contact information and the message details) and that the language and grammar used are correct. Use resources, if necessary, to ensure that the information is correct. For example, if there is a question about the spelling of a drug name, use a drug dictionary to look it up.

Complete Give the recipient all of the information needed to process and respond to a message efficiently. For example, if a patient calls for a medication refill, make sure that the details of the prescription (drug, dosage, frequency) are included in the message as well as the pharmacy contact information.

Concise Keep messages as short and simple as possible. While it is important to ensure that the information provided is complete, messages should focus on the key points to avoid confusion. In some cases, callers may veer off-topic when leaving messages, so it may be necessary to determine the relevance of information provided.

Courteous Messages should be respectful and courteous. Using language and tone to maintain professionalism and consideration is an important part of effective communication.

Coherent Ensure that communication has a logical flow and a consistent style, tone, and language so that it is coherent and understandable.

THINKING IT THROUGH 17.1

Consider the C's of communication. What are the potential consequences if messages are recorded inaccurately?

Taking an Effective Phone Message

Phone messages should be accurate, detailed, and understandable. Applying the C's of communication is a great framework for taking an effective message, but there are additional strategies to assist with taking the best messages. They include:

- Using good phone etiquette, such as answering by the third ring and asking patients before putting them on hold. Greet callers with a pleasant voice and a positive, respectful tone. Close the call by thanking the caller and asking if there is any other assistance that can be provided. Good phone etiquette sets the tone for a positive phone conversation.
- Be organized when recording the details of a call. In many cases, messages are recorded in electronic message systems, but it is sometimes necessary to gather thoughts and information so that they can be organized coherently in the electronic document. Take notes when necessary, and use resources, such as details found in the patient's chart or reference books for spelling.
- Record the most pertinent information for the message and read it back to the caller. It is a best practice to summarize a message for the caller to ensure that it is accurate and complete.
- Assess the message for urgency and escalate it accordingly. Messages should be prioritized and marked for priority so they can be addressed

in a timely manner. Not all messages can be marked as urgent; doing so defeats the purpose of prioritizing messages.

- Identify the caller. For example, a caller may be a patient, the patient's family member, or another provider calling about the patient. Remember that HIPAA prevents any sharing of patient information unless an authorization has been signed granting permission, although it is possible to take a message from someone on a patient's behalf.
- Obtain the caller's contact information. Although patient demographics, such as phone numbers, are listed in the EHR, the caller should always be asked to confirm the best number to call back. This prevents inefficiency when trying to respond to the message.
- Be courteous and helpful while giving the caller undivided attention. Use good listening skills, and avoid trying to do other tasks while taking messages over the phone.
- Avoid putting words into patient's mouths or rephrasing their own words without clarification. For example, if a patient states that his "head hurts," do not indicate in the message that he has a "headache." These may mean two different things to the patient. Always ask leading questions to get more accurate information from patients if anything is unclear.

Completing a Message

Once a message has been constructed, it is sent to the recipient for review. The message is then processed, and an appropriate action is determined. In some cases, for example, the provider may call the patient, or caller, back directly. In other cases, the provider may determine a course of action and send the message back to the person who originally sent it or forward it on to another person.

EXAMPLES

Electronic messages flow between various people in a medical practice until they are eventually resolved. Here are some examples of this flow:

- A patient calls asking for a prescription refill to be called in to an out-of-state pharmacy. The message is sent to the provider, who approves the refill and forwards it to the medical assistant. The medical assistant calls the prescription in, documents the refill, and signs and closes the message.
- A provider's colleague calls and leaves a message to inform the provider that he will be closing a clinic day due to a family emergency. The provider reviews the message and closes it.
- A pharmaceutical representative calls the office to schedule some time with a provider. The provider agrees to a day and time for the following week and sends the message back to the administrative medical assistant to schedule the appointment.
- A patient saw the provider for an appointment on Monday. On Wednesday, the patient calls and leaves a message to state that her symptoms have worsened. The provider calls the patient back to discuss this with her, documents the call, and then closes the message.

As shown in the examples above, each message moves through various stages to show its progress from beginning to end. The recipient of each stage of the message will document what has been done or indicate directions for the next recipient. Since messages–electronic or otherwise–are parts of the legal medical record, it is important that the date and time are recorded as the message moves through to completion. In an EHR, this information is typically recorded, along with the user's electronic signature, at each phase of the message's progress.

Messages in EHRclinic

In EHRclinic, emails and electronic telephone messages are initiated, sent, and responded to by using the same **messaging** system, which is similar to email functionality. Additionally, intra-office messages are sent using this messaging system, much like an internal email system. Both email and electronic telephone messages can have attachments added and link to patient charts. Figure 17.1 shows the following fields in the message screen:

messaging the sending and processing of messages through emails, texting, or other electronic means

subject line introduction that identifies the intent of a written communication

From Automatically generated based on the EHR user.

To Relates to the recipient. An email address can be added to this field, or a search can be conducted by typing the first three letters of the recipient's last name. More than one recipient can be included in the To field.

Subject The **subject line** provides an introduction that identifies the intent of the communication. The subject line should be clear, concise, and unique (to distinguish it from other messages).

Mark as urgent Triage the call to determine priority. If it is urgent, then the "Mark as urgent" box can be checked and the message will be displayed at the top of the recipient's message list. If the call is a medical emergency, then the caller

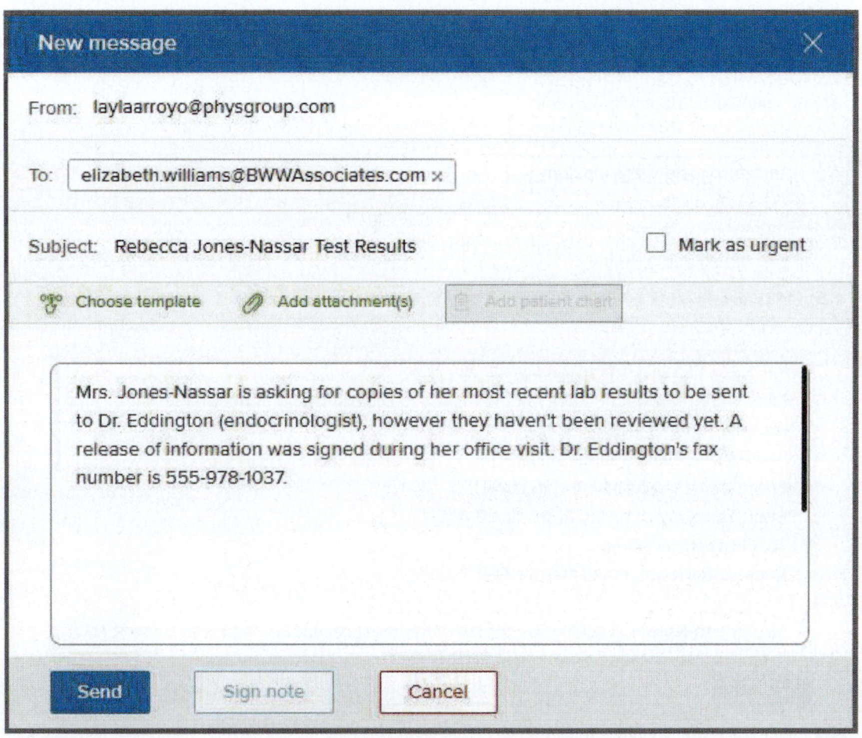

Figure 17.1 Message Initiated by Sender in EHRclinic

may be directed to hang up and call for emergency services (911 in the United States). Medical emergencies should not be sent to providers as messages.

Choose template Templates can be created by a practice and used for frequently used call types. For example, prescription refills may have a prescription refill template that asks all of the questions relevant to a prescription request. Click the Choose template button to select a specific template.

Add attachment(s) Attachments can be added to a message as needed. These are added as file uploads. For example, a patient may send a picture of a bug bite inside of the message.

Add patient chart If the call pertains to a patient, the patient's chart should be attached. Be sure to confirm the patient's name and date of birth, and then the chart can be linked to the message. When the message is complete, it will be documented in the patient's EHR.

body of a communication the main part of a written communication (message, email, letter, or memo); details the purpose of the communication

Message body The **body of a communication** or message refers to the main part of the written message. This is where the purpose of the communication is documented.

Send button Clicking Send electronically sends the message to the recipient.

Sign note Click the Sign note button after each stage in the message's progress to electronically sign it.

Cancel button Closes the message without saving the information. The message must be sent for any new information to be saved.

Once the message has been sent to at least one recipient, other fields become available for message processing, as shown in Figure 17.2.

Figure 17.2 Message Received by Recipient in EHRclinic

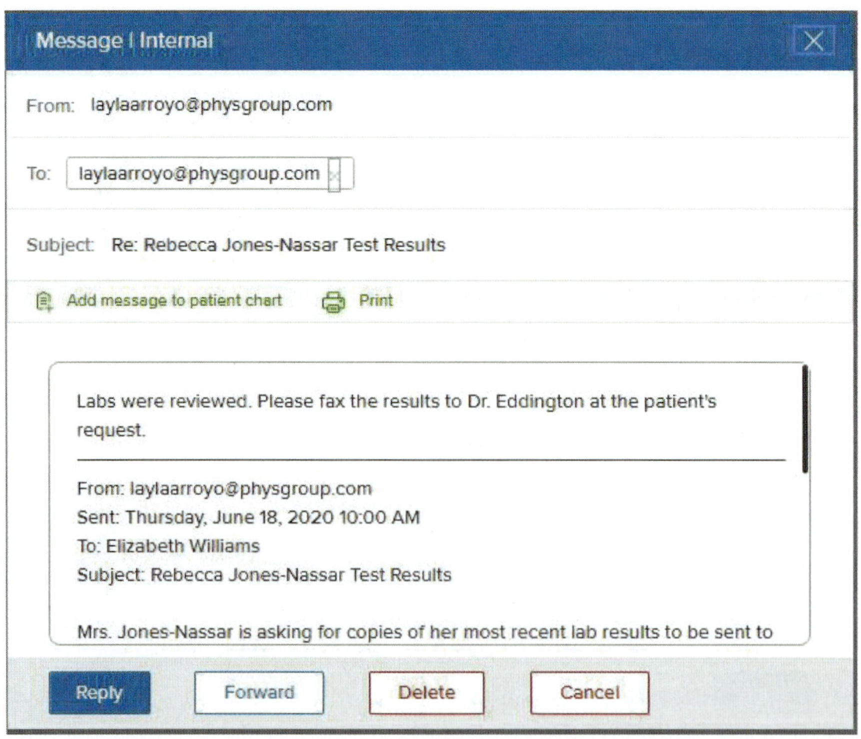

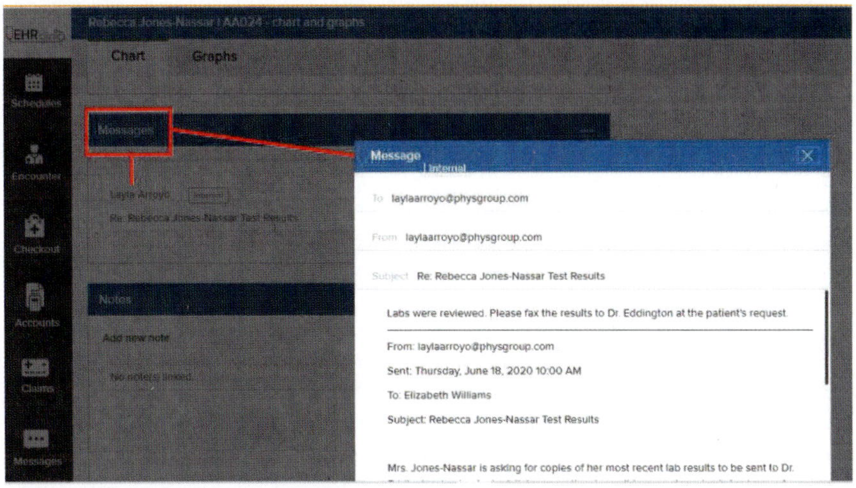

Figure 17.3 Completed Message in Patient's EHRclinic Chart

Reply Sends a reply to the original sender.

Forward Sends the message to a new recipient.

Add message to patient chart When the message is complete, click to select the correct patient and add it to the chart. Figure 17.3 shows an EHRclinic message that has been saved to the patient's chart and is accessible from the facesheet.

Print button If necessary, the message can be printed.

EXERCISE 17.1

Send an Email Communication to a Patient

A patient has indicated that their preferred method of contact is via email, including how they receive test results. Send the test results, along with Dr. Mancini's recommendations, to the patient.

Your instructor may assign this exercise to you in Connect. Exercise steps and EHRclinic Help Guides can be downloaded at http://www.mhhe.com/pmehr2.

EXERCISE 17.2

Create a Nonpatient Message

A representative of the AMA is calling to discuss Dr. Mancini's speaking engagement with her. Dr. Mancini is currently seeing a patient, so you will need to take a message.

Your instructor may assign this exercise to you in Connect. Exercise steps and EHRclinic Help Guides can be downloaded at http://www.mhhe.com/pmehr2.

EXERCISE 17.3

Create a Patient Message

A patient calls to leave a message for Dr. Cheng regarding something he forgot to mention in his office visit. Initiate the patient message and send it to Dr. Cheng.

Your instructor may assign this exercise to you in Connect. Exercise steps and EHRclinic Help Guides can be downloaded at http://www.mhhe.com/pmehr2.

EXERCISE 17.4

Resolve a Patient Message

EHRclinic

Dr. Cheng has received your message and responded to it. He sent it back to you with additional instructions. After you perform the tasks that Dr. Cheng requested, resolve the message by adding it to the patient's chart.

Your instructor may assign this exercise to you in Connect. Exercise steps and EHRclinic Help Guides can be downloaded at http://www.mhhe.com/pmehr2.

17.2 Written Communication

Creating and mailing letters are standard activities in medical practices. Letters are sent to patients, other providers, employers, insurance companies, and others. Patients are informed of test results and reminded about annual exams. Other providers, such as specialists, are asked to provide care to patients. Letters are sent to employers to document patients' absence from work. Insurance companies receive letters that state the medical necessity of care or follow up on denied insurance claims. The Letters feature in EHRclinic makes it easy for providers to create letters to and about their patients.

In addition to letters, medical practices may also send **memos.** Memos are generally used as a form of interoffice communication to present official information, such as communicating policies and procedures. Memos are brief and to-the-point in the presentation of information. A memo's heading includes who created the memo and who the recipients are, the subject, and the date. The body of a memo typically introduces the main subject, includes key points, and summarizes the topic. Memos should be professionally written with a formal tone. While some medical practices may print and distribute memos, EHRclinic memos can be sent using the messaging system.

memo brief written message typically sent to groups of people with the purpose of informing

written communication process of exchanging messages between a sender and receiver(s) by using written language

verbal communication speech-based communication; includes written communication because a particular language system is used in writing

nonverbal communication communication without the use of spoken language; includes gestures, facial expressions, and body language

one-way communication transfer of information or a message from the sender to the receiver without an opportunity for a response

Types of Communication

A letter is considered to be **written communication**, but many people do not realize that it is also a form of **verbal communication** because it uses a language system to communicate. While communicating through written language is an effective means of delivering information, it does lack the benefit of using **nonverbal communication**. For example, when nonverbal communication is used together with verbal communication, the sender and the recipient can use facial expressions, gestures, and body language to support the message and demonstrate intent. Since this is lacking in written communication, it is important to ensure that the message and tone of the letter are carefully conveyed to avoid miscommunication.

While emails and messages are forms of two-way communication, written communication, such as letter-writing, is considered to be **one-way communication** because the recipient does not have the opportunity to respond instantly by the same communication channel. It is important, therefore, to determine which form of communication is the most appropriate for a particular message.

Effective Letter-Writing

As in messaging, there are guidelines to effective letter-writing. The C's of communication still apply to letters, but there are other considerations that should be taken into account.

The following are some additional strategies for ensuring that letters are effective and well-written:

Know your audience A letter's audience is the person or group that the letter is intended for–the recipient. Understanding the recipients and their roles will help set the stage for the letter. For example, the way a letter is written to a provider about a patient will differ from tone and language used to communicate to a patient.

Organize the letter Take the time to organize the letter to present information in a way that is understandable and has the same basic elements, including a greeting, a main message, and a closing.

Use the right tone As mentioned earlier, written communication lacks the benefit of being accompanied by nonverbal communication. The tone of a letter, therefore, is essential to convey your attitude to the recipient. If the right tone is not carefully applied, the sender's intent can be misunderstood by the recipient. Consider the language used, how sentences are structured, and the thought that is put into the message. Knowing your audience is important for selecting the right tone as well.

Be mindful of writing mechanics Be sure to use proper grammar, punctuation, and spelling. When in doubt, resources such as dictionaries and spelling or grammar checkers should be used. In some cases, it might be helpful to ask another person to read the letter to provide feedback before you send it, as long as doing so would not violate HIPAA.

Letters in EHRclinic

In EHRclinic, letters are note-based in the same manner as patient histories and progress notes. Information can be entered by typing in the dialog box without the use of a template, although many practices use templates to save time when creating letters. Templates can be set up to automatically insert information in letters, such as the patient's name and address, the date of the last office visit, the name of a test performed, and so on.

Letters are created by clicking the Letters box in a patient's facesheet. Once this is opened, the Letter dialog box appears, as shown in Figure 17.4.

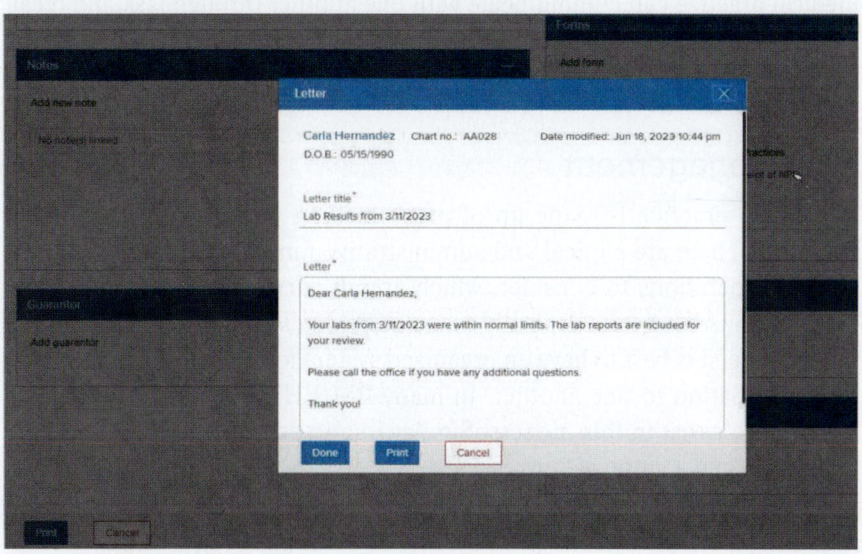

Figure 17.4 The Letter Dialog Box in EHRclinic

The patient's name, chart number, and date of birth are automatically filled in at the top of the Letter dialog box. Each letter should be given a descriptive and unique letter title so it will be clearly identifiable in the patient's chart. The details of the letter are added to the body. This is also the area a template would be added if one is being used. Once the letter is complete., it can be printed so a physical copy can be sent to the patient. Letters are also available within the patient portal, and patients can access them there. Upon completion of letters, they are electronically documented in the Letters section of the patient's facesheet.

EXERCISE 17.5

Create a Patient Test Result Letter EHRclinic

Dr. Mancini has reviewed today's incoming labs and has asked you to follow up by sending a test result letter to inform a patient of her high cholesterol results. Create a test result letter for the patient.

Your instructor may assign this exercise to you in Connect. Exercise steps and EHRclinic Help Guides can be downloaded at http://www.mhhe.com/pmehr2.

EXERCISE 17.6

Create an Excuse Note EHRclinic

A patient saw Dr. Cheng for a sore throat today. He was diagnosed with strep throat and is unable to work for the next few days. Create a work excuse note for this patient.

Your instructor may assign this exercise to you in Connect. Exercise steps and EHRclinic Help Guides can be downloaded at http://www.mhhe.com/pmehr2.

17.3 Task and Recall Lists

EHRs can be used to communicate with other health care professionals, patients, and outside sources through the use of emails, electronic telephone encounters, and letters. In terms of administrative workflow, members of a medical practice can communicate with one another through task and recall lists. These can help a practice run more efficiently by improving shared information.

Task Management

A medical practice is made up of many moving parts so that it can run smoothly. There are clinical and administrative functions, patient care, and practice operations to consider, which are all part of its day-to-day operations. Because there are typically many individuals responsible for running the practice, it is best to have an organized system for communicating details and information to one another. In many PM/EHR systems, **task lists** are available to assist in this process. Similar to a to-do list, a task list can help people to make note of any tasks they need to complete. As shown in Figure 17.5, task lists can be kept as personal reminders or assigned to others as task list items.

task list an EHR system of maintaining reminders and directives for various elements of operating a medical practice administratively and clinically

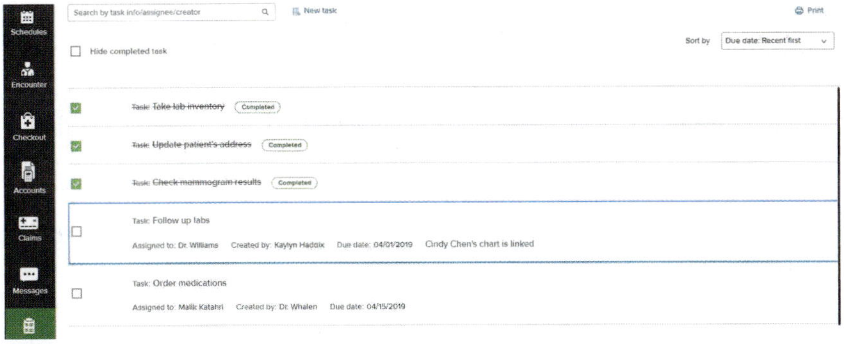

Figure 17.5 Task List in EHRclinic

EXAMPLES

Examples of tasks that can be assigned to others within a medical practice include:

- Dr. Williams assigns a task to the office manager, asking for more business cards to be ordered.
- Alex (the medical assistant) assigns a task to Dr. Mancini to remind her to check a patient's labs.
- The office manager assigns a task to Payton, a medical assistant, to stock the exam rooms.

In EHRclinic, the task list is accessed through Tasks on the menu bar (see Figure 17.5). Task items with green check marks are completed and will disappear from the task list when the user logs in next. An existing task can be clicked to update its details, such as setting a new due date or reassigning the task to another person. Alternatively, a new task can be initiated by clicking "New task." The details of a new task are shown in Figure 17.6 and include the following:

Task Add a task title; be clear and concise so it can be easily identified.

Assign to Add the recipient to the Assign to line. This is the person who will be responsible for completing the task.

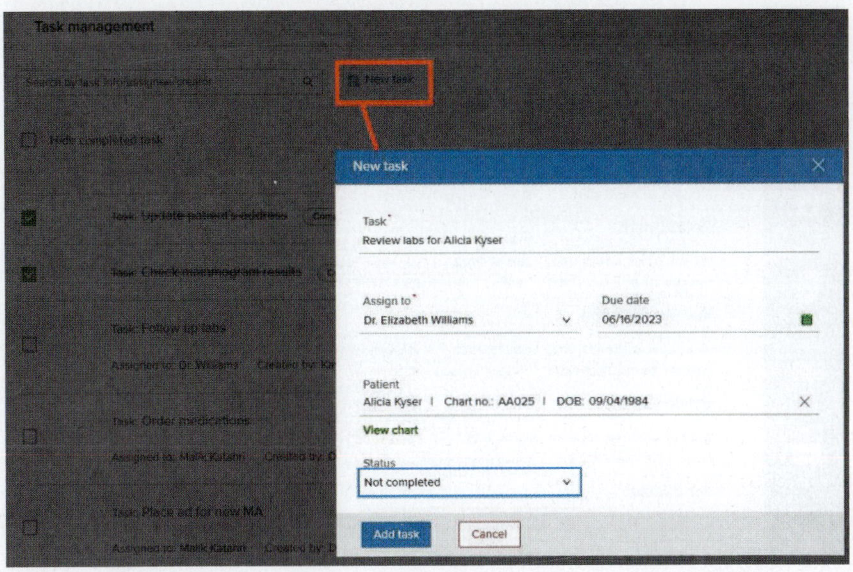

Figure 17.6 New Task Item in EHRclinic

Due date Assign a date that the task should be completed by. The date picker can be used, or the date can be entered into the date line.

Patient If the task relates to a patient, select the patient's chart to attach it to the list. Clicking View chart allows users to quickly reference the chart when completing the task.

Status The status of a task is assigned as either not completed or completed. The status can be changed within the task dialog box, or it will automatically update status when the box to the left of the task is checked. Completed tasks are identified by a green check and a strike through the task title.

EXERCISE 17.7 Assign and Complete Task Items

EHRclinic

You have roomed all of the patients who were waiting to be seen, and now you have some available time before the next patient arrives. Work on managing your task list by assigning and completing items.

Your instructor may assign this exercise to you in Connect. Exercise steps and EHRclinic Help Guides can be downloaded at http://www.mhhe.com/pmehr2.

The Recall List

recall list tool used to identify the status of patient reminders with the ability to update information as needed

Recall lists are used to help a practice to keep track of their patients' appointment-scheduling needs. This list acts like an electronic version of a traditional tickler file by reminding staff about patient accounts (see Figure 17.7). In EHRclinic, the Recall list can be managed, maintained, and updated as needed to ensure that patients are scheduling their follow-up appointments when they are due for them.

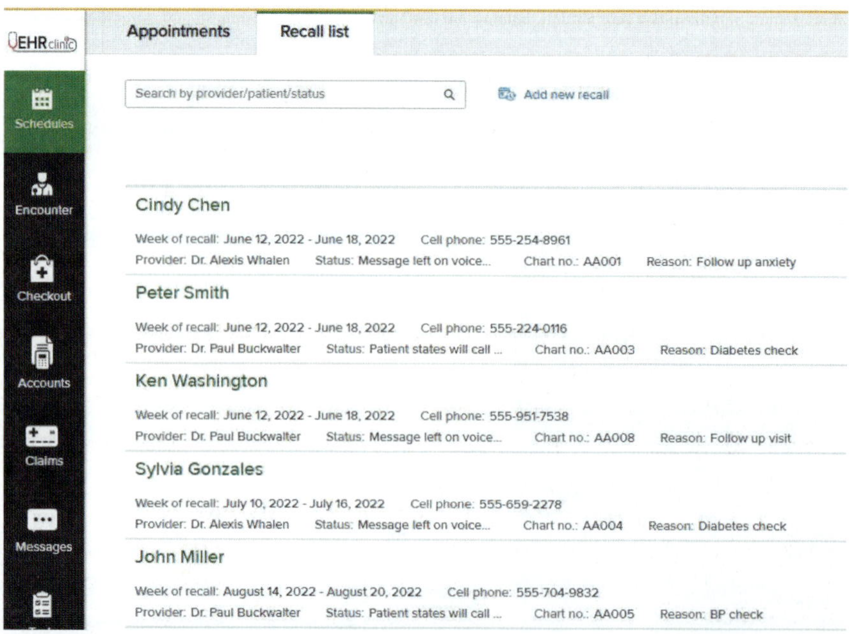

Figure 17.7 The Recall List in EHRclinic

EXAMPLES

A patient comes in for a complete physical exam. He is found to be in good health, and the provider recommends that he return in one year (sooner if needed) for his annual physical exam. When checking out at the front desk, the patient is told that appointments can only be scheduled six months ahead of time, so he will be placed on the recall list to receive a notification to make an appointment three months before his next physical is due.

The Recall list in EHRclinic is accessed in the Schedules section on the menu bar. Select the Recall list tab to see the list details. All of the patients who are currently in recall status will be shown on this list. Recall items can also be sorted by date or by provider, or they can be searched in the search bar. Click on the recall item to edit, update, or delete it. To initiate a new recall, click Add new recall at the top of the screen (see Figure 17.8). To create a new recall, complete the following information in the New Recall dialog box:

Patient Select a patient chart to assign a patient to the recall item.

Provider Select a provider. This is the provider with whom the patient should schedule the appointment.

Status Select a status from the drop-down. The status indicates whether it is a new recall with no action taken yet or whether it is in progress, and what action has been taken thus far.

Week of recall This is the estimated week when the patient should schedule a return visit.

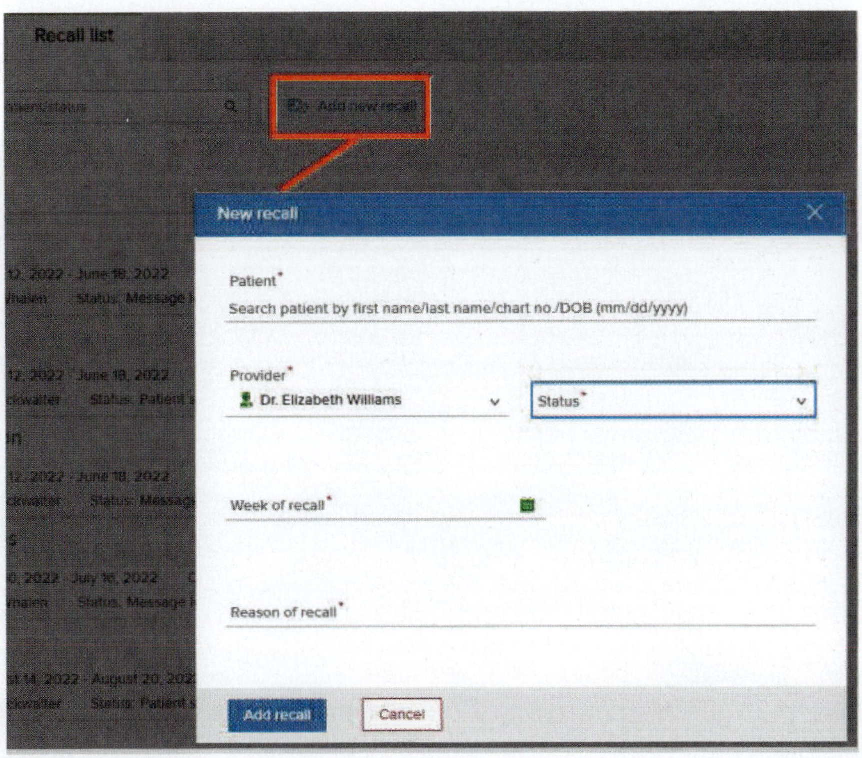

Figure 17.8 New Recall Item in EHRclinic

Reason for recall Add a reason for the appointment that should be scheduled.

Be sure to remind patients that they will be contacted at a later date to schedule their next appointment and that they can call to come in sooner if they need to be seen before their recall dates.

EXERCISE 17.8 Manage the Patient Recall List

EHRclinic

You are working at the front desk at Trilogy Family Care Center, and your supervisor has assigned you to the recall list. Contact the patients on the recall list and update the list as appropriate.

Your instructor may assign this exercise to you in Connect. Exercise steps and EHRclinic Help Guides can be downloaded at http://www.mhhe.com/pmehr2.

chapter 17 summary

KEY TERMS

body of a communication	nonverbal communication	subject line
electronic telephone message	one-way communication	task list
email	recall list	two-way communication
memo	recipient	verbal communication
messaging	sender	written communication

LEARNING OUTCOME	KEY CONCEPTS/EXAMPLES
17.1 Describe how emails and telephone encounters are used in electronic health records.	Messages are used to communicate internally with staff and externally with patients, vendors, and other outside providers or health systems. Messaging systems provide two-way communication, typically through email or electronic telephone messages. Effective message documentation includes the C's of communication: – Clarity – Correct information – Complete information – Concise language – Courteous tone and language – Coherent in flow and style Taking effective phone messages includes the following: – Using good phone etiquette – Being organized – Recording pertinent information and summarizing the message for the caller – Assessing the message for urgency – Identifying the caller – Obtaining the caller's contact information – Being courteous and helpful – Avoiding rephrasing the caller's statements without clarification The EHRclinic messaging system is similar to email functionality. Emails, electronic telephone messages, and intra-office communications use this messaging system within EHRclinic. Any patient-related messages can be linked to and documented within patients' charts.

<table>
<tr><th>LEARNING OUTCOME</th><th>KEY CONCEPTS/EXAMPLES</th></tr>
<tr><td>17.2 Demonstrate the professional use of written communications in an electronic health record.</td><td>In a medical practice, letters are often sent to patients, other providers, employers, insurance carriers, and other entities. The Letters feature in EHRclinic allows patient-related letters to be drafted and documented directly in the EHR.

Practices can also use memos to communicate with the staff. Memos are forms of interoffice communication, and they are used to present official information such as policies or procedures.

Letters are a form of one-way communication; they are considered to be both written communication and verbal communication because they use a language system to communicate. Letters lack nonverbal cues, so care should be taken to ensure that the tone of the letter is appropriate.

Effective letter-writing techniques include:
– Knowing the audience
– Organizing the letter
– Using the right tone
– Being mindful of writing mechanics</td></tr>
<tr><td>17.3 Explain how tasks and recall lists are used to communicate in a medical practice.</td><td>Task management functions within an EHR help a medical practice to communicate about tasks that need to be completed. These are effective because the tasks for the entire practice are located in one area within the EHR, and they can be assigned to specific persons. Tasks can be operations or patient-related, as well.

Recall lists are used to help practices keep track of their patients' appointment scheduling needs. Patients can be added to recall lists if they need to schedule a future appointment, in particular for a time when the provider's schedule is not yet available.</td></tr>
</table>

chapter 17 review

MATCHING QUESTIONS

Match the key terms with their definitions.

_____ 1. *[LO 17.1]* body

_____ 2. *[LO 17.3]* tickler

_____ 3. *[LO 17.1]* email

_____ 4. *[LO 17.3]* task list

_____ 5. *[LO 17.1]* subject line

_____ 6. *[LO 17.2]* memo

_____ 7. *[LO 17.1]* nonverbal communication

_____ 8. *[LO 17.2]* written communication

_____ 9. *[LO 17.1]* recipient

_____ 10. *[LO 17.2]* sender

a. Reminder to follow up on an account.

b. Introduction that identifies the intent of a written communication.

c. Individual who initiates a message to another person or entity.

d. EHR system of maintaining reminders and directives for a practice's operations.

e. Main part of a written communication that details the purpose.

f. Brief written message with the intent of informing.

g. Messages delivered electronically through a network.

h. Patient's description of the symptoms or reasons for seeking medical care.

i. Person, persons, or entity who receive a message.

j. Communication without the use of spoken language.

MULTIPLE CHOICE QUESTIONS

Select the letter that best completes the statement or answers the question.

1. *[LO 17.1]* Messages are considered to be forms of _________ communication.
   a. formal
   b. informal
   c. one-way
   d. two-way

2. *[LO 17.3]* What type of system is used to communicate operational and patient "to-do" items to staff within a medical practice?
   a. email system
   b. messaging system
   c. recall list
   d. task list

3. *[LO 17.2]* Letters are considered to be written and _________ communication.
   a. verbal
   b. two-way
   c. nonverbal
   d. three-way

4. *[LO 17.2]* What type of intra-office communication is generally used to present official information to a medical practice's staff?
   a. electronic telephone message
   b. email
   c. memo
   d. letter

5. *[LO 17.2]* What is nonverbal communication?
   a. speech-based communication
   b. communication without spoken language
   c. use of written language
   d. language-based communication

6. *[LO 17.3]* A reminder to follow up on a patient's account is known as a(n) ________.
   a. addendum
   b. task
   c. tickler
   d. note

7. *[LO 17.1]* What is a preformatted note that can be used in messages and office visits to work more efficiently?
   a. template
   b. tracker
   c. message
   d. recall list

8. *[LO 17.1]* Ensuring that a communication has a logical flow with a consistent style is part of which C of communication?
   a. Clear
   b. Complete
   c. Concise
   d. Coherent

9. *[LO 17.2]* Which of the following describes one-way communication?
   a. The sender and the recipient can communicate with one another.
   b. There is no opportunity for the recipient to instantly respond.
   c. It uses a particular language system.
   d. It ensures that the communication will be complete.

10. *[LO 17.3]* Recall lists are used to help a practice to keep track of which of the following?
    a. inventory
    b. cleaning schedule
    c. patients' appointment scheduling needs
    d. patient call logs

APPLYING YOUR KNOWLEDGE

Answer the questions below in the space provided.

17.1. *[LO 17.1]* What information should be obtained from a patient to ensure that a phone message is complete and accurate?

____

____

17.2. *[LO 17.2]* Explain what it means to be concise in written communication.

____

____

17.3. *[LO 17.3]* How can the use of a task list help to keep a medical practice organized?

____

____

17.4. *[LO 17.2]* What are three examples of unprofessional nonverbal communication?

____

____

chapter 18

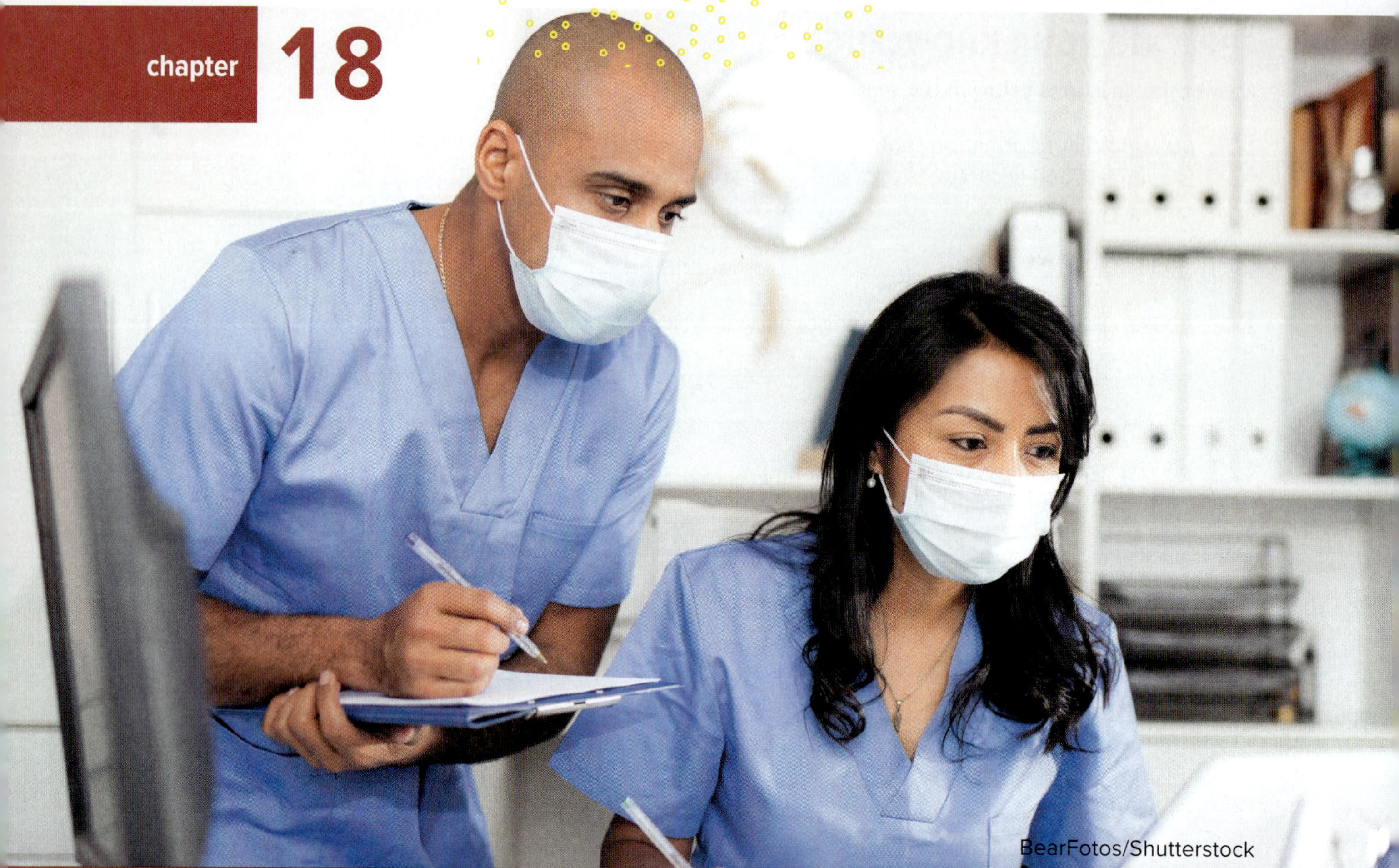

BearFotos/Shutterstock

Health Information Management Tasks

LEARNING OUTCOMES

When you finish this chapter, you will be able to:

18.1 Describe the use of practice databases for maintaining billing information, updating referral facilities, adding new employees, and developing patient education libraries.

18.2 Discuss the purpose of backing up and restoring PM/EHR data.

18.3 Describe the use of EHR for auditing patients' health records.

18.4 Discuss the use of data for practice analysis.

18.5 Describe the monitoring of coding compliance and why this is important.

Managing the Health Care Team

Trilogy Family Care Center is expanding! A new provider, medical assistant, and biller have been hired and will start work next week. The revenue cycle manager, Elrene, needs to add these new employees into the PM/EHR system.

As you read this chapter, consider the role of each new hire. Do you think that they should all have the same level of access to the PM/EHR system, EHRclinic? How can Elrene ensure that everyone has the appropriate access?

18.1 Maintaining Practice Databases

An important administrative function of any PM/EHR system is to maintain the practice's databases. **Databases** are structured sets of data within a computer system, and they are tools used to collect and organize information. For example, most medical practices have databases to store information related to their employees, patients, billing codes, medications, insurance carriers, fee schedules, and any number of other types of practice information. Having databases makes it easy to access the data when using the PM/EHR system.

database a collection of related bits of information

Maintaining Databases

Having a network of databases is essential for any practice, but databases are only useful to the extent that they are maintained. If a database's information has not been updated, then it is likely inaccurate and therefore useless. Typically, a designated person, such as an office manager or administrator, is assigned to maintain the practice databases. This includes making sure that current information is added and obsolete information is removed from each database. Databases should be reviewed for relevance and accuracy.

Using Databases

Databases can be accessed in a variety of ways. Each PM/EHR system usually has one area in which all of the databases are found (see Figure 18.1). Additionally, databases can be accessed when performing a variety of tasks in the PM/EHR system.

EXAMPLES

Examples of accessing databases while performing PM/EHR tasks include:

- Patient education, medication, and referring provider databases can be accessed directly during a patient's office visit. This allows for easy selection of these resources, as well as automatic documentation within the encounter.
- ICD and CPT databases are accessed when completing the patient's billing and claim submission.
- Patient databases are accessed when scheduling appointments.
- Drug databases are accessed when initiating E-Prescribing.

Figure 18.1 List of EHRclinic Databases

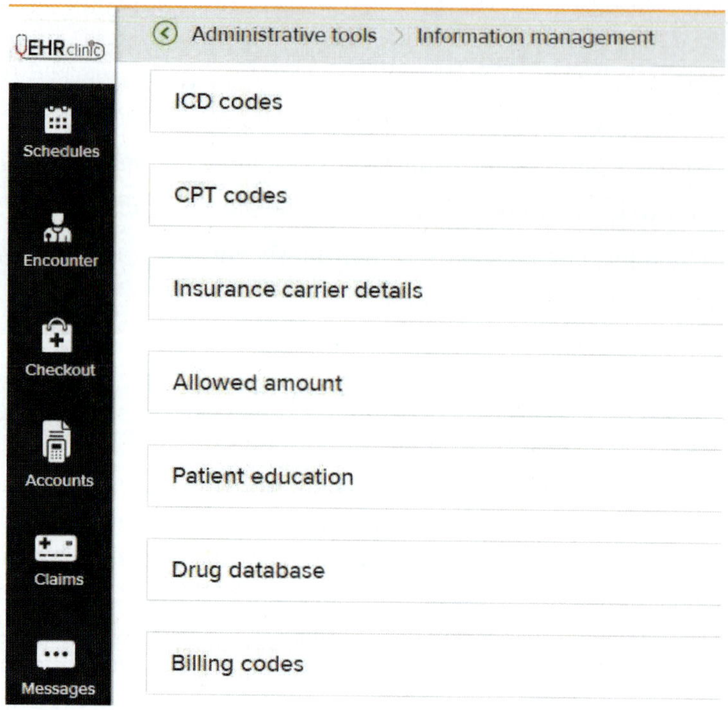

Databases in EHRclinic

As shown in Figure 18.1, EHRclinic relies on a number of databases for day-to-day operations. EHRclinic databases can be accessed through Tools in the menu and then clicking on “Manage practice data” in the “Information management” tile (see Figure 18.2).

The databases used in EHRclinic are typical of most PM/EHR systems and include the following:

Patient information New patients can be added to the patient information database, and patient demographic and insurance information can be edited.

Provider information All providers within a practice are included in the provider information database. Demographic and provider information, such as credentials, DEA, NPI, and license numbers are kept in this database.

Staff information Information for all practice staff is kept in the staff information database. New staff should be added to the database upon hire, and any staff member who terminates employment should be removed from the database.

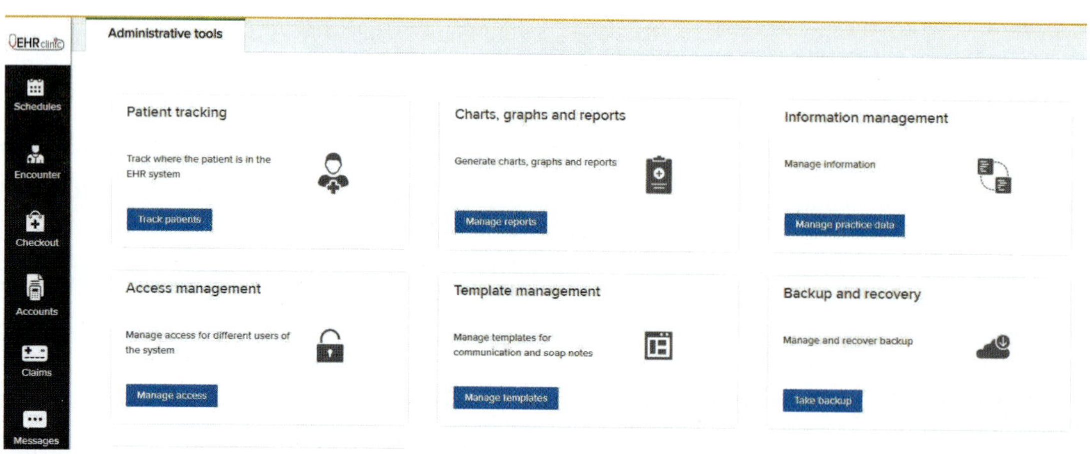

Figure 18.2 EHRclinic Tools Menu

ICD codes The ICD (diagnosis) code database houses ICD-10-CM codes so they can be easily accessed. This should be updated with the annual ICD code updates.

CPT codes The CPT (procedure) code database keeps CPT codes that are often used within a practice. This database should be updated with the annual CPT code updates. This database also includes the practice's fee schedule (charges) for each CPT code.

Insurance carrier details Many practices participate in and accept a variety of insurance plans. Maintaining a database of insurance carriers facilitates access to this information.

Allowed amount The allowed amount database keeps records of the amounts allowed by insurance carriers for the procedure codes listed in the CPT code database. When posting insurance payments, the allowed amount database can be accessed, ensuring ease and accuracy of making adjustments when balance billing is not allowed.

Patient education The patient education database is customizable and contains patient education based on a practice's patient population. For example, a pediatrician's office will have patient education related to children, whereas an internal medicine practice may have a variety of educational materials related to acute and chronic conditions, treatments and procedures, and medications.

Drug database Frequently prescribed medications are kept in the drug database. These lists include the most common doses, frequencies, and drug forms so they are accessible for E-Prescribing and recording medications in the patient's facesheet.

Billing codes Billing codes refer to commonly used codes for billing. For example, in EHRclinic, PATCHK is the billing code used to describe a patient's payment by check and PATCSH is used when a patient makes a cash payment.

Practice information The practice information database keeps a record of the practice's address, contact information (phone and fax), website, and primary contact, such as the office manager. More than one practice can be listed here in the case of multispecialty clinics. The practice information database can be updated as needed.

Referring providers Name, provider information, and provider specialties for referring providers are maintained in the referring providers database. This database is helpful for identifying providers who are referring patients to a practice or for referring patients to other providers.

Referring labs Practices typically refer to specific labs, imaging, and diagnostic centers. This information is housed in the referring labs database. It can be printed and provided to patients or will be added to a patient's electronic order when the facility is selected.

TIP

Provider and Staff Access Levels

Once provider and staff information is entered into their respective databases, it is important to identify their staff access levels. The various health care professionals in a medical practice have different access levels within the PM/EHR based on their scopes of practice. In other words, access is only granted on a need-to-know basis to protect HIPAA and the security of patient records.

For example:

- A provider typically cannot access claims management.
- Medical assistants do not have access rights to prescribe medications.
- Coders cannot edit office visits, but they can view them.

THINKING IT THROUGH 18.1

Why do you think that it is important to maintain databases? What can happen if they are not kept up to date?

EXERCISE 18.1

Maintain the Diagnosis Code Database

EHRclinic

There have been some updates to ICD-10-CM. Add, delete, and revise diagnosis codes within the ICD database.

Your instructor may assign this exercise to you in Connect. Exercise steps and EHRclinic Help Guides can be downloaded at www.mhhe.com/pmehr2.

EXERCISE 18.2

Maintain the Procedure Code Database

EHRclinic

The annual CPT updates are available! Maintain the CPT database by adding, deleting, and revising procedure codes as needed.

Your instructor may assign this exercise to you in Connect. Exercise steps and EHRclinic Help Guides can be downloaded at www.mhhe.com/pmehr2.

EXERCISE 18.3

Add a Provider to the Database

EHRclinic

Trilogy Family Care Center is expanding and has hired a new provider. Add the provider to the database, and assign the appropriate access rights.

Your instructor may assign this exercise to you in Connect. Exercise steps and EHRclinic Help Guides can be downloaded at www.mhhe.com/pmehr2.

EXERCISE 18.4

Add a New Employee to the Database

EHRclinic

As Trilogy Family Care Center begins to grow with the addition of new providers, new staff is also being hired. Add a new medical assistant to the database, and assign the appropriate access rights.

Your instructor may assign this exercise to you in Connect. Exercise steps and EHRclinic Help Guides can be downloaded at www.mhhe.com/pmehr2.

EXERCISE 18.5

Manage the Fee Schedule and Allowed Amounts

EHRclinic

Trilogy Family Care Center has added a new procedure to the services offered to patients. Add the procedure to the CPT database, including the fee schedule charges. Then add the procedure to the allowed amount database to identify the amount each insurance carrier will pay for the procedure.

Your instructor may assign this exercise to you in Connect. Exercise steps and EHRclinic Help Guides can be downloaded at www.mhhe.com/pmehr2.

EXERCISE 18.6

Add a Testing Facility

EHRclinic

There's a new lab in town! Add the lab to the Trilogy Family Care Center's referring labs database.

Your instructor may assign this exercise to you in Connect. Exercise steps and EHRclinic Help Guides can be downloaded at www.mhhe.com/pmehr2.

EXERCISE 18.7

Add a Referring Provider to the Database

EHRclinic

Trilogy Family Care Center often refers patients to a specialty clinic, and they have announced that a new provider has been hired. Add the new provider to the referring providers database.

Your instructor may assign this exercise to you in Connect. Exercise steps and EHRclinic Help Guides can be downloaded at www.mhhe.com/pmehr2.

EXERCISE 18.8

Maintain the Practice Billing Code Database

EHRclinic

Trilogy Family Care Center is going digital and has decided to accept cryptocurrency. Add the new form of payment to the practice's billing code database.

Your instructor may assign this exercise to you in Connect. Exercise steps and EHRclinic Help Guides can be downloaded at www.mhhe.com/pmehr2.

EXERCISE 18.9

Manage the Practice Information

EHRclinic

Trilogy Family Care Center has a new office manager.
Update the contact information in the practice information database.

Your instructor may assign this exercise to you in Connect. Exercise steps and EHRclinic Help Guides can be downloaded at www.mhhe.com/pmehr2.

EXERCISE 18.10 **Add to the Patient Education Database** EHRclinic

Trilogy Family Care Center's new provider would like to update the patient education database. Add new patient education materials to the database.

Your instructor may assign this exercise to you in Connect. Exercise steps and EHRclinic Help Guides can be downloaded at www.mhhe.com/pmehr2.

EXERCISE 18.11 **Maintain the Drug Database** EHRclinic

Some new drugs have recently been approved by the FDA. Add them to the practice's drug database.

Your instructor may assign this exercise to you in Connect. Exercise steps and EHRclinic Help Guides can be downloaded at www.mhhe.com/pmehr2.

18.2 Data Backup and Recovery

With the widespread use of PM/EHR systems, physician practices are more dependent on information technology than ever before. This increased reliance on technology, coupled with the HIPAA Security Rule, has forced practices to develop and implement disaster recovery plans. A **disaster recovery plan** is a plan for resuming normal operations after a disaster such as a fire or a computer malfunction.

disaster recovery plan plan for resuming normal operations after a disaster such as a fire or a computer malfunction

backing up making a copy of data files at a specific point in time that can be used to restore data

cloud storage saving data securely online so that it can be shared and accessed at any time from any location

restoring process of retrieving data from a backup storage device

Backing Up Files

Disaster recovery plans require practices to back up computer data. **Backing up** refers to the process of saving a copy of files on a regular schedule to facilitate file recovery if data loss occurs. During a backup, files are copied from their normal location to a different location. The files may be copied to portable media, such as discs or USB drives, or they may be transferred over a computer network or to **cloud storage.** Most practices back up data on a daily basis; they store one copy of the backup in the office, and the other at an off-site location. Using an off-site location for storage protects the data should a natural disaster such as a fire or flood occur at the office. While paper records can be physically destroyed, it is also possible that electronic records can be lost. In fact, computerized records are subject to additional threats, such as computer viruses and hardware malfunctions.

In EHRclinic, backup and recovery of the practice database can be done at any time by accessing "Backup and recovery" in the Tools menu (see Figure 18.3). EHRclinic's backup files are stored in the cloud, so the risk of loss due to a natural disaster is eliminated.

Restoring Files

Files that are properly backed up can be restored. **Restoring** is the process of copying backup files onto the office's computer systems, facilitating a return to normal business activities. The process to restore a backup file is very similar to the steps used to back up a file. Each backup is given a file name, and the data can be restored to any previous point by selecting a specific file name (see Figure 18.4).

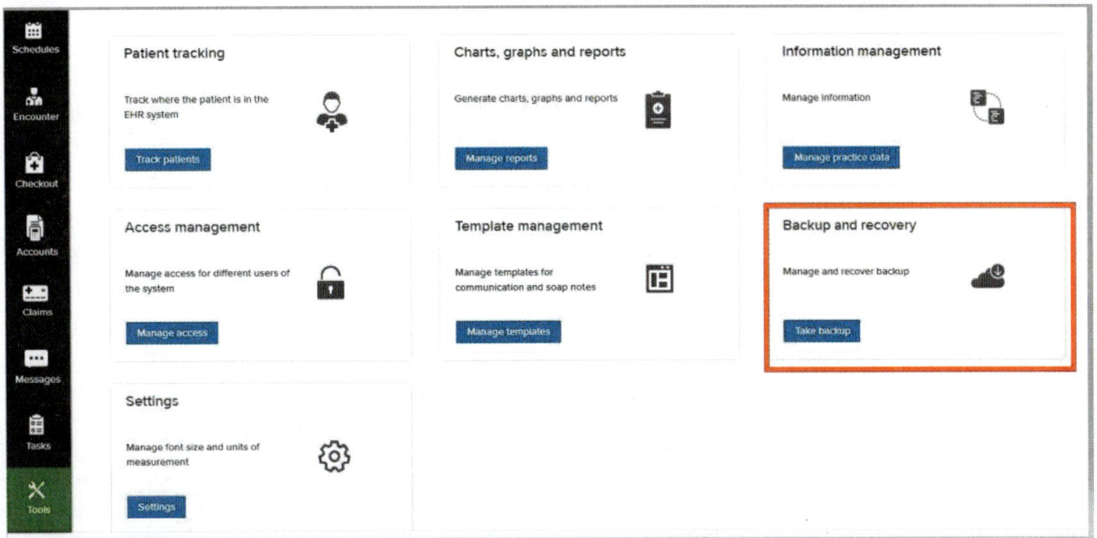

Figure 18.3 EHRclinic Backup and Recovery in Tools

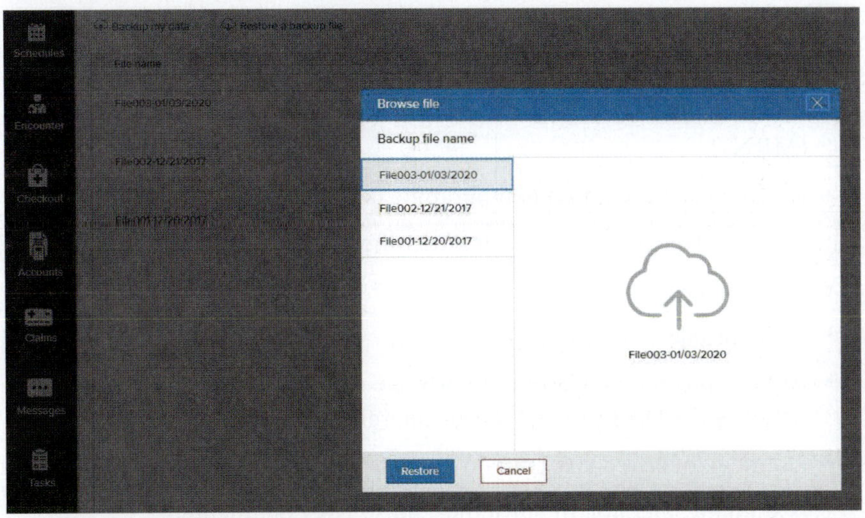

Figure 18.4 Restoring a Backed-Up File in EHRclinic

EXERCISE 18.12

Back Up and Restore to the EHR

EHRclinic

The office manager of Trilogy Family Care Center is training you to open and close the practice. Back up and restore the practice files as part of your training.

Your instructor may assign this exercise to you in Connect. Exercise steps and EHRclinic Help Guides can be downloaded at http://www.mhhe.com/pmehr2.

18.3 Auditing Health Records

A medical record audit is a lengthy process, but it's a necessary process for the office. Precise clinical documentation in medical records is crucial to delivering the highest quality care to patients, and disorganized medical records can easily hinder this. As discussed later in this chapter, medical record auditing can determine areas that need attention before they result in fraudulent claims and billing activities or identify areas needing support for quality care of the patient.

Medical Record Audits

A medical record audit includes internal or external reviews of what processes are being conducted accurately and what needs to be improved. This includes reviews of medical billing and coding accuracy (discussed later in this chapter), procedures of documenting, policies, and any other components that affect the efficiency and effectiveness of detailed documentation in the office.

Medical record auditing is a preventive measure to catch potential errors that can result in liabilities and investigations. For example, audits can catch overlooked compliance issues that could affect revenue, HIPAA regulations, and the quality of care delivered to patients.

Many offices have a clinical documentation improvement department (CDI). This department reviews documentation within 24 to 48 hours of completion and requests corrections as needed. You will find these departments in both inpatient and outpatient settings. They will review documentation to support medical necessity, quality of care, and whether or not the documentation meets specific guidelines.

The following checklist itemizes what should be reviewed in the office's ongoing audit of medical records at the point of care.

- Do the patient records have an accurate medical record number (MRN)?
- Do the records contain demographic data?
- Is the person(s) providing care identified on each chart entry?
- Are all chart entries dated?
- Is the problem list complete?
- Are any prominent allergies or adverse drug reactions documented or noted as NKDA (no known drug allergies)?
- Do the patient records contain appropriate past medical HX?
- Is smoking, alcohol, or substance abuse HX documented?
- Were lab and other tests ordered as appropriate?
- Are the contents of a history and physical examination available?
- Are plans of action/treatment consistent with diagnosis(es)?
- Were problems from previous visits addressed?
- Is there any documented evidence of appropriate use of consultants?
- Is there any documented evidence of continuity and coordination of care between primary and specialty physicians?
- Are consultant summaries, lab, and imaging study results included to reflect primary care physician review?
- Is there a completed immunization record on file as needed?
- Are all prescriptions and refills noted?
- Is there a med sheet used and appropriately located?
- Is the chronology maintained?
- Is informed consent noted for all procedures and appropriate prescriptions?

- Are there documentation of patient education and follow-up instructions about procedures?
- Is there a history of missed or canceled appointments?

THINKING IT THROUGH 18.2

What are the potential consequences of failure to perform medical record or chart audits?

18.4 Analyzing Data

Medical data analysis refers to the collection, analysis, and interpretation of **data** from a variety of sources, such as medical histories, electronic health records, billing claims, cost reports, and **surveys.** The purpose of performing medical data analysis is to help health institutions with process improvement, efficient operations, and strategic decision making. The end result is cost reduction and improved patient experiences.

medical data analysis application of statistical techniques to improve outcomes and reduce costs in health care

data information in a digital form that can be transmitted or processed

survey a method of gathering information using relevant questions from a sample of people

dashboard a visualization tool that allows a practice to review user performance and performance metrics

Accounts Receivable (A/R) Aging Report shows all current unpaid charges and health care claims including the amount owed and their duration

Using Reports for Analysis

As discussed in Chapter 16, running practice management reports on a regular basis is a key factor in maintaining a healthy revenue cycle. Reports and **dashboards** provide data to identify areas where the office may be unknowingly losing income. Although there are many types of reports, each providing a different lens through which to view the financial health of a practice, there are three in particular that should be analyzed to provide data for financial decision making. These include the Accounts Receivable (A/R) Aging report, the Key Performance Indicators (KPI) report, and the Insurance Analysis/Charging report.

Accounts Receivable (A/R) Aging Report

The **Accounts Receivable (A/R) Aging report** is used to track how long claims take to process. This is important because it directly relates to the practice's accounts receivable (monies coming in), which is necessary to maintain a healthy cash flow.

Consider a practice's accounts payable, which are monies going out of a practice. Accounts payable cover payment of staff, building lease or rent, utilities, facilities, and supplies and equipment. These expenses are standard and expected, meaning that they occur continually. With inconsistent accounts receivable, the practice will not have adequate cash coming in to maintain the accounts payable.

The A/R Aging report breaks each claim down to the number of days they've been unpaid. Typically, claims take an average of a month and ideally no longer than 45 days for remittance of payment. There are, of course, some circumstances in which payment takes a bit longer than 45 days, but this should be the exception to the rule. An A/R Aging report can help identify trends if certain insurance carriers continually take longer to pay or if there are internal issues such as inefficient billing practices. In any case, the information learned from analyzing this report helps practice managers to determine if there is a potential issue with cash flow and what steps need to be taken to increase efficiency.

key performance indicators (KPI) the critical indicators of progress toward a desired result with a focus on operational improvement

performance measure processes, experience, and/or outcomes of patient care, observations, or treatment that relate to one or more quality aims for health care, such as effective, safe, efficient, patient-centered, equitable, and timely care

Key Performance Indicator (KPI) Report

Key performance indicators (KPI) are linked to the overall goals of a medical practice. They are quantifiable by comparable metrics, such as showing an increase or decrease of a factor between two (or more) time periods. KPIs are important in a medical practice because they provide clear and identifiable goals with the following benefits:

- Providing measurable targets
- Promoting learning
- Receiving important information
- Encouraging accountability
- Boosting morale through measurable targets

Key Performance Indicator (KPI) reports are then used to measure if those goals have been met or to compare the metrics over time. The KPI report is a valuable tool for identifying key areas in a practice's revenue cycle management process. Specifically, the indicators determine **performance measures,** such as where performance is critical, establish goals for those areas, and measure the practice's progress against those goals. For example, using KPI reports can help identify any breakdowns in the claims process as well as determining which CPT codes are the most profitable for the practice.

EXAMPLES

Some examples of information that can be tracked by KPI reports include:

- Total encounters for a specified time period
- Total number of procedures
- Total charges
- Total collections
- Outstanding accounts receivable (A/R)
- Total adjustments made by the practice

Practice managers can analyze the trends in the KPI report to evaluate performance and identify any red flags, such as a sudden drop in collections. These reports are then used to make process improvement decisions for the future.

Insurance Analysis/Charging Report

The Insurance Analysis/Charging report shows the average charge amount billed and payment amount received from each payer by CPT code. Cross-checking the average payment received across payers gives the practice a side-by-side comparison of the payment amounts from each insurance carrier. This comparison allows the practice to determine if their fees are set too low. When fees are set below payer allowable amounts, the office is losing revenue. This report should be reviewed yearly to ensure that the fee schedule is in alignment with the insurance carrier's allowed charges (see Chapter 12). Analyzing this report is vital in the success of the office. If a payer's average payment amount equals the office's charge, this is an indicator that the office should increase the fee.

EXAMPLES

Vaccines are often undercharged. Practices have a tendency to set vaccine prices based on their out-of-pocket costs, such as how much they paid to buy them. They do not realize that many payers allow substantially higher payments than the practice's purchase price.

Using an Insurance/Analysis/Charging report helps to ensure that a practice's charges align with the amount that payers are willing to pay; otherwise the practice can lose potential revenue.

THINKING IT THROUGH 18.3

How do accounts receivable and accounts payable relate to a practice's overall cash flow? Why is this important?

Using Surveys for Analysis

While financial reports are integral to the financial health of a practice, surveys can be used to provide information about the patients' experiences. The data gathered in surveys is important because it measures patient satisfaction and provides opportunities for improvement through the lens of the patient. Specifically, surveys provide a link between patients and providers, they serve as quality improvement tools, and they improve patient retention.

Patient satisfaction surveys often include questions related to their encounters, and they include a variety of aspects to each visit, such as:

- Scheduling–Were you able to make an appointment that was convenient? Were you satisfied with the provider's availability? Did you receive an appointment reminder?
- Wait time–How long did you wait to be taken to your exam room? How long did you wait for the provider to see you?
- Office personnel–Was the front office staff courteous and friendly? Were they able to answer your questions?
- Providers and medical staff–Did the provider explain information to you clearly? Did the provider listen to your concerns? Were all of your questions answered? Did the provider involve you in decisions related to your treatment? Do you feel that it is easy to speak to your provider during office hours? Was the medical staff courteous and friendly? How likely are you to recommend this provider to family or friends?

Surveys are typically conducted using a **Likert scale,** in which there is a five-point scale ranging from Strongly Agree to Strongly Disagree, as shown in Figure 18.5. The midpoint of a Likert scale is typically neutral, such as "Neither Agree nor Disagree." The range of response options allows patients to closely match their responses to their opinions. There is usually an N/A option for questions that are not applicable, as well. Using a Likert scale, the practice can gather data from patients in a measurable and meaningful way. In addition to the Likert scale responses, patients are also provided with a Comments section in which they can share specific experiences or opinions.

Likert scale used in surveys to allow individuals to express the extent that they agree or disagree with a particular statement

Figure 18.5 Example of a Survey Question and Likert Scale for Responses

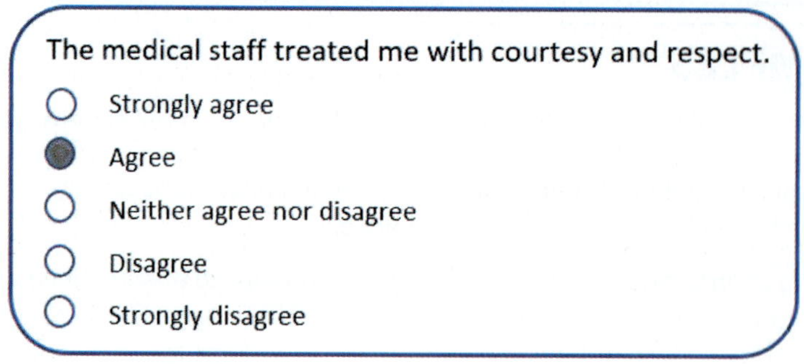

The medical staff treated me with courtesy and respect.

- Strongly agree
- Agree (selected)
- Neither agree nor disagree
- Disagree
- Strongly disagree

Microsoft Corporation

EXAMPLES

A patient survey asks patients to rate "The provider listened to my concerns" using a Likert scale of Strongly Agree to Strongly Disagree.

When the results are collated, data show this statement was rated at an average of Disagree, indicating that most of the patients surveyed felt that the provider did not appear to listen to their concerns.

Once this is identified, practice managers can determine why patients may feel that way. Perhaps the provider is typing in the EHR and not maintaining eye contact during patient encounters, or maybe there is an opportunity for the provider to show more empathy when communicating with the patient. Whatever the case, knowing this can help providers to make adjustments in their encounters so they can better address how patients perceive their visits.

THINKING IT THROUGH 18.4

Why is patient satisfaction important? What are the consequences of poor patient satisfaction?

18.5 Monitoring Coding Compliance

monitoring coding compliance process that ensures that the coding of diagnoses and procedures follows all coding rules and guidelines to minimize the risk of fraud

compliance adhering to a written, adopted, or required set of rules

Monitoring coding processes helps health care organizations to stay compliant with federal and state regulations. **Monitoring coding compliance** is a process for finding, correcting, and preventing illegal medical office practices. The goal is to prevent fraud and abuse (intentional and unintentional), to ensure **compliance** with federal, state, and local laws, and to help defend providers if they are investigated or prosecuted for fraud by showing that efforts are made to ensure compliant behavior. When compliance monitoring processes are in place, it demonstrates to payers that honest, ongoing attempts have been made to find and fix areas of weakness.

The compliance department of any practice should have a coding compliance plan in place explaining and documenting the following (at minimum):

- Audit coding by performing internal and external audits and correcting any errors, when found.
- Provide ongoing training to staff on coding regulations and guidelines.

Compliance Audits

As discussed in Chapter 2 and Chapter 14, audits are formal reviews, such as examinations of accounts, records, or processes. In coding compliance, audits serve to evaluate a medical practice's coding process to ensure compliance and minimize the risk of fraud. Internal and external audits are typically performed to monitor coding compliance.

Internal Audits

Internal audits are reviews of a medical office's coding, conducted by the practice's compliance department. **Prospective audits** (prior to submitting for billing) and **retrospective audits** (after submission for billing) should be conducted internally. These audits should be performed according to the audit schedule identified in the compliance plan, such as monthly, bimonthly, or quarterly.

From the PM/EHR system, a report is pulled for a date range for each provider and/or coder. The compliance department will review the sample and provide feedback to the coders or providers. This depends on who captured the coding because providers can code their own services. Results should be kept for tracking of trends.

Corrections should be made for any errors that are found during the internal audits. If these are found prospectively, the corrections can be made before submitting the claim. If errors are found retrospectively, then a corrected claim will be made and resubmitted to the payer. Adjustments to the patient's account will be made as well. If the payer or patient has made a payment on the service, any necessary refunds will be submitted for processing.

internal audit review of a medical office's coding that is conducted by the practice's compliance department

prospective audit review of billing and coding prior to claim submission

retrospective audit review of billing and coding after claim submission

external audit formal review that is conducted by an independent entity not associated with the medical practice

External Audits

External audits are completed by an agency outside of the health care system or medical practice. These can be government entities (such as Medicare and Medicaid), managed care organizations, private payers, or an agency hired by the health care system. Government entities and payers may want to investigate the medical records further and will request a date range from a provider or request a random sample. The PM/EHR can pull the records for the requested accounts, and medical records can be sent electronically for review.

If payers or government entities find errors, then refunds and fines may have to be paid. Results of the audit will be reviewed with the compliance department, and they will have an opportunity to dispute the findings. If the audit shows an intent of fraud, then the practice will face fines and possibly a deeper investigation.

As part of the compliance plan, health care systems or medical practices may hire a private agency to perform an external coding audit for a nonbiased review. Agencies can objectively analyze operations, detect holes in the system, and uncover deficiencies that an internal audit program may miss. This outside review helps strengthen future internal audits by discovering how and why internal audits may have overlooked findings. A health system should conduct an external audit every five years, and the timing of external audits should be documented in the compliance plan. The agency will review a sample and provide feedback on accuracy and any areas of strength or opportunity. If errors are found within the coding and/or claims, refunds and corrections to the patient's account must be made.

THINKING IT THROUGH 18.5

How can coding compliance plans prevent fraud and abuse?

Training of Staff

Coding changes quarterly and yearly; CPT is updated yearly at the first of the year, and ICD-10-CM is updated yearly on October 1. Amendments are made to ICD-10-CM throughout the year as needed, usually in April. Compliance plans indicate ongoing staff training. Documentation of appropriate training on coding changes should be recorded in each coding staff member's file. This demonstrates that office staff have been trained properly on required federal and state laws and internal procedures in the health system or medical practice. Documentation of staff compliance training is essential to submitting clean claims for proper reimbursement.

chapter 18 summary

KEY TERMS

Accounts Receivable (A/R) Aging report
backing up
cloud storage
compliance
dashboard
data
database
disaster recovery plan
external audit
internal audit
key performance indicators (KPI)
Likert scale
medical data analysis
monitoring coding compliance
performance measures
prospective audits
restoring
retrospective audits
survey

LEARNING OUTCOME	KEY CONCEPTS/EXAMPLES
18.1 Describe the use of practice databases for maintaining billing information, updating referral facilities, adding new employees, and developing patient education libraries.	Databases are structured sets of data within computer systems that are used to collect and store information. Databases must be maintained to keep the information they contain up to date. Databases within EHRclinic include: – Patient, provider, and staff information – ICD and CPT codes – Insurance carrier details – Allowed amounts – Patient education – Drugs – Billing codes – Practice information – Referring providers and labs
18.2 Discuss the purpose of backing up and restoring PM/EHR data.	Disaster recovery plans are developed to assist in resuming normal operations after a disaster. Data files are backed up regularly so they can be restored if a disaster occurs. Files should be backed up off-site or to the cloud to ensure the safety of the backed-up files.
18.3 Identify the use of EHR for auditing patients' health records.	Medical record audits are needed to ensure that clinical documentation is accurate. Audits identify areas of strength and opportunities to avoid fraud and abuse. Medical record auditing is a preventive measure to catch potential errors that can result in liabilities and investigations. Clinical documentation improvement departments review documentation for adherence to specific guidelines within 24 to 48 hours and request corrections as needed.

LEARNING OUTCOME	KEY CONCEPTS/EXAMPLES
18.4 Discuss the use of data for practice analysis.	Medical data analysis refers to the collection, analysis, and interpretation of data from sources such as medical histories, electronic health records, billing claims, cost reports, and surveys. The three key reports for practice analysis include: – Accounts Receivable (A/R) Aging Report – Key Performance Indicator (KPI) Report – Insurance Analysis/Charging Report Patient satisfaction surveys are also used to provide information about the patients' experiences. They provide a link between patients and providers, serve as quality improvement tools, and improve patient retention.
18.5 Describe the monitoring of coding compliance and why this is important.	Monitoring coding compliance is a process for finding, correcting, and preventing illegal medical office practices with the goal of preventing fraud and abuse, ensuring compliance, and providing defense in the event of an investigation. The two elements of a coding compliance plan include: – Auditing coding by performing internal and external audits and correcting errors – Providing ongoing training to staff on coding regulations and guidelines The various types of audits include: – Internal: conducted by the medical practice – External: conducted by an agency outside of the medical practice (government entities, insurance carriers, or other outside agencies) – Prospective: conducted prior to billing – Retrospective: conducted after submission for billing

chapter 18 review

MATCHING QUESTIONS

Match the key terms with their definitions.

_____ 1. *[LO 18.4]* dashboard

_____ 2. *[LO 18.5]* prospective audit

_____ 3. *[LO 18.5]* retroactive audit

_____ 4. *[LO 18.5]* internal audit

_____ 5. *[LO 18.5]* external audit

_____ 6. *[LO 18.5]* compliance

_____ 7. *[LO 18.2]* backing up

_____ 8. *[LO 18.1]* database

_____ 9. *[LO 18.4]* Likert scale

_____ 10. *[LO 18.4]* key performance indicators

a. Reviewing claims that have already been submitted to insurance carriers so that adjudication results can be analyzed.

b. Adhering to a written, adopted, or required set of rules.

c. A visualization tool that allows a practice to review user performance and performance metrics.

d. Used in surveys to allow individuals to express the extent to which they agree or disagree with a particular statement.

e. Formal review that is conducted by an independent entity not associated with the medical practice.

f. The critical indicators of progress toward a desired result with a focus on operational improvement.

g. Making a copy of data files at a specific point in time that can be used to restore data.

h. Review of billing and coding prior to claim submission.

i. A collection of related bits of information.

j. Review of a medical office's coding that is conducted by the practice's compliance department.

MULTIPLE CHOICE QUESTIONS

Select the letter that best completes the statement or answers the question.

1. *[LO 18.2]* Medical practices should develop a _________ plan to assist in resuming normal operations in the event that something catastrophic happens.
   a. restoration
   b. backup
   c. disaster recovery
   d. storage and retrieval

2. *[LO 18.1]* Access levels are assigned to employees based on which factor?
   a. Length of employment at the facility
   b. Scope of practice
   c. Background check results
   d. Completing PM/EHR education modules

3. *[LO 18.5]* One of the goals of monitoring coding compliance is to _________.
   a. ensure that the highest revenue is captured
   b. protect providers against medical malpractice
   c. prevent HIPAA violations
   d. prevent fraud and abuse

4. *[LO 18.1]* Which of the following is an example of a database in a PM/EHR system?
   a. Drug database
   b. Rejected claims database
   c. Petty cash fund database
   d. Emergency protocol database

5. *[LO 18.2]* Saving data securely online is done through which method?
   a. USB drive
   b. Computer network
   c. Cloud storage
   d. Internal storage drive

6. *[LO 18.3]* Preventive measures to catch potential errors that can result in liabilities and investigations are conducted through _________.
   a. account review processes
   b. patient satisfaction surveys
   c. provider reviews
   d. medical record audits

7. *[LO 18.4]* Which report is used to track how long claims take to process?
   a. Accounts Payable (A/P) Aging report
   b. Key Performance Indicator (KPI) report
   c. Accounts Receivable (A/R) Aging report
   d. Procedure Code Analysis report

8. *[LO 18.2]* What process is used to copy backup files into an office's computer systems?
   a. Recovery
   b. Restoring
   c. Regenerating
   d. Reversal

9. *[LO 18.5]* Which coding audits are performed by the practice's compliance department prior to submission for billing?
   a. External and retrospective
   b. External and prospective
   c. Internal and retrospective
   d. Internal and prospective

10. *[LO 18.4]* Key Performance Indicator reports are used to measure if certain goals have been met and to determine _________.
    a. coding compliance
    b. performance measures
    c. outstanding account aging
    d. Title VII compliance

SHORT ANSWER QUESTIONS

Define the following abbreviations.

1. *[LO 18.4]* A/R ____________________
2. *[LO 18.4]* A/P ____________________
3. *[LO 18.4]* KPI ____________________

APPLYING YOUR KNOWLEDGE

Working with HIPAA

18.1 *[LO 18.3, LO 18.5]* Describe how you would develop a coding compliance plan. What schedule would you set for your audits and staff training?

____

____

18.2 *[LO 18.1]* Provide an example of how each of the following databases would be used.

a. Patient education

____

____

b. Staff information

____

____

c. Insurance carrier details

____

____

18.3 *[LO 18.2]* Why is it recommended that medical practice files be backed up to a location outside of the medical practice? How can this be done?

____

____

18.4 *[LO 18.4]* What are the benefits to conducting patient surveys? How can these be used to improve practice operations?

____

____

part five

PM and EHR Practical Applications

chapter 19

Putting It All Together

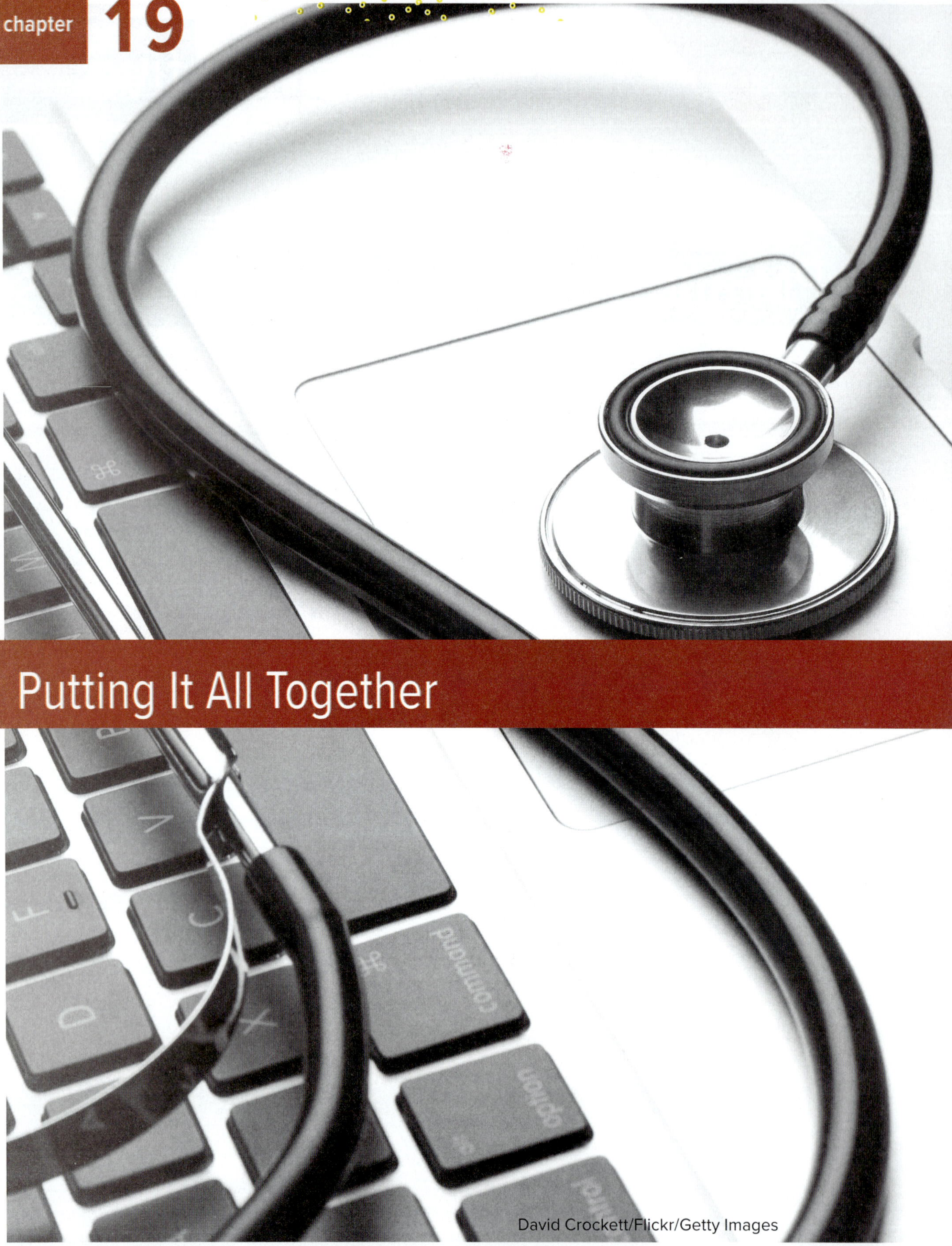

David Crockett/Flickr/Getty Images

LEARNING OUTCOMES

When you finish this chapter, you will be able to:

19.1 Demonstrate the application of practice management and electronic health record software using EHRclinic.

A Total Patient Encounter

In this chapter, you will have the opportunity to apply your knowledge of practice management and electronic health record systems as you complete a scenario that will take you through the entire medical documentation and billing process.

Using source documents and references to earlier chapters, you will use your critical thinking skills to complete the simulated exercises related to the following scenario:

Ciara Dylan walked into Trilogy Family Care Center to schedule a new patient appointment to see one of the providers for abdominal pain. Dr. Mancini had some cancellations, so Ciara was added to the afternoon schedule.

You will use the following source documents, located after this chapter, to help you complete several of the exercises:

- Source Document A: Patient Registration Form
- Source Document B: Insurance Card
- Source Document C: Patient Intake Sheet
- Source Document D: Office Visit Notes
- Source Document E: Patient Payment—Check
- Source Document F: Provider Notes
- Source Document G: Message Notes
- Source Document H: Remittance Advice (RA)

19.1 Practice Management and Electronic Health Record Applications

EXERCISE 19.1

Schedule the New Patient

EHRclinic

Refer to Chapter 4 for guidance.

Ciara Dylan walks into Trilogy Family Care Center and asks if she can schedule a new patient appointment to see one of the providers because she is experiencing a sore throat, ear pain, and voice loss. There have been some cancellations, so she can be added to the afternoon schedule.

Using the patient registration form found in Source Document A and the insurance card in Source Document B, create a new patient account for Ciara and schedule her appointment.

Your instructor may assign this exercise to you in Connect. Exercise steps and EHRclinic Help Guides can be downloaded at http://www.mhhe.com/pmehr2.

EXERCISE 19.2

Record the Receipt of Patient Documents

EHRclinic

Refer to Chapter 5 for guidance.

Ciara has received the Notice of Privacy Practices. Document the signed acknowledgement of receipt in her EHR.

Your instructor may assign this exercise to you in Connect. Exercise steps and EHRclinic Help Guides can be downloaded at http://www.mhhe.com/pmehr2.

EXERCISE 19.3

Build the New Patient's Facesheet

EHRclinic

Refer to Chapter 6 for guidance.

Using the completed patient intake sheet found in Source Document C, begin building Ciara's new patient facesheet.

Your instructor may assign this exercise to you in Connect. Exercise steps and EHRclinic Help Guides can be downloaded at http://www.mhhe.com/pmehr2.

EXERCISE 19.4

Add Allergies to the Patient's Facesheet

EHRclinic

Refer to Chapter 6 for guidance.

Using the completed patient intake sheet found in Source Document C, add Ciara's allergies to her facesheet.

Your instructor may assign this exercise to you in Connect. Exercise steps and EHRclinic Help Guides can be downloaded at http://www.mhhe.com/pmehr2.

EXERCISE 19.5

Add Medications to the Patient's Facesheet

EHRclinic

Refer to Chapter 6 for guidance.

Using the completed patient intake sheet found in Source Document C, add Ciara's medications to her facesheet.

Your instructor may assign this exercise to you in Connect. Exercise steps and EHRclinic Help Guides can be downloaded at http://www.mhhe.com/pmehr2.

EXERCISE 19.6

Maintain the Immunization Record

EHRclinic

Refer to Chapter 6 for guidance.

Using the completed patient intake sheet found in Source Document C, add Ciara's historical immunizations to her facesheet.

Your instructor may assign this exercise to you in Connect. Exercise steps and EHRclinic Help Guides can be downloaded at http://www.mhhe.com/pmehr2.

EXERCISE 19.7

Record the Patient's Vitals

EHRclinic

Refer to Chapter 6 for guidance.

Ciara has been brought back to the exam room, and you have taken her vital signs.

Using the office visit notes found in Source Document D, add the vitals to the office visit.

Your instructor may assign this exercise to you in Connect. Exercise steps and EHRclinic Help Guides can be downloaded at http://www.mhhe.com/pmehr2.

EXERCISE 19.8

Build the Office Visit Note

EHRclinic

Refer to Chapter 7 for guidance.

During patient intake, you record Ciara's CC and HPI. Acting as a scribe, you also assist the provider by documenting the remainder of the office visit.

Use the office visit notes found in Source Document D to record the office visit details.

Your instructor may assign this exercise to you in Connect. Exercise steps and EHRclinic Help Guides can be downloaded at http://www.mhhe.com/pmehr2.

EXERCISE 19.9

Mark the Order Status

EHRclinic

Refer to Chapter 10 for guidance.

Mark Ciara's order status for the procedures ordered during the office visit.

Your instructor may assign this exercise to you in Connect. Exercise steps and EHRclinic Help Guides can be downloaded at http://www.mhhe.com/pmehr2.

EXERCISE 19.10

Document the Point-of-Care Results

EHRclinic

Refer to Chapter 10 for guidance.

Using the office visit notes found in Source Document D, document the patient's point-of-care test results.

Your instructor may assign this exercise to you in Connect. Exercise steps and EHRclinic Help Guides can be downloaded at http://www.mhhe.com/pmehr2.

EXERCISE 19.11

Create the Patient's Excuse Note

EHRclinic

Refer to Chapter 17 for guidance.

The provider recommends that the patient not return to work for a few days folllowing her office visit.

Using the office visit notes found in Source Document D, create a work excuse note for Ciara.

Your instructor may assign this exercise to you in Connect. Exercise steps and EHRclinic Help Guides can be downloaded at http://www.mhhe.com/pmehr2.

EXERCISE 19.12 Create the Clinical Visit Summary

EHRclinic

Refer to Chapter 10 for guidance.

Ciara is preparing to check out. Create a clinical visit summary for her office visit.

Your instructor may assign this exercise to you in Connect. Exercise steps and EHRclinic Help Guides can be downloaded at http://www.mhhe.com/pmehr2.

EXERCISE 19.13 Create the Electronic Routing Slip (Encounter Form)

EHRclinic

Refer to Chapter 11 for guidance.

As Ciara checks out, create an electronic routing slip.

Your instructor may assign this exercise to you in Connect. Exercise steps and EHRclinic Help Guides can be downloaded at http://www.mhhe.com/pmehr2.

EXERCISE 19.14 Post the Patient Copayment

EHRclinic

Refer to Chapter 11 for guidance.

Before leaving the office, Ciara stops at the front desk to make her copayment.

Using the patient check found in Source Document E, document payment of the patient's copay and print a receipt.

Your instructor may assign this exercise to you in Connect. Exercise steps and EHRclinic Help Guides can be downloaded at http://www.mhhe.com/pmehr2.

EXERCISE 19.15 Create the Insurance Claim

EHRclinic

Refer to Chapter 13 for guidance.

Create an insurance claim for Ciara's office visit.

Your instructor may assign this exercise to you in Connect. Exercise steps and EHRclinic Help Guides can be downloaded at http://www.mhhe.com/pmehr2.

EXERCISE 19.16 Submit the Insurance Claim

EHRclinic

Refer to Chapter 13 for guidance.

Submit the insurance claim to Ciara's insurance carrier.

Your instructor may assign this exercise to you in Connect. Exercise steps and EHRclinic Help Guides can be downloaded at http://www.mhhe.com/pmehr2.

Add the Test Results to the Patient's Chart

EHRclinic

EXERCISE 19.17

Refer to Chapter 8 for guidance.

Ciara's test results are complete and have been scanned into EHRclinic. Add the test results to the patient's EHR so Dr. Williams can review them.

Your instructor may assign this exercise to you in Connect. Exercise steps and EHRclinic Help Guides can be downloaded at http://www.mhhe.com/pmehr2.

Create the Patient Test Result Letter

EHRclinic

EXERCISE 19.18

Refer to Chapter 17 for guidance.

Using the provider notes found in Source Document F, create a letter to notify the Ciara of her test results.

Your instructor may assign this exercise to you in Connect. Exercise steps and EHRclinic Help Guides can be downloaded at http://www.mhhe.com/pmehr2.

Create the Patient Message

EHRclinic

EXERCISE 19.19

Refer to Chapter 17 for guidance.

Ciara called with questions about her office visit and test results.

Using the message notes found in Source Document G, create a new message in EHRclinic and send it to the provider.

Your instructor may assign this exercise to you in Connect. Exercise steps and EHRclinic Help Guides can be downloaded at http://www.mhhe.com/pmehr2.

Resolve the Patient Message

EHRclinic

EXERCISE 19.20

Refer to Chapter 17 for guidance.

The provider has responded to Ciara's message and sent it back to you for follow-up.

Using the message notes found in Source Document G, complete the patient's message and document it in her EHR.

Your instructor may assign this exercise to you in Connect. Exercise steps and EHRclinic Help Guides can be downloaded at http://www.mhhe.com/pmehr2.

Manage the Patient Recall List

EHRclinic

EXERCISE 19.21

Refer to Chapter 17 for guidance.

The provider wants Ciara to return to the clinic in two months. Add her to the patient recall list.

Your instructor may assign this exercise to you in Connect. Exercise steps and EHRclinic Help Guides can be downloaded at http://www.mhhe.com/pmehr2.

EXERCISE 19.22 Post the Insurance Payments Using an RA

EHRclinic

Refer to Chapter 14 for guidance.

The remittance advice and insurance payment have come in for Ciara's claim.

Using the remittance advice found in Source Document H, post payments for the patients listed.

Your instructor may assign this exercise to you in Connect. Exercise steps and EHRclinic Help Guides can be downloaded at http://www.mhhe.com/pmehr2.

EXERCISE 19.23 Assign and Complete Daily Task Items

EHRclinic

Refer to Chapter 17 for guidance.

Manage the task list by completing task items. The office manager has also requested that tasks be created to order business cards for the new provider and place an ad for a new medical assistant.

Your instructor may assign this exercise to you in Connect. Exercise steps and EHRclinic Help Guides can be downloaded at http://www.mhhe.com/pmehr2.

EXERCISE 19.24 Add a New Provider to the Database

EHRclinic

Refer to Chapter 18 for guidance.

A new provider is starting at Trilogy Family Care Center. Add Adrian Zaman to the new provider database and assign provider access rights to their account.

Your instructor may assign this exercise to you in Connect. Exercise steps and EHRclinic Help Guides can be downloaded at http://www.mhhe.com/pmehr2.

part six

Source Documents

SOURCE DOCUMENTS

A Patient Registration Form

B Insurance Card

C Patient Intake Sheet

D Office Visit Notes

E Patient Payment—Check

F Provider Notes

G Message Notes

H Remittance Advice (RA)

source documents

A PATIENT REGISTRATION FORM

Trilogy Family Care Center

REGISTRATION FORM

(Please Print)

Today's date: *July 28, 2023* **Care Provider:** *Dr. Williams*

PATIENT INFORMATION

Patient's last name:	**First:**	**Middle:**	❑ Mr. ❑ Mrs.	❑ Miss ☒ Ms.	**Marital status (circle one)**
Dylan	*Ciara*	*Marie*			(Single) / Mar / Div / Sep / Wid

Is this your legal name?	**If not, what is your legal name?**	**(Former name):**	**Birth date:**	**Age:**	**Gender assigned at birth:**
☒ Yes ❑ No			*09/21/1996*	*26*	❑ M ☒ F

Street address:	**Social Security no.:**	**Home phone:**	**Cell phone:**
4519 Roselawn Drive	*303-86-1857*	*586-555-9898*	*586-555-0701*

P. O. Box:	**City:**	**State:**	**ZIP Code:**
	Shelby	*MI*	*48315*

Occupation:	**Employer:**	**Employer phone no.:**
Medical coder	*Summit Bay Health Center*	*567-555-2378*

E-mail address: *cdylan@patient.com*

Race: *Caucasian* **Ethnicity:** *Not Hispanic or Latino* **Primary language:** *English* **Religion:** *Catholic*

Other family members seen here: *none* **Preferred gender pronouns:** ❑He/him/his ☒ She/her/hers ❑ They/them/their ❑ Ze/hir/hirs, ze/zir/zirs

INSURANCE INFORMATION

(Presentation of Insurance Card is required at time of each visit)

Person responsible for bill:	**Date of birth:**	**Address:**	**Home phone:**	**Cell phone:**
Ciara Marie Dylan	*09/21/1996*	*4519 Roselawn Drive, Shelby, MI 48315*	*586-555-9898*	*586-555-0701*

Is this person a patient here? ☒ Yes ❑ No

Occupation:	**Employer:**	**Employer address:**	**Employer phone no.:**
Medical coder	*Summit Bay Health*	*831 Hayes Road, Clinton Township, MI 48035*	*586-555-6875*

Is this patient covered by insurance? ☒Yes ❑ No

Please indicate primary insurance ☒ Med-Plus ❑ BlueCross/ Blue Shield ❑ Ameri-Access ❑ Fulton Health ❑ Aetna

❑ Medline Plus ❑ Workers' Compensation ❑ Medicare ❑ Medicaid *(Please provide card)* ❑ Other

Subscriber's name:	**Subscriber's S.S. no.:**	**Date of birth:**	**Group no.:**	**Policy no.:**	**Co-payment:**
Ciara Marie Dylan	*303-86-1857*	*09/21/1996*	*819*	*CMD428036455*	*$ 30.00*

Patient's relationship to subscriber: ☒ Self ❑ Spouse ❑ Child ❑ Other Effective Date: *01/01/2023*

Name of secondary insurance (if applicable):	**Subscriber's name:**	**Group no.:**	**Policy no.:**
None			

Patient's relationship to subscriber: ☒Self ❑ Spouse ❑ Child ❑ Other

IN CASE OF EMERGENCY

Name of local friend or relative (not living at same address):	Relationship to patient:	Home phone no.:	Work phone no.:
Angela Dylan	*Mother*	*(586) 555-5346*	*(586) 555-4310*

The above information is true to the best of my knowledge. I authorize my insurance benefits be paid directly to the physician. I understand that I am financially responsible for any balance. I also authorize [Name of Practice] or insurance company to release any information required to process my claims.

Patient/Guardian signature: Ciara Dylan *Date:* 7/28/23

B INSURANCE CARD

MED-Plus®

Subscriber Name:
Ciara Marie Dylan

Identification Number:
CMD428036455

Group Number: 819
Coverage Date: 01/01/2023

SINGLE

Office Copay	$30
Emergency Copay	$250
RX Generic Copay	$30
RX Brand Copay	$50

RxID: 062491
RxNFP: 30798

PPO℞

C PATIENT INTAKE SHEET

Trilogy Family Care Center
Patient Intake Sheet

Date: 7/28/2023 Provider: Dr. Williams

Patient Name: Ciara Marie Dylan DOB: 9/21/1996 Chart #: AA050

Personal Health Information

Allergies (List all allergies and reactions)
Levofloxacin, difficulty breathing and swelling of lips, tongue and throat. Reaction date 12/1/2012.

Medications (all prescription and over-the-counter)
Levothyroxine 0.25 mg one daily
Multivitamin one daily

Family Medical History (list age and health history)
Mother: 54 years old, asthma, at age 22
Father: 60 years old, hypertension, at age 55
Sister(s): 29 years old, diabetes Type 1, at age 11
Brother(s): 21 years old, in good health
Other:

Past Medical History	Yes	No	If yes, when?
Asthma		√	
Bronchitis		√	
Cancer		√	
Diabetes		√	
Gout		√	
Heart Disease		√	
Hernia		√	
High Blood Pressure		√	
High Cholesterol		√	
HIV Positive		√	
Kidney Disease		√	
Liver Disease		√	
Migraines		√	
Pneumonia	√		12/1/2012
Thyroid Problems	√		hypothyroidism
Other			
Other			

Surgeries (list below)
Rotator cuff surgery (left) 2017

Past Immunizations (from immunization records)
Pneumovax 0.5 mL by Dr. Alamant, left deltoid
Mfr: Pharmapro Labs Lot: 79811 Exp: 12/1/2020

Social History (Check all that apply)
Tobacco Use: (Choose one) Yes √ No ___
Current – every day? _____ some days? √
Former smoker? _____ Never smoked? _____
Heavy tobacco? _____ Light tobacco? _____
Exercise? Occasional **Sleep:** 8 hours per day
Illicit drugs? Yes __ No √ Details Never
Alcohol Use: (Choose one) Yes √ No _____
Frequency? Monthly Details? 2-3 Mixed drinks
Caffeine Use: Yes √ No__ Frequency? daily
Marital Status: Single ______ Married √
Divorced ____ Widowed ____ Never Married____
Living Arrangements: With partner **Seatbelt use:** always
Sexually Active?: Yes √ No __ Use Protection? never
 # Partners in 12 mo? 1 **Gender of partners?** male
STI History? Yes __ No √ Details________________
Education: Student ___ High School__ College grad √
Occupation: Medical coder (healthcare)

Language
Preferred language English

Current Medical Problems	Yes	No	Details
Unexplained weight loss		√	
Headaches		√	
Pain	√		right ear
Dental problems		√	
Arthritis		√	
Diarrhea/Constipation		√	
Urinary problems		√	
Menstrual problems		√	
Fatigue	√		
Problems with eating		√	
Problems with memory		√	
Chronic coughs/colds		√	
Back problems		√	
Other	√		sore throat/ voice loss

D OFFICE VISIT NOTES

Trilogy Family Care Center
Office Visit Notes

Date: 7/28/2023	Provider: Dr. Williams
Patient Name: Ciara Marie Dylan DOB: 9/21/1996	Chart #: AA050
CC:	C/o right ear pain, fatigue, sore throat, and voice loss
PI:	Pt states that she developed a sore throat with voice loss and Ⓡ ear pain about three days ago. She also says that she has increased fatigue and a fever of 101°F. She has been treating her symptoms with OTC pain relievers, allergy medications, and throat spray with minimal relief.
ROS:	ROS Normal and pt reports no signs of cough or chest congestion, no nausea/vomiting or chills/sweats, no recent changes in weight, no headaches. Abnormals: + difficulty swallowing and throat pain, + voice loss + Ⓡ ear Pain, + fatigue.
Vitals:	T: 102.8 °F oral R: 18 P: 94 bpm BP: 118/82 mmHG Ⓡ arm, sitting Ht: 66 in Wt: 158#
Exam:	26 y/o female in no apparent acute distress, well nourished, well developed, alert, cooperative Exam: bilateral lymph nodes in the neck, slight redness of throat and tonsils, + hoarseness. Abdomen soft, nontender without distension. No notable splenic or hepatic enlargement or tenderness. Eyes: PERRLA Ears: Ⓛ external auditory canal and tympanic membrane is clear. + erythema of Ⓡ middle ear. Nose: No nasal discharge. Lungs: Clear to auscultation and percussion. Cardiac: Regular rhythm, no peripheral edema, cyanosis, or pallor, no bruits.
Dx:	Acute laryngitis and pharyngitis; otitis media (right); fatigue; fever
Labs:	Strep screen; CBC
Results:	POC strep screen: negative with valid controls
Rx:	Amoxicillin 500 mg, one tab by mouth three times daily until gone Ibuprofen 200 mg, two tabs by mouth every 6 hours as needed
F/U	Return to clinic in one week
RTW Note:	Patient was seen by Dr. Williams on 7/28/2023. She is excused from work from 7/28/2023 through 8/2/2023 and may return to work on 8/3/3023 with no restrictions.
Signed	Karlisha Williams, MD 7/28/23

E PATIENT PAYMENT—CHECK

Ciara Dylan **1983**

4519 Roselawn Dr
Shelby, MI 48315
(586) 555-0701

DATE July 28, 2023 1222/6359

PAY: Trilogy Family Care Center **$** 30.00
TO THE ORDER OF

Thirty and 00/100 **DOLLARS**

Ascension Bank & Trust
20571 Engelburg St
Macomb, MI 48035

FOR OV Copay Ciara Dylan

F PROVIDER NOTES

Letter Title – Test Results from 7/28/23

Letter – Your CBC indicated an elevated white blood cell count, which is not unusual during an infection. Continue to take your antibiotics until they are gone and call the office if your symptoms persist. Thank you!

G MESSAGE NOTES

Subject – Question about Test Results

Add Ciara Dylan's patient chart.

Message from Ciara Dylan to Dr. Williams –

Ciara called and stated that she received her test results in the mail. She is asking if she needs to return to have her CBC tested again after she finishes the antibiotics.

Reply from Dr. Williams –

Please let Ciara know that she does not need to repeat her CBC blood test, but she should be sure to make an appointment if she is still not feeling well.

Resolve the Patient Message

Patient was informed and verbalizes understanding.

After adding the resolution, sign the note with the password *1234* then click *send.* Click on the final message and add the message to Ciara Dylan's chart.

H REMITTANCE ADVICE (RA)

MED-Plus®

PROVIDER REMITTANCE

THIS IS NOT A BILL

Trilogy Family Care Center

PAGE: 1 OF 1
DATE: 09/13/2023
ID NUMBER: CMD428036455

PROVIDER: KARLISHA WILLIAMS, M.D.

PATIENT: Ciara Dylan CLAIM: 072823AA050

FROM DATE	THROUGH DATE	PROC CODE	UNIT	AMT BILL	AMT ALLOW	AMT PAID	DED	COPAY	ADJ	COIN	PROV PAID	REASON CODE*
07/28/23	07/28/23	85025	1	62.00	46.56	46.56	0.00	0.00	15.44	0.00	46.56	PR2
07/28/23	07/28/23	87880	1	22.00	16.52	16.52	0.00	0.00	5.48	0.00	29.69	PR2
07/28/23	07/28/23	99201	1	56.00	42.06	12.06	0.00	30.00	13.94	0.00	12.06	PR2
CLAIM TOTALS				140.00	105.14	75.14	0.00	ADJ	34.86	0.00	75.14	

PAYMENT SUMMARY		TOTAL ALL CLAIMS		EFT INFORMATION	
TOTAL AMOUNT PAID	75.14	AMOUNT CHARGED	140.00	NUMBER	4280316042011
PRIOR CREDIT BALANCE	.00	AMOUNT ALLOWED	105.14	DATE	09/13/23
CURRENT CREDIT DEFERRED	.00	DEDUCTIBLE	0.00	AMOUNT	75.14
PRIOR CREDIT APPLIED	.00	COPAY	30.00		
NEW CREDIT BALANCE	.00	COINSURANCE	0.00		
NET DISPERSED	75.14				

*REASON CODES

PR1 - Deductible PR2 – Paid PR3 – Co-pay PR4 – Denied V – VOID ADJ - Adjustment

glossary

a

abuse: actions that improperly use another person's resources

accept assignment: participating physician's agreement to accept the allowed charge as full payment

access levels: security option that determines the areas of the program a user can access, and whether the user has rights to enter or edit data

accounts payable (A/P): monies going out of a business or medical practice, such as to pay staff, lease/rent, utilities, supplies, and equipment

accounts receivable (A/R): monies that are coming into a practice

Accounts Receivable (A/R) Aging Report: shows all current unpaid charges and health care claims including the amount owed and their duration

Acknowledgment of Receipt of Notice of Privacy Practices: form accompanying a covered entity's Notice of Privacy Practices; covered entities must make a good-faith effort to have patients sign it

addendum: information provided in an EHR that is not available in the original entry; adding to an original entry or correcting an erroneous entry

adjudication: series of steps that determine whether a claim should be paid

adjustments: changes to a patient's account

advance beneficiary notice of noncoverage (ABN): Medicare form used to inform a patient that a service to be provided is not likely to be reimbursed by Medicare

adverse effects: undesired harmful effects resulting from a medication

aging: classification of accounts receivable by length of time

aging report: a report that lists the amount of money owed to the practice, organized by the amount of time the money has been owed

allowed charge: maximum charge a plan pays for a service or procedure

Alphabetic Index: section of ICD-10-CM alphabetically listing diseases and injuries with corresponding diagnosis codes

analog: stored on paper and unable to be read by a computer

appeal: request for reconsideration of a claim adjudication

appellant: person who appeals a claim decision

assignment of benefits: authorization by a policyholder that allows a health plan to pay benefits directly to a provider

audit: formal examination or review, such as a review to determine whether an entity is complying with regulations

auto log-off: feature of PM/EHR systems that automatically logs a user out of the program after a period of inactivity

autoposting: software feature enabling automatic entry of payments from a remittance advice

b

backing up: making a copy of data files at a specific point in time that can be used to restore data

balance billing: collecting the difference between a provider's usual fee and a payer's lower allowed charge

bankruptcy: declaration that a person is unable to pay his or her debts

benefits: the amount of money a health plan pays for services covered in an insurance policy

billing cycle: steps that establish financial responsibility, check-in, check-out, and coding, the professional medical staff gathering clinical information

birthday rule: guideline that determines which of two parents with medical coverage has the primary insurance for a child; the parent whose day of birth is earlier in the calendar year is considered primary

Blue Cross Blue Shield Association (BCBS): a federation of 35 separate United States health insurance companies that provide health insurance in the United States to more than 106 million people

body (of a communication): the main part of a written communication (message, email, letter, or memo); details the purpose of the communication

breach: under the HIPAA Privacy Rule, impermissible use or disclosure that compromises the security or privacy of PHI that could pose a significant risk of financial, reputational, or other harm to the affected person

breach notification: document used by a covered entity to notify individuals of a breach in their protected health information required under the new HITECH breach notification rules

bundled code: two or more related procedure codes combined into one

c

capitated plan: insurance plan in which prepayments made to a physician cover the physician's services to a plan member for a specified period of time

capitation: a prepayment covering provider's services for a plan member for a specified period

capitation (cap) rate: periodic prepayment to a provider for specified services to each plan member

capitation payments: payments made to physicians on a regular basis for providing services to patients in a managed care plan

cash flow: the movement of monies into and out of a business

Category I codes: procedure codes found in the main body of CPT

Category II codes: optional CPT codes that track performance measures

Category III codes: temporary codes for emerging technology, services, and procedures

CCI column 1/column 2 code pair edits: Medicare code edit in which CPT codes in column 2 will not be paid if reported for same day of service, for the same patient, and by the same provider as the column 1 code

CCI edits: CPT code combinations that are used by computers to check Medicare claims

CCI modifier indicator: number showing whether the use of a modifier can bypass a CCI edit

CCI mutually exclusive code (MEC) edits: edits for codes for services that could not have reasonably been done during one encounter

Centers for Medicare and Medicaid Services (CMS): federal agency in the Department of Health and Human Services that runs Medicare, Medicaid, clinical laboratories, and other government health programs; responsible for enforcing all HIPAA standards other than the privacy and security standards

certification: a nationally recognized designation that acknowledges that an individual has mastered a standard body of knowledge and meets certain competencies

charge capture: process of recording billable services

charge: amount a provider bills for performed health care services

chart number: unique alphanumeric code that identifies a patient

chief complaint (CC): a brief description of the patient's current problem in his or her own words

Civilian Health and Medical Program of the Department of Veterans Affairs (CHAMPVA): health care plan for families of veterans with 100 percent service-related disabilities and the surviving spouses and children of veterans who die from service-related disabilities

claim adjustment group code (CAGC): used on an RA/EOB to indicate the general type of reason code for an adjustment

claim adjustment reason code (CARC): used on an RA/EOB to explain why a payment does not match the amount billed

claim control number: unique number assigned to a claim by the sender

claim scrubber: software that checks claims to permit error correction

claim status category codes: used to report the status group for a claim

claim status codes: used to provide a detailed answer to a claim status inquiry

claim turnaround time: time period in which a health plan must process a claim

claimant: person or entity exercising the right to receive benefits

clean claim: a claim that has no edits and can go directly to the payer

clearinghouse: company that processes electronic health information and executes electronic transactions such as insurance verification and claim submission for providers

clinical check-out: performing the final steps of a patient's encounter or office visit; includes initiating orders such as lab work or radiology, providing referrals, administering in-office medications, and any other task designated by the provider as part of the encounter

clinical decision support (CDS): provides timely information to help inform decisions about a patient's care, including preventive care reminders, alerts about drug interactions, and so on

clinical visit summary: provides patients with relevant information and instructions pertaining to an encounter

cloud storage: saving data securely online so that it can be shared and accessed at any time from any location

CMS-1500 (08/05) claim: the mandated paper insurance claim form

code linkage: clinically appropriate connection between a provided service and a patient's condition or illness

coinsurance: the portion of charges that an insured person must pay for health care services after payment of the deductible amount; usually stated as a percentage

collection agency: outside firm hired to collect on delinquent accounts

collection list: tool for tracking activities that need to be completed as part of the collection process

collection tracer report: tool for keeping track of collection letters that were sent

companion guide: guide published by a payer that lists its own set of claim edits and formatting conventions

compliance: adhering to a written, adopted, or required set of rules

compliance plan: a process for finding, correcting, and preventing illegal medical office practices. It is a written document prepared by a compliance officer and committee that sets up the steps needed to (1) audit and monitor compliance with government regulations, especially in the area of coding and billing, (2) have policies and procedures that are consistent, (3) provide for ongoing staff training and communication, and (4) respond to and correct errors

compliant billing: billing actions that satisfy official requirements

computerized provider order entry (CPOE): a provider's use of computer software to enter medical orders (medication, lab, or radiology orders) directly from a computer or mobile device

continuity of care: coordination of care received by a patient over time and across multiple health care providers

controlled substance: drug whose use and possession is regulated by law

coordination of benefits (COB): clause in an insurance policy that explains how the policy will pay if more than one insurance policy applies to the claim

coordination of care: deliberate organization of patient care between a patient and at least one other participant, such as a health care provider

copayment (copay): an amount that a health plan requires a beneficiary to pay at the time of service for each health care encounter

Correct Coding Initiative (CCI): computerized Medicare system that prevents overpayment

covered services: medical procedures and treatments that are included as benefits under an insured's health plan

crossover claim: claim billed to Medicare and then submitted to Medicaid

Current Procedural Terminology (CPT): the standardized classification system for reporting medical procedures and services

d

dashboard: a visualization tool that allows a practice to review user performance and performance metrics

data: information in a digital form that can be transmitted or processed

data element: smallest unit of information in a HIPAA transaction

data mining: the process of analyzing large amounts of data to discover patterns or knowledge

data warehouse: a collection of data that includes all areas of an organization's operations

database: a collection of related bits of information

day sheet: a report that provides information on practice activities for a twenty-four-hour period

deductible: an amount that an insured person must pay, usually on an annual basis, for health care services before a health plan's payment begins

demographics: various identifying characteristics of an individual, such as a patient's name, date of birth, address, telephone number, and gender

determination: payer's decision about the benefits due for a claim

development: process of gathering information to adjudicate a claim

diagnosis code: a code that represents the physician's determination of a patient's primary illness

diagnostic statement: the medical term describing the condition for which a patient is receiving care

dictation: the process of recording spoken words that will later be transcribed into written form

digital: stored on electronic media that can be read by a computer

digital dictation: the process of dictating using a microphone, a headset connected to a computer, a smartphone, or a PDA

disability compensation programs: programs that provide partial reimbursement for lost income when a disability prevents an individual from working

disaster recovery plan: plan for resuming normal operations after a disaster such as a fire or a computer malfunction

discounted fee-for-service: payment schedule for services based on a reduced percentage of usual charges

documentation: the record created when a physician provides treatment to a patient

drug interaction checker: tool to identify potentially harmful and unsafe combinations of prescription medications

drug–diagnosis warning: a warning given by an E-Prescribing system when a patient's reported diagnosis does not support the drug being prescribed

drug–drug interactions: reaction between two or more drugs in which the efficacy and/or side effects of at least one of the drugs in increased or decreased

dual-eligible: Medicare–Medicaid beneficiary

e

E-Prescribing (ERX): a provider's ability to electronically send accurate and understandable prescriptions directly to a pharmacy from the point-of-care, such as the provider's practice during an office visit

electronic encounter form (EEF): an electronic version of the form that lists procedures and charges for a patient's visit

electronic funds transfer (EFT): electronic routing of funds between banks

electronic health record (EHR): a computerized lifelong health care record for an individual that incorporates data from all sources that provide treatment for the individual

electronic medical record (EMR): computerized record of one physician's encounters with a patient over time

electronic remittance advice (ERA): electronic document that lists patients, dates of service, charges, and the amounts paid or denied by the insurance carrier

electronic signature: symbols or other data in a digital form attached to an electronically transmitted document as verification of the sender's intent

electronic telephone message: communication that is transmitted by telephone and entered into an electronic health record for response and resolution

email: messages delivered electronically through a network to one or more recipients

Employee Retirement Income Security Act of 1974 (ERISA): law providing incentives and protection for companies with employee health and pension plans

encounter: the meeting of a patient with a physician or other medical professional for the purpose of providing health care (also known as a visit)

encryption: process of converting electronic information into an unreadable format before it is distributed

Equal Credit Opportunity Act (ECOA): law that prohibits credit discrimination on the basis of race, color, religion, national origin, sex, marital status, or age, or because a person receives public assistance

established patient (EP): patient who has received professional services from a provider (or another provider with the same specialty in the same practice) within the past three years

evaluation and management (E/M) codes: codes that cover physicians' services performed to determine the optimum course for patient care

expiration date: date after which a drug or vaccine should not be administered

explanation of benefits (EOB): document showing how the amount of a benefit was determined

external audit: formal review that is conducted by an independent entity not associated with the medical practice

f

Fair Debt Collection Practices Act of 1977 (FDCPA): federal law regulating collection practices

False Claims Act: prohibits submitting a fraudulent claim or making a false statement or representation in connection with a claim; encourages reporting suspected fraud and abuse by protecting and rewarding people involved in qui tam (whistleblower) cases

family history (FH): a detailed record of medical events among members of the patient's family, including the ages, living status, and diseases of siblings, children, parents, and grandparents

Federal Employees Health Benefits (FEHB): health care program that covers federal employees

fee schedule: document that specifies the amount the provider bills for services

fee-for-service: health plan that repays the policyholder for covered medical expenses

filter: a condition that data must meet to be selected

financial policy: practice's rules governing payment for medical services from patients

formulary: list of a plan's selected drugs and their proper dosages

fraud: intentional act of deception to take financial advantage of another person

g

global period: days surrounding a surgical procedure when all services relating to the procedure are considered part of the surgical package

group health plan (GHP): plan of an employer or employee organization to provide health care to employees, former employees, and/or their families

guarantor: person who is the insurance policyholder for a patient of the practice; agrees to financial responsibility for a patient

h

Health Care Fraud and Abuse Control Program: government program to uncover misuse of funds in federal health care programs; run by the Office of the Inspector General

health informatics: knowledge required to optimize the acquisition, storage, retrieval, and use of information in health and biomedicine

health information technology (HIT): the use of computers and electronic communications to manage medical information and its secure exchange

Health Information Technology for Economic and Clinical Health (HITECH) Act: provisions in the American Recovery and Reinvestment Act (ARRA) of 2009 that extend and reinforce HIPAA and contain new breach notification requirements for covered entities and business associates, guidance on ways to encrypt or destroy PHI to prevent a breach, requirements for informing individuals when a breach occurs, higher monetary penalties for HIPAA violations, and stronger enforcement of the Privacy and Security Rules

Health Insurance Portability and Accountability Act of 1996 (HIPAA): legislation that protects patient's private health information, ensures health care coverage when workers change or lose jobs, and uncovers fraud and abuse in the health care system

health maintenance organization (HMO): managed health care system in which providers offer health care to members for fixed periodic payments

health plan: an individual or group plan that either provides or pays for the cost of medical care; includes group health plans, health insurance issuers, health maintenance organizations, Medicare Part A and B, Medicaid, TRICARE, and other government and nongovernment plans

Healthcare Common Procedure Coding System (HCPCS): procedure codes and supplies for Medicare claims

Hierarchical Condition Category Coding (HCC): a risk-adjustment model based on ICD-10-CM coding to assign risk scores to patients to estimate health care cost and give a picture of the patient's complexity

HIPAA Breach Notification Rule: law that requires HIPAA covered entities and their business associates to provide notification following a breach of unsecured protected health information

HIPAA National Identifiers: HIPAA-mandated identification systems for employers, health care providers, health plans, and patients; national provider system and employer system are in place; health plan and patient systems have not been created

HIPAA Privacy Rule: law that regulates the use and disclosure of patients' protected health information

HIPAA Security Rule: law that requires covered entities to establish administrative, physical, and technical safeguards to protect the confidentiality, integrity, and availability of health information

HIPAA Transaction and Code Set Standards: HIPAA–mandated standardization in health care e-commerce, the standard requires the provider to submit information electronically, always in the same format

HIPAA X12 276/277 Health Care Claim Status Inquiry/ Response: electronic format used to ask payers about claims

HIPAA X12 837 Health Care Claim: HIPAA standard format for electronic transmission of the claim to a health plan

history of present illness (HPI): a description of the course of the present illness, including how and when the problem began, up to the present time

i

indemnity plan: type of medical insurance that reimburses a policyholder for medical services under the terms of its schedule of benefits

individual health plan (IHP): medical insurance plan purchased by an individual

insurance aging report: a report that lists how long a payer has taken to respond to insurance claims

internal audit: review of a medical office's coding that is conducted by the practice's compliance department

International Classification of Disease 10th Revision, Clinical Modification (ICD-10-CM): the source of the codes used for reporting diagnoses, since October 1, 2015

interoperability: allows computer applications or software to share and exchange information

k

key components: factors documented for various levels of evaluation and management services

key performance indicators (KPI): the critical indicators of progress toward a desired result with a focus on operational improvement

l

Likert scale: used in surveys to allow individuals to express the extent that they agree or disagree with a particular statement

lot number: a number given to a specific batch of drug or vaccine as it was manufactured; used for identification of a drug or vaccine

m

managed care: system that combines the financing and delivery of appropriate, cost-effective health care services to its members

manufacturer: a company that makes drugs or vaccines

Master Patient Index (MPI): a database that links patient records from multiple financial and administrative source systems

meaningful use: the utilization of certified EHR technology to improve quality, efficiency, and patient safety in the health care system

means test: process of fairly determining a patient's ability to pay

Medi-Medi beneficiary: person eligible for both Medicare and Medicaid

Medicaid: federal and state assistance program that pays for health care services for people who cannot afford them

medical assistant (MA): health care professional who performs both administrative and certain clinical tasks in physician offices

medical biller: health care professional who performs administrative tasks throughout the medical billing cycle

medical coder: medical office staff member with specialized training who handles the diagnostic and procedural coding of medical records

medical coding: the process of applying the HIPAA-mandated code sets to assign codes to diagnoses and procedures

medical data analysis: application of statistical techniques to improve outcomes and reduce costs in health care

medical documentation and billing cycle: a ten-step process that results in timely payment for medical services

medical insurance: financial plan that covers the cost of hospital and medical care

medical malpractice: the provision of medical services at a less than acceptable level of professional skill that results in injury or harm to a patient

medical necessity: treatment that is in accordance with generally accepted medical practice

medical necessity denial: refusal by a plan to pay for a procedure that does not meet its medical necessity criteria

medical record: a chronological health care record that includes information that the patient provides, such as medical history, as well as the physician's assessment, diagnosis, and treatment plan

medically unlikely edits (MUEs): units of service edits used to lower the Medicare fee-for-service paid claims error rate

Medicare: federal health insurance program for people sixty-five or older and some people with disabilities

Medicare Access and CHIP Reauthorization Act (MACRA): legislation that created the Quality Payment Program that changes the way that Medicare rewards clinicians, streamlines quality programs under MIPS, and provides bonuses for participation in eligible alternative payment models

Medicare Part A: program that pays for hospitalization, care in a skilled nursing facility, home health care, and hospice care

Medicare Part B: program that pays for physician services, outpatient hospital services, durable medical equipment, and other services and supplies

Medicare Part C (Medicare Advantage): managed care health plans under the Medicare program

Medicare Part D: Medicare prescription drug reimbursement plans

Medicare Physician Fee Schedule (MPFS): allowed fees based on the resource-based relative value scale that are the basis for Medicare reimbursements

medicaton reconciliation: the process of identifying the most accurate and current list of all medications taken by a patient; includes name, dosage, frequency, and route and compares medical records to external lists of medications (such as from the patient or the pharmacy)

Medigap: plan offered by a private insurance carrier to supplement Medicare coverage

memo: brief written message typically sent to groups of people with the purpose of informing

Merit-Based Incentive Payment System (MIPS): program that determines Medicare payment adjustments through the Quality Payment Program

messaging: the sending and processing of messages through emails, texting, or other electronic means

modifier: number appended to a code to report particular facts

monitoring coding compliance: process that ensures that the coding of diagnoses and procedures follows all coding rules and guidelines to minimize the risk of fraud

n

National Provider Identifier (NPI): under HIPAA, system for identifying all health care providers using unique ten-digit identifiers

National Uniform Claim Committee (NUCC): organization responsible for claim content

new patient (NP): a patient who has not received professional services from a provider (or another provider with the same specialty in the same practice) within the past three years

noncovered services: medical procedures that are not included in a plan's benefits

nonparticipating (nonPAR) provider: a provider who chooses not to join a particular government or other health plan

nonsufficient funds (NSF): check or debit that is not honored by the bank because the account lacks funds to cover it

nonverbal communication: communication without the use of spoken language; includes gestures, facial expressions, and body language

Notice of Privacy Practices (NPP): a HIPAA-mandated document stating the privacy policies and procedures of a covered entity

O

office visit (OV): an encounter between a patient and provider in which new or existing health issues, concerns, or symptoms can be discussed

one-way communication: transfer of information or a message from the sender to the receiver without an opportunity for a response

Original Medicare Plan: Medicare fee-for-service plan

out-of-network: a provider that does not have a participation agreement with a plan; using an out-of-network provider is more expensive for the plan's enrollees

out-of-pocket: expenses the insured must pay before benefits begin (deductible) or as a portion of cost-sharing (coinsurance)

overpayment: improper or excessive amount received by provider from payer

P

package: combination of services included in a single procedure code

participating (PAR) provider: a provider who agrees to provide medical services to a payer's policyholders according to the terms of the plan's contract

password: confidential authentication information

past medical history (PMH): the patient's history of medical problems, including chronic conditions, surgeries, and hospitalizations

past, family, and social history (PFSH): patients' answers to physicians' questions about their personal medical histories, medical events in their families, and factors relating to their social environments

patient aging report: a report that lists a patient's balance by age, date and amount of the last payment, and telephone number, grouping unpaid bills by the length of time they remain due

patient day sheet: a summary of patient activity on a given day

patient examination: an examination of a person's body in order to determine his or her state of health

patient flow: the progression of patients from the time they enter the office for a visit until they exit the system by leaving the office after a visit

patient information form: form that includes a patient's personal, employment, and insurance data needed to complete a health care claim; also known as a registration form

patient ledger: a report that lists the financial activity in each patient's account

patient portal: secure website that enables communication between patients and health care providers for tasks such as scheduling, completing registration forms, and making payments

patient refund: money owed to patient

patient registry: method of reporting clinical data to payers using an online service rather than claim-based reporting

patient statement: list of the amount of money a patient owes, the procedures performed, and the dates the procedures were performed

patient tracking features: function attached to the electronic scheduler that is used during a patient encounter to track where the patient is during the different steps of the encounter

payer: health plan or program

payment day sheet: a report that lists all payments received on a particular day, organized by provider

payment plan: agreement between a patient and a practice in which the patient agrees to make regular monthly payments over a specified period of time

payments: money paid by patients and health plans

pending: claim status in which the payer is waiting for information before making a payment decision

performance measures: processes, experience, and/or outcomes of patient care, observations, or treatment that relate to one or more quality aims for health care, such as effective, safe, efficient, patient-centered, equitable, and timely care

personal health record (PHR): private, secure electronic health care files that are created, maintained, and owned by the patient

personal identification number (PIN): unique number that is assigned to or selected by an individual; in EHRs, the use of a PIN often serves as an electronic signature

physical exam (PE): examination of the bodily functions and condition of an individual; typically reported as a body system assessment

place of service (POS) code: location where medical services were provided

point-of-care (POC): ability of providers to document clinical information while interacting with the patient during the patient encounter

point-of-service (POS) plan: managed care plan that permits patients to receive medical services from nonnetwork providers

policyholder: person who buys an insurance plan; the insured, subscriber, or guarantor

postpayment audit: review conducted after a claim is adjudicated

practice analysis report: a report that analyzes the revenue of a practice for a specified period of time

practice management (PM) program: program used to perform administrative and financial functions in a medical office

preauthorization: prior authorization from a payer for services to be provided; if preauthorization is not received, the charge is usually not covered

preexisting condition: illness or disorder of a beneficiary that existed before the effective date of insurance coverage

preferred provider organization (PPO): managed care network of health care providers who agree to perform services for plan members at discounted fees

premium: money the insured pays to a health plan for a health care policy; usually paid monthly

preregistration: the process of gathering basic contact, insurance, and reason for visit information before a new patient comes into the office for an encounter

preventive medical services: care that is provided to keep patients healthy or to prevent illness, such as routine checkups and screening tests

primary care physician (PCP): physician in a managed care organization who directs all aspects of a patient's care

primary diagnosis: the patient's major illness or condition for an encounter

primary insurance plan: health plan that pays benefits first when a patient is covered by more than one plan

procedure code: a code that represents the particular service, treatment, or test provided by a physician

procedure day sheet: a report that lists all the procedures performed on a particular day, in numerical order

progress note: note documenting the care delivered to a patient, and the medical facts and clinical thinking relevant to diagnosis and treatment

prompt payment laws: state laws that mandate a time period within which clean claims must be paid; if they are not, financial penalties are levied against the payer

prospective audit: review of billing and coding prior to claim submission

protected health information (PHI): individually identifiable health information transmitted or maintained by electronic media or in any other form or medium

provider: person or entity that supplies medical or health services and bills for or is paid for the services in the normal course of business; may be a professional member of the health care team, such as a physician, or a facility, such as a hospital or skilled nursing home

q

Quality Payment Program (QPP): the Medicare value-based reimbursement system

query: request for more information from a provider

r

real-time claim adjudication (RTCA): process used to contact health plans electronically to determine visit charges

recall list: tool used to identify the status of patient reminders with the ability to update information as needed

recipient: a person, persons, or entity who receives a message

records retention schedule: a plan for the management of records that lists types of records and indicates how long they should be kept

Recovery Audit Contractor (RAC): entity that audits Medicare claims to determine where there are opportunities to recover incorrect payments from previously paid but noncovered services, erroneous coding, and duplicate services

referral: transfer of patient care from one provider to another

referral number: authorization number given by a referring physician to the referred physician

referring provider: physician who refers the patient to another physician for treatment

registration: process of gathering personal and insurance information about a patient before an encounter with a provider

relative value scale (RVS): system of assigning unit values to medical services based on their required skill and time

release of information (ROI): process followed by employees of covered entities when releasing patient information

remainder statements: statements that list only charges that are not paid in full after all insurance carrier payments have been received

remittance advice (RA): document describing a payment resulting from a claim adjudication

remittance advice remark code (RARC): code that explains a payer's payment decision

resource-based relative value scale (RBRVS): relative value scale for establishing Medicare charges

restoring: process of retrieving data from a backup storage device

retrospective audit: reviewing claims that have already been submitted to insurance carriers so that adjudication results can be analyzed

revenue cycle management (RCM): management of the activities associated with a patient encounter to ensure that the provider receives full payment for services

review of systems (ROS): an inventory of body systems in which the patient reports signs or symptoms he or she is currently having or has had in the past

s

schedule matrix: schedule framework that provides parameters for scheduling appointments, such as blocking schedule times for office closures, meetings, or lunch

schedule of benefits: list of the medical expenses that a health plan covers

secondary insurance plan: health plan that pays benefits after the primary plan pays when a patient is covered by more than one plan

self-insured health plans: health insurance plans paid for directly by the organization, which sets up a fund from which to pay

self-pay patients: patients with no medical insurance

sender: an individual who initiates a message to another person or entity

signs: objective evidence of a disease or condition

small-balance account: overdue patient account in which the amount owed is less than the cost of pursuing payment

SOAP: format used to enter progress notes; it stands for subjective, objective, assessment, and plan

social history (SH): information about the patient's tobacco use, alcohol and drug use, sexual history, relationship status, and other significant social facts that may contribute to the care of the patient

sponsor: in TRICARE, the active-duty service member

standard statements: statements that show all charges regardless of whether the insurance carrier has paid on the transactions

standards: statements of expected quality in the performance of a health care activity

status: relates to the progress of a patient's orders

subject line: introduction that identifies the intent of a written communication

Supplementary Medical Insurance (SMI): also known as Medicare Part B; program that pays for physician services, outpatient hospital services, durable medical equipment, and other services and supplies

survey: a method of gathering information using relevant questions from a sample of people

suspended: claim status when the payer is developing the claim

symptoms: subjective indication of a disease or conditon as experienced by an individual

t

Tabular List: section of ICD-10-CM listing diagnosis codes numerically

takeback: balance that a provider owes a payer following a postpayment audit

task list: an EHR system of maintaining reminders and directives for various elements of operating a medical practice administratively and clinically

Telephone Consumer Protection Act of 1991: federal law regulating collection practices

template: preformatted note that contains selections appropriate to the medical condition or type of visit

third-party payer: private or government organization that insures or pays for health care on behalf of beneficiaries

tickler: reminder to follow up on an account

timely filing: health plan's rules specifying the number of days after the date of service that the practice has to file the claim

transaction: an electronic exchange of information between two parties to carry out financial or administrative activities related to health care

treatment, payment, and health care operations (TPO): under HIPAA, three conditions under which patients' protected health information may be released without their consent

TRICARE: government health program serving dependents of active-duty service members, military retirees and their families, some former spouses, and survivors of deceased military members

Truth in Lending Act: part of the federal Consumer Credit Protection Act that regulates collection practices related to finance charges and late fees

two-way communication: when one person is the sender of a message that is transmitted to another person (the receiver)

u

unbundling: incorrect billing practice of breaking a panel or package of services/procedures into component parts

uncollectible account: account that does not respond to collection efforts and is written off the practice's expected accounts receivable

US Department of Health and Human Services (HHS): government agency that mandates laws to enhance the health and well-being of all Americans, by providing for effective health and human services and by fostering sound, sustained advances in the sciences underlying medicine, public health, and social services; the agency that has mandated the HIPAA Privacy Rule to implement the requirements of HIPAA

username: name that an individual uses for identification purposes when logging onto a computer or an application

usual fees: normal fees charged by a provider

usual, customary, and reasonable (UCR): fees set by comparing usual fees, customary fees, and reasonable fees

v

Vaccine Information Statement (VIS): information sheets produced by the Centers for Disease Control and Prevention (CDC) that explain both the benefits and risks of a vaccine to vaccine recipients

verbal communication: speech-based communication; includes written communication because a particular language system is used in writing

vital signs: measurements of a patient's temperature, respiratory rate, pulse, and blood pressure

voice recognition software: software that recognizes spoken words

w

walkout receipt: report that lists the diagnoses, services provided, fees, and payments received and due after an encounter

workers' compensation insurance: state or federal plan that covers medical care and other benefits for employees who suffer accidental injury or become ill as a result of employment

write off: balance that has been removed from a patient's account

written communication: process of exchanging messages between a sender and receiver(s) by using written language

x

X12 835 Remittance Advice Transaction: electronic transaction for payment explanation

index

a

b

C

d

e

f

g

h

i

k

l

m

n

O

P

q

r

S

t

U

V

W

X